psychotherapeutic efforts, while the diversity of disciplines could well foster mutual learning and maturation, far too often the advocates of these models collapse into divisiveness and competitions that impoverish our opportunities to learn from one another. In these two volumes, Kevin Smith places ethics at the heart of these professional debates, examining and critiquing the values that divergent models of psychotherapy hold, both explicitly and implicitly, arguing that each represents a practice that promotes a particular vision of the good life. As a psychotherapist often drawn quite passionately into taking sides in these theory wars, I found in Smith's book a quiet, deeply resourced perspective that allowed me to take a more reflective stance with regard to both the differences and the commonalities of contemporary models of psychotherapy. These books will be of great value to practitioners, researchers, scholars and teachers who value the reflective practice of the art, the science, and the philosophies of psychoanalysis and psychotherapy."

William F. Cornell, author of *Self-Examination in Psychoanalysis and Psychotherapy*

evin Smith's work is essential. Every single practitioner of psychotherapy uld be familiar with Smith's message, and should be aware of the issues ises for their work, every moment of every day. Psychotherapy, Smith us, is not a technical exercise in the amelioration of problems. The aims onduct of psychotherapy are not adequately described or measured in rms of evidence-based practice. Every aspect of psychotherapy, from y problems are defined to the means by which they are addressed, xpression, often inadvertent, of what we believe makes life good. herapy of every variety is a social practice, and like all such practices, otes an ethic. Whether they are used to thinking of their work as an ndeavor or not, all psychotherapists spend their entire professional uencing those with whom they work to live in certain ways and not Psychotherapists are far too little aware of what is, after all, the al) ground under their feet.

two books should be assigned in every psychotherapy training d should be required reading for those who have finished for-, regardless of their theoretical orientation (yes, I do mean to ntire spectrum, from psychoanalysis to CBT) or the profession lants. Psychologists, psychiatrists, social workers, counselors, atric nurses, marriage and family therapists—all really do need h the issues presented here."

Donnel B. Stern, Ph.D., William Alanson White Institute, author of *The Infinity of the Unsaid*

Endorsements

"A pleasure to read from start to finish, this short book is packed [with inter]esting insights and arguments. A compelling case is made for [understanding] psychotherapy as a set of social practices in Taylor's sense, sha[ped by ideals] whose capacity to empower and give meaning to life often esca[...]. By making these ideals explicit and placing them in the history [of Western] identity, Smith helps us to see what's fundamentally at stake [...] and in disputes between the various schools. Smith cuts thr[ough the] polemics typical of those disputes and points the way forw[ard to con]structive debate."

Nicholas Smith, Professor of Philosophy, [...] author of *Charles Taylor: Meaning, [...]*

"How can we better understand psychotherapy's et[hical thera]pies—drawing on particular pictures of human flou[rishing that] involves ethical visions? In this very perceptive b[ook ... relates psy]chotherapy's ethical visions to the intuitions and [... of the] client, to therapists' gentle interrogation and "i[...] cal visions, and to the history of Western tho[ught .... In examining] psychotherapy's contemporary ethical visio[ns ... however] deeply and implicitly they may not even be[... In addressing] the diversity of extant ethical visions, he e[ncourages ... respect]ful, open-minded conversation among di[fferent ... Psychotherapy in] *Context and in Dialogue* provides invalu[able ... for] developing richer, more sophisticated [...]"

Alan Tjeltveit, Profess[or ...] auth[or ...]

"All too often our contemporary [...] social, ethnic, or professional, [...] and claims of rightness and s[...]"

Therapeutic Ethics in Context and in Dialogue

The standard view of psychotherapy as a treatment for mental disorders can obscure how therapy functions as a social practice that promotes conceptions of human well-being. Building on the philosophy of Charles Taylor, Smith examines the link between therapy and ethics, and the roots of therapeutic aims in modern Western ideas about living well.

This volume builds on a complementary volume (*The Ethical Visions of Psychotherapy*), to explore therapeutic conceptions of human flourishing. Smith illustrates how therapeutic aims implicitly promote ideas about a good life, even though therapists rarely tell their patients how they should live. Taylor's history of the modern identity provides a framework to examine the historical and cultural origins of therapeutic ethics. Utilizing Taylor's work on practical reasoning and ethical debate, Smith considers the prospects for dialogue between the divergent ethical visions promoted by different psychotherapies.

A key text for upper-level undergraduates, postgraduate students, and professionals in the fields of psychotherapy, psychoanalysis, theoretical psychology, and philosophy of mind.

Kevin R. Smith is Adjunct Associate Professor of Psychology at Duquesne University, USA. He is a psychotherapist in private practice in Pittsburgh, USA, and supervises the psychotherapy training of psychiatry residents and doctoral students in clinical psychology. He has published papers on psychotherapy and phenomenological psychology.

Advances in Theoretical and Philosophical Psychology
Series Editor
Brent D. Slife
Brigham Young University

Editorial Board

Brian Schiff
Situating Qualitative Methods in Psychological Science

Brent D. Slife and Stephen Yanchar
Hermeneutic Moral Realism in Psychology: Theory and Practice

Jeff Sugarman and Jack Martin
A Humanities Approach to the Psychology of Personhood

Bethany Morris, Chase O'Gwin, Sebastienne Grant, Sakenya McDonald
Subjectivity in Psychology in the Era of Social Justice

Kevin R. Smith
The Ethical Visions of Psychotherapy

Kevin R. Smith
Therapeutic Ethics in Context and in Dialogue

https://www.routledge.com/psychology/series/TPP

Therapeutic Ethics in Context and in Dialogue

Kevin R. Smith

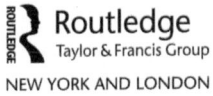
Routledge
Taylor & Francis Group

NEW YORK AND LONDON

First published 2021
by Routledge
52 Vanderbilt Avenue, New York, NY 10017

and by Routledge
2 Park Square, Milton Park, Abingdon, Oxon OX14 4RN

Routledge is an imprint of the Taylor & Francis Group, an informa business

Library of Congress Cataloging-in-Publication Data
Names: Smith, Kevin R., 1953- author.
Title: Therapeutic ethics in context and in dialogue / Kevin R. Smith.
Description: New York, NY: Routledge, 2020. | Series: Advances in theoretical
and philosophical psychology | Includes bibliographical references and index. |
Identifiers: LCCN 2020011015 (print) | LCCN 2020011016 (ebook) |
ISBN 9780367480332 (hardback) | ISBN 9780367524975 (paperback) |
ISBN 9781003039167 (ebook)
Subjects: LCSH: Psychotherapy–Moral and ethical aspects. | Psychotherapist
and patient.
Classification: LCC RC455.2.E8 S64 2020 (print) | LCC RC455.2.E8 (ebook) |
DDC 616.89/14–dc23
LC record available at https://lccn.loc.gov/2020011015
LC ebook record available at https://lccn.loc.gov/2020011016

ISBN: 978-0-367-48033-2 (hbk)
ISBN: 978-1-003-03916-7 (ebk)

Typeset in Times New Roman
by Deanta Global Publishing Services, Chennai, India

For Beth, my only "one"

Contents

Acknowledgments

Many people and institutions have provided direct and indirect support for this work. My philosophical thinking about therapy was initially formed in my graduate training at Duquesne University. My understanding of therapy as a practitioner has been shaped by many supervisors, colleagues, supervisees, and patients over the years, as well as my own experience of being a patient in humanistic, psychoanalytic, and Jungian therapy. At the Western Psychiatric Institute and Clinic in Pittsburgh I had the good fortune to be introduced to therapy research through my work as a therapist in multisite studies examining the efficacy of cognitive-behavioral and psychodynamic therapies. Paul Pilkonis modeled how psychotherapy researchers can be appreciative of the depth and complexity of therapeutic process while trying to formulate and answer well-defined research questions. Both the Pittsburgh Psychoanalytic Institute and the seminars of the "Keeping Our Work Alive" group in Pittsburgh organized by Bill Cornell have been crucial to deepening my understanding and practice of therapy. Brent Slife has offered much-needed encouragement.

Many people have been kind enough to read and comment on portions of this work. I am particularly indebted to four people who have given extensively of their time, reading all (or most) of the book: Beth Knapp, Mark Kroll-Fratoni, Jane Matz, and Jeff McCurry. They have corrected numerous errors and made important recommendations regarding the substance and style of the argument. I am deeply grateful for their advice and support.

Series Foreword

Brent D. Slife, Editor

Psychologists need to face the facts. Their commitment to empiricism for answering disciplinary questions does not prevent pivotal questions from arising that cannot be evaluated exclusively through empirical methods, hence the title of this series: *Advances in Theoretical and Philosophical Psychology*. Such moral questions as, "What is the nature of a good life?" are crucial to psychotherapists but are not answerable through empirical methods alone. And what of the methods themselves? Many have worried that our current psychological means of investigation are not adequate for fully understanding the person (e.g., Schiff, 2019). How do we address this concern through empirical methods without running headlong into the dilemma of methods investigating themselves? Such questions are in some sense philosophical, to be sure, but the discipline of psychology cannot advance even its own empirical agenda without addressing questions like these in defensible ways.

How then should the discipline of psychology deal with such distinctly theoretical questions? We could leave the answers exclusively to professional philosophers, but this option would mean that the conceptual foundations of the discipline, including the conceptual framework of empiricism itself, are left to scholars who are *outside* the discipline. As undoubtedly helpful as philosophers are and would be, this situation would mean that the people doing the actual psychological work, psychologists themselves, are divorced from the people who formulate and re-formulate the conceptual foundations of that work. This division of labor would not seem to serve the long-term viability of the discipline.

Instead, the founders of psychology — thinkers such as Wundt, Freud, and James — recognized the importance of psychologists in formulating their own foundations. These parents of psychology not only did their own theorizing, in cooperation with many other disciplines; they realized the significance of psychologists continuously *re*-examining these theories and philosophies.

This re-examination process allowed for the people most directly involved in and knowledgeable about the discipline to be the ones to decide *whether* changes were needed and *how* such changes would best be implemented. This book series is dedicated to that task, the examining and re-examining of psychology's foundations.

1 Introduction

Sources of Therapeutic Ethics and the Prospects for Dialogue

There are many types of psychotherapy and different ways to sort them. Therapies differ in terms of their practices or techniques and in terms of their theories of psychopathology. Therapies also differ in their conceptions of human well-being, of what people can hope for in life, what sorts of problems interfere with their flourishing, and how those problems are best addressed. Therapies are distinct from one another in that they promote, implicitly or explicitly, different ethics, different visions of a good life. This is not to deny that therapies can also be distinguished as different means to more specific therapeutic ends, like a decrease in symptoms or the treatment of disorders. But they also point toward different ideas about which ends are most worth pursuing, ends that go beyond these circumscribed goals. Indeed, the central task of evidence-based practice, determining which therapies work best to treat specific disorders, includes an implicit conception of well-being as independent, self-directed agency, unencumbered by psychological symptoms.

A number of therapists have claimed that specific ethical ideals can be among the benefits of psychotherapy. Ethical views are present in Ellis' (1962) promotion of self-enhancing rationality, Thompson's (2004) argument for an ethic of honesty in psychoanalysis, Rogers' (1951) aim to protect the organismic values of individuals from the distorting influences of family and society, McWilliams' (2005) claim that therapy can foster self-understanding, authenticity, empathy, and compassion, and Yalom's (1980) effort to assist patients therapeutically by helping them to face the existential realities of death, meaninglessness, and solitude.

In another work (*The Ethical Visions of Psychotherapy*) I look more closely at a few therapies, demonstrating how even technical therapies intended to treat well-defined disorders can include broader ethical aims. Exposure therapy for anorexia (Glasover et al., 2016) promotes courage in facing one's fears in order to develop a sense of self-efficacy and autonomy. Cognitive therapy of depression (Beck et al., 1979) promotes an ethic of scientific detachment and autonomous individualism in pursuing one's freely chosen ends, combined with a skeptical attitude toward anything that cannot be empirically verified.

I also explore in this companion volume how even closely related therapies, like different versions of psychoanalysis, can be distinguished by their different visions of human flourishing. Paul Gray's (1994) ego-psychology promotes intrapsychic spontaneity, increased autonomy, voluntary control over impulses, and a rational capacity for reflective self-observation. The Lacanian analysis of Bruce Fink (1995, 1997, 2004, 2007, 2014a, 2014b, 2016, 2017) promotes different aims: not the increased autonomy of a reflective ego, but freedom from an ego that has been built up out of the impositions of others, a freedom that allows one to pursue one's satisfaction. Fink's freedom is not that of autonomous self-direction but that of liberated Eros. The relational analysis of Stephen Mitchell (Greenberg and Mitchell, 1983; Mitchell, 1988, 1993, 1997, 2000, 2002; Mitchell and Black, 1995) promotes openness to the complexity and depth of human experience in the context of relationships, where we inevitably shape one another to be the particular persons we are.

Given the pervasive role of ethics in the therapies, the effort to assess them simply in terms of differential efficacy in changing the symptoms of disorders neglects much of what distinguishes them. Further, as many have noted (Lambert, 2013; Wampold and Imel, 2015), most research evidence suggests that there is little difference in efficacy between different therapeutic orientations, even when using standard measures of symptomatic change.

What would it mean to directly engage the different ethics of different therapies? To do so requires a deeper explication of therapeutic ethics. Paradoxically, one might begin by looking at how psychotherapy has often been understood to be critical of ethics. Most therapists are adamant that there is no room in therapy for telling people how they should live their lives. However, this reluctance to persuade is built upon the value that therapists accord to fostering the uniqueness and autonomy of individuals. Beyond these two core values the therapies also promote more specific ideas about living well. In Chapter 2 I outline the significance of therapists' reticence to persuade, and offer a provisional sorting of therapeutic ethics into four distinct pictures of human flourishing.

A therapeutic view of flourishing may sometimes appear to be the work of a particular theorist. But ideals for how to live well are not the inventions of individuals. Even when an ethical vision has something novel in it, it is not created out of whole cloth but partakes of the socio-cultural world in which it arises. In Chapter 3 I look at the roots of therapeutic ethics in modern Western ideals for living well, building upon Charles Taylor's (1989, 2007) history of the modern identity. Taylor articulates the rise and transformations of various modern practices and theories that promote particular visions of what is essential to being human, and to human well-being. I link these modern ethics to the aims of contemporary therapies. Exploring the cultural context for psychotherapy helps to clarify what is at stake between contrasting therapeutic ethics, and what constitutes the appeal of divergent therapeutic aims.

I am not interested in explicating the contrasting ethics of different therapies only for descriptive purposes, but in order to lay the groundwork for dialogue and debate among them. How does one argue for one ethical vision in relation to another? This is a hotly contested question, with some claiming that there can be no real reasoning about such matters, for ethics are not capable of rational grounding. On this view, all one can ultimately do is to follow non-rational preferences built up out of personal and cultural predilections. Others claim to be able to ground ethics in a scientific analysis of what constitutes human well-being. Neither of these approaches seem satisfactory to me, nor to accurately reflect what happens when people debate ethics. Utilizing Taylor's (1989, 1995a) work on practical reasoning, I explore in Chapter 4 the nature of ethical argument, the role of ethical intuitions, and the value of framing ethical debate as ongoing dialogue. Applied to therapeutic ethics, I argue that the value of dialogue lies in its role in strengthening particular ethical positions and in preventing the presumptive dominance of one perspective. I conclude that it is neither feasible nor desirable to understand the psychotherapies without considering the ethical proposals that are present in their theories and practices.

2 Therapy Against Ethics and the Ethics of Therapy

Easing Ethical Demands

In this chapter I want to address one obvious difficulty with the idea that the therapies enact distinctive visions of a good life. Many therapists repudiate any effort to persuade patients to subscribe to ideas about what would be good for them. Beck et al.'s (1979) cognitive therapy does not involve talking patients into a particular perspective on their depression, or even on how to be less depressed. Instead, patients are encouraged to think for themselves about what worsens and improves their depressions, to become investigators of and interveners in their own difficulties, based on what makes sense to them from their own experience.

Likewise, Gray (1994) warns against depth interpretation and personal influence (such as using rather than interpreting transference) because he wants to respect patients' autonomy. He wants to help them come to a better understanding of their own defensive processes so they can choose to do something different with their libidinal and aggressive inclinations. He does not want them to feel better about themselves by taking on his values or identifying with his presumably less punitive superego.

As a relational analyst, Mitchell (1997) does not believe that patient and analyst can avoid influencing each other, but he too is concerned about patient autonomy. The way to safeguard autonomy on his view is not to try to avoid influence (which is impossible anyway) but to pay attention to it and discuss it with the patient. Discussed influence is not surreptitiously enacted in a way that leaves the patient subject to it.

Fink's (2007) elusive oracular interpretations are intended to set patients to work following the trail of the unconscious, not to provide knowledge about who they are, let alone who they should be.

None of these therapies attempt to convert patients to a set of "aims for better living." But, in fact, they go further. Therapists not only eschew talking patients into any ideals, they often aim to free patients from the burdens of ethical demands that they bring with them into therapy. Cognitive-behavioral therapy can involve strengthening patients' capacity to challenge the ideals ("shoulds" and "musts") that have been imposed upon them by family and society. Carl Rogers (1951) wants to protect patients' organismic values from being pushed aside by what others have told them they should want or value. Fink (2014b) is quite explicit: "As Freud discovered very early in his work with hysterics, neurosis results precisely from the repeated attempt to squelch one's own desire in order to do good, to do what one believes to be the right thing" (p. 56). Analysis is not about offering the patient yet another set of ideas about the "right thing," but to undo the damage already done by such ideas.

As Fink notes, this line of thinking was present from the beginning in psychoanalysis. For example, in "'Civilized' sexual morality and modern nervous illness", Freud (1908/1959) writes that "all who wish to be more noble-minded than their constitution allows fall victims to neurosis; they would have been more healthy if it could have been possible for them to be less good" (p. 191). In *Civilization and Its Discontents* (1930/1961a) he compares the individual's superego to cultural commands to do what is right. In his view, both aim too high.

> Consequently, we are very often obliged for therapeutic purposes, to oppose the super-ego, and we endeavor to lower its demands. Exactly the same objections can be made against the ethical demands of the cultural super-ego. It, too, does not trouble itself enough about the facts of the mental constitution of human beings ... If more is demanded of a man, a revolt will be produced in him or a neurosis, or he will be made unhappy.
>
> (p. 143)

It is clear that a common focus of psychotherapy is the easing or undoing of the ill effects of various prescriptions to do good, or to follow a set of ideals or obligations promoted by one's family, social group, or the larger society. However, I am claiming that the psychotherapies promulgate ethics; that they are guided by, promote, or enact particular pictures of human flourishing. Don't such ethics include ideas regarding what one should do in order to live well? Doesn't that contradict the claim that the psychotherapies aim to free patients from the deleterious effects of the demands of externally imposed values and ideals? Are the therapies simply replacing one set of ideals with another?

One way to answer such questions is to look more closely at therapeutic aims, at the benefits that therapies intend to bring to patients. For many schools of therapy, the critique of standard ethical and moral injunctions aims not to abolish such standards, but to modify or critically re-assess them so that the person has a different relationship to these ideals.

Certainly, Freud makes it plain that he is not advocating the abolition of the superego, or of all cultural restrictions and checks upon behavior. His picture of "homo homini lupus" ("man is a wolf to man," Freud, 1930/1961a, p. 111) makes plain his view that, without restraints (both internal and external), we would live in an even more violent and sexually predatory world than we already do. The uniting force of Eros provides a counter to our destructive impulses, but Freud remains skeptical about the prospects for that force carrying us into more utopian social arrangements of mutual tolerance and beneficence.

Nevertheless, Freud is clear that the socially instituted restrictions on sex and aggression, particularly in their internalized form as superego, often exact a high price, constricting human vitality and engagement in life. The benefit psychoanalysis can bring is to free up energy squandered in unnecessarily strict prohibitions of the expression of sexual and aggressive drives. The blanket denial or repression of such desires is rarely successful (they will show up anyway in disguised symptomatic form) and risks turning vibrantly alive human beings into "well-behaved weaklings" (Freud, 1908/1959, p. 197).

If Freud is critical of common morality, it is in order to free people to accept aspects of themselves that were widely censured in his day. Analysis provides an alternative to the self-destructive, neurosis-inducing project to fully conform to social ideals. One central benefit of analysis is the freedom to make a more reasoned decision about how to handle the conflict between desire and social expectation, rather than simply repress desire in order to "be good." Prior to analysis, neurotics cannot be seen as straightforward ethical actors aiming at the good, for too much of who they are is operating behind their backs, giving the lie to consciously intended aims.

Built into the therapies is a wariness about ethics, a caution about the risk of psychological harm that can arise from self- and other-imposed obligations to live according to ethical norms or ideals. This wariness may be one reason why therapists do not typically consider another possible relationship between therapy and ethics. One could frame therapeutic action as an aid to ethics, and not simply in the sense that the therapies implicitly promote their own ethics, like the freedom to re-think societal expectations that Freud recommends. Ethical injunctions can cause psychological problems, but psychological problems can also undermine ethics. Consider a man who is crushed with guilt over his perceived moral failures and believes he simply needs to try harder to be good, when in fact there are psychological factors at play that will frustrate his efforts. His determination to be kind or thoughtful may be acting as a defense against bitterness, rage, or hostility that feels too dangerous to acknowledge and has roots he doesn't understand. Perhaps the disavowed rage is evident to others in the violence with which he castigates himself for moral faults he believes are inexcusable. In this case, the unacknowledged rage or aggression will continually interfere with his ethical aims. Therapy might well help this man undo the psychological problems caused by the way he has turned against his anger and aggression. But addressing those psychological problems might enable greater success in his efforts to be ethical. Therapy might then not simply be against ethics, but clear psychological impediments to being ethical. It is true that therapeutic change here need not take the form of the substitution of one set of ethical aims for another. A therapist is not likely to dogmatically assert to this patient that restraint on all aggressive impulses is wrong. Therapeutic work is more likely to effect a different relationship to his ethical strictures, so that his ethical action might be freer, less constricted, and compulsively enacted. Nevertheless, implicit in this change is the idea that openness, nuance, and flexibility in living ethically are important components of a good life. Yet therapists rarely frame therapy as including ethical benefits.[1]

In the passages cited above Freud explicitly takes up the implications of psychoanalysis for ethics. In therapies that offer concrete techniques to address specific symptoms the ethical implications may not be so obvious, but they are still present. Glasover et al.'s (2016) case study describing an exposure-based therapy for eating disorders outlines an effort to change the patient's sense of where the threat to her well-being lies. She comes to therapy afraid of her desire to eat. She fears that unless she guards against this desire, it will take over and she will be doomed to endless weight gain. She is moved through the practices of the therapy to focus on a different danger: not weight gain, but fear of weight gain. Fear is what is really controlling her, rendering her subject to the symptoms of anorexia. By overcoming this fear she can feel freer to make choices about eating based on her appetite or practical considerations regarding healthy eating. She will thus be freed from a fear that pushes her into a corner, where she can't assess what would be good or bad for her, but is simply running from a fantasied dire outcome of ever-ballooning obesity.

There is a surface-level change here in the shift regarding where to locate the danger to living well (not weight gain, but fear of weight gain). But there is something more as well. The patient is brought to experience a greater sense of mastery over her life through the courage necessary to face her fears. The case description does not spell this out, but it is easy to imagine that one source of the patient's fear may be current societal views regarding the attractiveness of a slender body type for women. To the extent that this is so, the offer of courageous self-mastery is also offered as an alternative to that social ideal. At the very least, in helping the patient to be less afraid of the possibility that she might fail to meet that ideal, she is being encouraged to loosen its hold upon her. She then has the option to re-examine this ideal, and to decide about whether or to what extent she might endorse or reject it, instead of continuing to fearfully and compulsively act in service to it.

While this therapy offers a new perspective on where the patient can find greater well-being, there is little in the way of explicitly arguing for this new perspective. Nor is there an explicit critique of the societal expectation that women be thin. It is this lack of formal advocacy for an ethic that can lead to doubts about the idea that therapies promote ethics. Most therapists do not preach to their patients about how to live well. Some do, Ellis (1962) being a well-known example. But most do not. And with those who do advocate for the therapist's role in addressing moral issues directly there is also the recognition that this is not a matter of dictating moral rules to patients (see Doherty, 1995). Nancy McWilliams (2005) has argued that psychotherapy provides a significant social benefit in its promotion of specific values or ideals, such as authenticity, self-understanding, empathy, growth in personal responsibility, and respect for others. However, she does not suggest that therapists are to argue for such values or try to persuade patients to subscribe to them. Such values are the by-product of therapeutic work that has nothing to do with proselytizing. While McWilliams acknowledges that there can be educative messages in therapists' comments, she also notes that "psychoanalytic therapists tend to avoid being explicitly didactic because their concern is to help patients find their own answers" (2004, p. 244). The general reticence about overt proselytizing says something important about therapeutic ethics. But it does not render therapy ethics-free. To think that it does would be to overlook a fundamental aspect of ethics, namely, that it is first (and sometimes primarily) promulgated through practices rather than articulated rules or maxims.

Ideals for living well come in many forms, some closer to common moral rules (for example, "don't manipulate people") and some having to do with nuances of how we are to behave toward or position ourselves with others. As an example of the latter, consider the ideal of "being cool" as it arose for white American college students in the 1950's who were listening to jazz musicians like Miles Davis and reading Beat poets. There's a style of dress, an attitude of detached aloofness, even a way of smoking a cigarette that is labelled cool. It is not defined, and certainly no one is proselytizing for it—either you get it or you don't. Proselytizing is decidedly too sincere, not ironic or knowing enough to be cool. One would see cool in certain ways of talking or positioning oneself with others, and come to admire it and adopt it oneself. But cool is not primarily a concept one argues for or against, though social commentators and critics may have done so. It is first of all seen, implicitly understood, and lived.

Cool is a good example to illustrate the broad meaning I am giving to ethics. Ethics are visions for how to live well that include more than rules regarding obligations to others. Clearly, 1950's cool cannot be easily assimilated to fundamental moral injunctions (don't lie, cheat, or steal) or moral recommendations like the golden rule. Instead, cool belongs to another (although related) side of ethics, views about what is truly worthwhile in life.[2] A New York financial salesman of the 1950's who went to jazz clubs after his day at the office may have done so out of a sense that simply meeting his obligations to job and family was unfulfilling. That does not mean that he had developed cool into a fully articulated philosophy of life, or that this ethic didn't have any limitations. A leftist friend might have argued with him that this wasn't enough, that his dilatant dabbling in the Greenwich Village world of cool neglected far more sweeping critiques of corporate capitalism and the need for fundamental socio-political change. The salesman might have agreed with his friend, while still maintaining that he had found something personally meaningful in the world of jazz that he did not want to forego.

The enactment of ethics prior to or apart from its articulation or explicit verbal promotion is a commonplace of social and historical analysis. Charles Taylor (2016) references examples of machismo (enacted in a swaggering walk and contempt for sentimental songs) and of children in some cultures learning respect for elders through bodily postures like bowing or learning not to look their elders in the eye. Machismo and respect for elders are contested views of what constitutes a good life in our culture, where patriarchal attitudes and hierarchical social arrangements are often the target of critique. But this is a critique that aims to correct what are seen as problematic ethical views and to replace them with better ones. They are still recognized as ethics, as views about how men should behave in relation to one another and to women, or about how youth should properly position themselves with elders.

So the fact that most therapists rarely actively promote verbally articulated ethical principles, ideals, or injunctions does not mean they are not promoting an ethic. Encouraging patients to face their fears in exposure exercises does enact an ethic of courage in the service of self-mastery.

What about non-directive therapies like psychoanalysis? Patients aren't told to do anything. There are no "exercises" to engage in, behavioral or cognitive, that might enact an ethic without explicitly promoting it. Isn't psychoanalysis outside of this idea of promoting ethics, for it neither preaches nor enacts?

Psychoanalysis does enact, it is a social practice. Patients are instructed to talk freely, and their attention is directed by the analyst to their defensive processes, their speech, or their relational enactments, in order that they may be "set free" in some sense. This is a freedom from compulsive constrictions of sexual and aggressive wishes, from the ways their lives have been overwritten by the social-symbolic world, or from repetitive interpersonal positions. Patients learn in Gray's (1994) ego psychological analysis (perhaps without ever being told as much) that they have been inhibiting themselves, turning against certain aspects of their affective experience in ways that leave them hobbled, interfering with a more vital pursuit of their aims in their social, sexual, or work lives.

Patients in Fink's (2007) analysis learn that they are not masters in their own house, cannot think their way out of their dilemmas or symptoms, cannot be freed by modeling themselves on or competing with others (including with the analyst). They come to sense that they are actively participating in their enslavement to symbolic impositions that create and shape their desires, and can only be freed through an analytic process that unsettles and destabilizes their devotion to an imaginary self and the endless pursuit of that which will never fulfill their desire (for it is the nature of desire never to be satisfied). Patients certainly don't learn this as a set of ideas. But, if analysis is successful, they are freed to live in such a way as to get off the merry-go-round of desire and seek their satisfaction. They live differently, enacting a differently configured set of aims. They are not taught or encouraged to do this. It simply happens in the process of analysis. But it is offered to patients as a better way to live, and the experience of this shift will speak for itself. Patients will sense in how they now live their lives that something is better, even if they might not frame the change as their analysts would, as a freedom from previously imprisoning impositions of the social-symbolic world.

The ethic that is opposed in this case is in one sense less specific than with the behavioral treatment of anorexia, which may loosen the grip upon the patient of a particular ideal (thin is beautiful). Fink's analysis is an alternative to any ethic that says one should live one's life in accordance with the expectations, demands, and injunctions of one's family, social class, church, culture, etc. But in another sense, the ethic that is opposed here is *more* specific. For each patient there will be particular expectations or demands that are not derived from general cultural expectations, but were fashioned in childhood by the patient through an idiosyncratic reading of ambiguous messages coming from the family.

Fink's Lacanian analysis subverts the pressure to act in conformity with both broad cultural expectations and the more specific demands that patients perceived or imagined were coming from their families. The liberation from such demands is done for the sake of something else. Fink frames this in several ways: to further the patient's Eros (Fink, 1995, p. 146); for the sake of life, and against death (Fink, 2016, p. 147); so that patients may live out their own particularity as individuals rather than be subsumed within the "normal" (Fink 2017, p. 250). It is true that particularity does not have a specific content like cognitive-behavioral therapy's idealization of rational self-transformation or some Freudians' idealization of genital sexuality.[3] Nevertheless, the aim of releasing the patient's particularity from being submerged or overwritten by the desires of others still operates as a guidepost. By way of analogy, consider that it is difficult to give a specific content to Buddhist concepts like Enlightenment or Nirvana. But these terms are clearly central to Buddhist ideas about what is worth aiming for in life. Moreover, comparing Lacanian particularity with Buddhist Enlightenment indicates that these concepts are not so empty. They take on the different significances that they have from the very different set of practices and histories of theorizing from which they originate.

The Ethics of Therapy

The fact that the practice of therapy enacts ideals without directly promoting them says something important about the content of those ideals. Therapeutic ideals entail the valuing of something specific to the patient, something to be fostered or discovered in the patient which makes the patient more unique or particular, or which renders the patient more capable of self-direction. At the risk of simplification, one might characterize these aims as enhancing individual uniqueness or particularity and promoting autonomy. Some therapies clearly emphasize one over the other, but many are concerned with both. Of course, much more specific aims are present in many therapies, especially in those that directly focus on reducing the severity and frequency of symptoms. Such therapies are more likely to have as a distal goal the fostering of autonomy rather than particularity, for they often frame symptoms as interfering with patients' abilities to live their lives as they would like, as obstructing autonomy. But there is no reason that respect for particularity could not be an added component of such treatments.

There are a number of objections one could raise to a summary of therapeutic ethics in terms of the two themes of particularity and autonomy. One objection is that no ethical ideal, no picture of flourishing, can be boiled down to a simple principle or rule ("be the particular person you are," or "work to assert your autonomy"). Ideas about what constitutes a good or full life only come alive in context, and different contexts give such ideals different connotations. Aaron Beck and Paul Gray are not necessarily promoting the same ethical aim when they both write about the importance of respecting patient autonomy. Particularity takes the form of authenticity for some humanistic and analytic therapists, with the aim being to discover one's true self. Other therapists would avoid such language, holding that persons are not unitary and coherent, that they are too fluid to be contained in *a* true self. Fink would find such an aim to be alienating.

I do not intend to subsume all therapeutic ethics under these two headings of particularity and autonomy, even if I believe there is evidence that they operate as consistent themes across many of the psychotherapies. But these two ethical ideals do help to explain the reticence of therapists to explicitly promote ethical ideals with more specific content.

The absence of more explicitly articulated ethical conceptions in therapy is seen as a limitation by some. For example, Robinson (2010) has written an extended analysis of the connection between cognitive-behavioral therapy and ancient Stoic philosophy. He expresses disappointment that "modern CBT seems to fall short of explicitly endorsing a system of positive values of the kind found in Stoicism, although they are clearly assumed in its prescriptions" (p. 160).

However, therapeutic ideas about human well-being are not always restricted to an implicit form in therapeutic practices. For example, Robinson's work is an attempt to provide more detailed content to the ethical aims of cognitive-behavioral therapy. At the end of their survey of psychoanalytic theory, Mitchell and Black (1995) briefly reference each of the clinical cases they have used to illustrate the psychoanalytic theories they have summarized. In doing so, they point to various benefits that were brought to each of these patients. In addition to authenticity and autonomy, there are benefits of: (1) the integration of wildly disparate parts of the person, without the "bad" (hostile, envious, murderous) parts of the person destroying the "good"; (2) a greater capacity for interpersonal intimacy; (3) a capacity to be "in" one's experience rather than coldly detached from it, and hence to increase the depth and range of experience. Humanistic therapists (Task Force for the Development of Practice Recommendations for the Provision of Humanistic Psychosocial Services, 2004) aim to promote a conception of psychological development which is defined in terms of several of the ideals listed above, but also as "the strengthening of relational bonds [and] the promotion of an environment of mutual care and empathy" (p. 5).

In session, psychoanalysts rarely recommend specific ethical aims directly to patients, even if values like personal honesty or liberated Eros are implicitly present in the practices of free association, attention to dream and fantasy, and interpretations of sexual or aggressive wishes. Outside the consulting room, however, some psychoanalytic writers are quite explicit about their ideas of human flourishing. One of the more detailed examples can be found in *The Psychodynamic Diagnostic Manual, 2nd Edition* (Lingiardi and McWilliams, 2017—hereafter referred to as PDM2). Chapter 2's "Profile of Mental Functioning" lays out in some detail several features of psychological health. What is clear from even a casual perusal of these standards for the assessment of mental functioning is that they present a rich and complex picture of human well-being. The highest level of psychological health in this system includes such things as the capacity to "use, express, communicate, and understand a wide range of subtle emotions effectively" (p. 85), to "think about self and others in subtle and sophisticated ways" (p.89), to "have a deep, emotionally rich capacity for intimacy, caring, and empathy" (p. 95), to "maintain a stable sense of well-being, confidence, vitality, and realistic self-esteem in varying contexts and even under stress" (p. 99). The psychologically healthy "are highly motivated to observe and understand themselves in relation to others and to reflect on the full range of their own and others' experiences and feelings (including subtle variations in feelings)" (p. 111). The general spirit of these ideals would suggest that psychological health is evident when people are motivated to do what they would be encouraged to do in psychodynamic therapy.

So one can find explicit formulations of therapeutic ethics, even if these are seldom directly promulgated by therapists in the practice of therapy. Summarizing these ethics is not an easy task. There are many psychotherapies, each of which embodies certain notions of well-being in particular ways. In fact, the situation is even more complicated. Each practitioner, even each instance of therapeutic practice, instantiates a variation on therapeutic aims and the picture of well-being they enact. In the effort to summarize I am forced to synthesize and assume the consistency of themes that, in practice, branch out in multiple directions. Nevertheless, I think there are themes that recur in the various therapies and provide the basis for generalizations regarding therapeutic pictures of human flourishing. Below I outline four distinct therapeutic ethics derived from the examination of different therapies summarized above (and examined in more detail in *The Ethical Visions of Psychotherapy*). These ethics are not necessarily school-specific. That is, while some schools of therapy seem to emphasize one ethic, an ethical theme can appear in different therapies, albeit often modified to fit a particular therapy's conceptual environment.

The following is a provisional list of ideals for living well that are endorsed, practiced, or promoted by the psychotherapies.

1) *Rational Self-Mastery.* Human flourishing is most securely attained through self-mastery based upon careful empirical assessment of one's problems, broken down into manageable sub-problems that can be addressed through specific interventions directed to their causes or maintaining factors. This ethic is most clearly embodied not only in some schools of therapy (behavioral and cognitive-behavioral) but in research into the efficacy of specific interventions. However, one can see elements of this ethic in other therapies, for example, in Paul Gray's effort to enhance patients' autonomy by helping them to develop skills for identifying their defensive operations.

2) *Honest Self-Exploration.* Human flourishing is to be found in an open, curious, and honest exploration of who one is, an exploration that does not turn away from what is unpleasant, unflattering, or disturbing, which

involves a willingness to face that which may have been previously disa-vowed. As Freud (1900/1953) puts it in *The Interpretation of Dreams*: "It cannot be denied that to interpret and report one's dreams demands a high degree of self-discipline. One is bound to emerge as the only villain among the crowd of noble characters who share one's life" (p. 485). Part of the point of this is a sort of personal honesty (Thompson, 2004). But the aim can also be framed in terms of freeing up energies previously spent on repressing unsavory truths about oneself, thus mak-ing it easier to live life in a more vitally engaged way. Sometimes this can be given a predominantly biological spin, as Freud sometimes did, and Rogers did with his "organismic" values. At other times, this vital-ity has a broader meaning that involves capacities for creativity and the exploration of meaningful possibilities for engagement with others (as in Stephen Mitchell).

3) *Particularity Liberated from Social Expectation.* Human flourishing is to be found in freeing oneself from social expectations, from fixed errands of self-fashioning or desire that have been taken on despite the constrictions they impose, or perhaps precisely because such constric-tions seem to offer an illusory dream of completion. The aim is for peo-ple to give up such dreams and let their Eros take them where it will. All the rest, the expectations of the social world, the effort to figure out how to do life "right," or to earn approval, is a sort of dead end that frustrates the only thing that can truly matter: a satisfaction that exceeds any framing in terms of what is "good for you." I have given this picture of liberation from expectations, from self- and other-imposed templates for how to live, a Finkian/Lacanian spin. But there are other ways to conceptualize that which exceeds a socially shaped self-fashioning, for example, in some of Bollas' writing on personal idiom (Bollas, 1992). Freud clearly saw deleterious psychological effects coming from com-mon social expectations regarding sex and hoped psychoanalysis would provide some measure of relief. Rational-emotive therapy aims to help patients escape the tyranny of the "should." And many contemporary psychotherapies have been influenced by broad political movements that advocate for recognition of those who do not fit a culturally valued sexual orientation, gender identity, race, etc.

4) *Development of and Attunement to a Complex Inner Life in Relationship with Others.* A flourishing life is to be found in the development of particular human capacities: a rich inner life that involves an attune-ment to the nuances of one's own emotional and motivational complex-ity, nuances that can be articulated for oneself and to others as the basis for personal intimacy in relationships that are rooted in empathy and an

appreciation for the ambiguities of care and desire. Particularity here consists of the specific way this life is realized, rather than what remains after the impositions of others are subtracted. This picture of flourishing is present in various forms in humanistic and psychodynamic therapies (see for example various works by Stephen Mitchell and Nancy McWilliams, as well as the PDM2 and the Task Force for the Provision of Humanistic Psychological Services, 2004).

I want to emphasize that some variation on any one of these pictures of flourishing can be found in a number of different psychotherapies, and several of them may be combined in a given therapy. Most schools of therapy have been influenced by more than one of these aims. I am separating them here in order to illustrate central themes of therapeutic ethics. Further, this list is hardly exhaustive. These ideas about flourishing could be added to or modified by looking at other therapies (systemic, solution-focused, mindfulness-based, etc.) or at other examples of humanistic, cognitive-behavioral, and psychodynamic therapies. My aim here is not to spell out every variation on therapeutic ideas about flourishing but to point to a few of the more common themes.

Understanding Therapeutic Ethics

Many therapists may not even realize that they are implicitly promoting particular ethics because they seem obvious—these are "our" ethics, those of modern citizens of Western or North Atlantic societies. For example, valuing what is unique or particular to each person is so common for us that we find it hard to see that we are promoting it, or to conceive of a worthwhile alternative. Could any therapy imagine itself as working toward helping people to become just like everyone else? In fact, this is one of the critiques that some therapeutic schools bring against others (for example, in Fink's paper on the ethics of psychoanalysis, 2014b). Notice how this version of the alternative is formulated: becoming just like everyone else, "normal." We have a similar unquestioned assumption that autonomy is a fundamental good, so fundamental that it doesn't even require comment—except when charging others with undermining it, as Gray (1994) does when criticizing analysts who use patients' positive feelings about their analysts to get them to endorse the truth of an interpretation. For Gray, such emotional influence brings us close to the dreaded realms of suggestion and hypnosis. We so much take for granted the value of particularity and autonomy that we imagine the alternatives to be dangerous and destructive, producing obedient conformists. We don't imagine alternatives framed in such terms as, for example, affirming and valuing our place in family and community, a place that helps to define us, provides a secure base from which to venture forth, and where we depend upon others to whom we owe some debt.

In fact, ideals like particularity and autonomy are not universally valued as essential to human flourishing. The cultural support for such ideals in the West is not matched in other cultures. Gish Jen's *The Girl at the Baggage Claim: Explaining the East–West Culture Gap* (2017) illustrates the ways that the modern Western self is not like that of the East. One is individualistic and independent, the other collectivistic and interdependent (to greatly simplify her more nuanced discussion). Cross-cultural work like this is helpful in illustrating that many of the fundamental assumptions about human flourishing that are pervasive in the psychotherapies are far from universal. Multicultural critique of standard therapeutic practice relies upon such cultural comparisons (Roland, 1988; Sue and Sue, 2003).

Besides cross-cultural examination there have been numerous efforts to explain therapeutic ethics in terms of the social, political, and economic forces that shape them. Dalal (2018) describes how a distorted picture of cognitive-behavioral therapy as a set of techniques for happiness has been promoted through official health care policies in Britain. The result has been a denial of meaningful treatment in a capitalist program that runs public services on the model of a private business. Rose's (1990) Foucault-inspired analysis explores psychotherapy as a technology of the self that produces individuals whose "freedom" consists of an obligation to make choices of self-management and commodity consumption in order to be happy. As a result, they act in compliance with "political values of consumption, profitability, efficiency, and social order" (p. 10). Cushman (1995) argues that therapy often unwittingly serves consumerist capitalism, and urges therapists to help patients push back against such economic forces.

I believe that cross-cultural and political-economic analyses of the roots and consequences of therapeutic ideas about flourishing are important. I am going to take a different approach, however, examining these ethics in the context of their historical origins in modern Western culture. It is not just cultures in Asia or Africa that have contrasting ideas about human well-being. The therapeutic visions of flourishing listed above would have sounded alien to Europeans of an earlier era as well. Looking at the rise of the modern Western ethics that provide the matrix for therapeutic visions of a good life can reveal their historical-cultural contingency. But exploring their origins can also clarify aspects of their appeal. Modern ideas about who people are and what they need in order to live well arose in the context of broad changes in human self-understanding and social practice. These changes have resulted from efforts to address perceived problems or limitations in prior self-understandings and practices. Modern ideas about what constitutes human flourishing reflect a history of attempts to see human existence in a new way in order to live better. These efforts were partly shaped by influences outside the conscious grasp of the participants (by various structural changes, be these social, political, or economic). But the rise of distinctively modern ethics was also motivated by a more deliberate search for a better understanding of people as a way to help them live more fully, freely, capably, authentically, etc. Understanding modern ethics in the context of this search will help to clarify the appeal of therapeutic aims. It is to this historical-cultural context that I turn in the next chapter.

Notes

1 One could read Lear (2005) as an exception. In describing how neurosis undermines the ethical enterprise, he suggests that psychoanalysis can serve as a supplement to ethics, although he believes that it does not offer patients an alternative set of ethical principles.
2 For discussion of the relationship between basic moral obligations and ideas about living well, see the second chapter of *The Ethical Visions of Psychotherapy*.
3 Lear (2000) makes a similar point about the lack of ethical content to psychoanalysis. He speaks of analytic mindedness as an openness to new possibilities outside of any specific ethical structure (p. 128). Nevertheless, this openness, while not giving principles to live by, functions like particularity as a recommended constituent of living well.

3 Therapeutic Ethics and Charles Taylor's History of the Modern Identity

Introduction

Ideas about living well are not the inventions of individuals working in isolation. Even innovative ideals arise in response to a larger social world. In this chapter, I consider how the socio-historical context for therapy sheds light on its various ethics, clarifies why and how those ethics are important, and provides a framework for understanding the differences, overlap, and conflicts among them. The frame of reference I use to describe this social context is the history of modern ideas about a good life in Charles Taylor's work, especially his *Sources of the Self: The Making of the Modern Identity* (1989). Taylor's history of the modern West begins circa 1500 with the rise of early modern science and philosophy, the Protestant Reformation, and various changes in personal, cultural, and political life. He focuses on north Atlantic countries, with the bulk of his examples being drawn from England, France, and Germany in the early period, later adding Anglophone North America, Australia, and New Zealand. He is well aware of the limitations of such boundaries, pointing at times to examples of similar developments in other countries and to variations within the bounds of his focal analysis. But his survey of slow cultural change over several centuries in several countries already relies upon careful attention to details of social history, history of ideas, and cultural studies that would become yet more complex if even nearby countries were added, let alone other regions.

Taylor's history is built around a few key themes: the sense of inwardness central to the modern experience of self, the affirmation of ordinary life, and the new value attributed to the voice of nature. In explicating these themes, Taylor describes the development of various modern conceptions of knowledge, reason, human motivation, personal and social relations, and the place of humanity in the rest of the natural world. These ideas have implications for any modern Westerner's understanding of what is possible and optimal in the effort to live well. Although he describes some links between ethical ideals and the social structures and institutions that helped to engender and support them, his primary intent is not to provide a causal explanation of the modern identity. Instead, he asks:

> What drew people to it? ... What gave it its spiritual power? ... What this question asks for is an interpretation of the [modern] identity ... which will show why people found (or find) it convincing/inspiring/moving, which will identify what can be called the "idées-forces" it contains.
>
> (Taylor, 1989, p. 203)

As I summarize Taylor's account of the rise of modern ethics, I point to links with the contemporary psychotherapeutic ethics summarized in the last chapter. These connections to contemporary psychotherapy are my interpretations of Taylor's history (he only occasionally links his exposition of the modern identity to therapy). My intention is to provide the cultural-historical context for therapeutic aims in order to highlight the ethical aspirations of therapy that go beyond the scientific treatment of disorders.

Inwardness as Rational Self-Mastery: The Influence of Descartes and Locke

Many of the psychotherapies depend upon the idea of a personal inner realm, whether this is conceived of as unnoticed cognitive assumptions or the depths of the unconscious. But the idea of an inner theater of the mind is not a universal way of framing the nature of persons. The modern notion of personal inwardness involves a division between inside and outside, with thoughts, ideas, feelings, and wishes being inside, and the objects in the world that mental states bear upon being outside. There is a version of the inner–outer distinction that is present in many cultures. This is the distinction between what is felt or thought but remains private because it is not spoken, and that which is shared with others. This take on the inside–outside difference does not capture what is specific to the modern distinction, however. In order to illustrate what is unique to the modern view, Taylor turns to Plato's picture of the soul in *The Republic* to present a contrasting picture of the relation between mind and world. Taylor looks at Plato's distinctions between the soul and the body, the immaterial and the material, the eternal and the changing, and notes that these do not map neatly onto a division between inner and outer.

It is Plato's view that the rational part of the soul should rule over both the appetites and the passionate, spirited part of the soul (thumos). This does not sound alien to moderns. We know various versions of the idea that the rational part of the mind (as we would call it) should rule in life. Even if many moderns (the Romantics, for example) critique some versions of the idea, we are familiar with it. Cognitive-behavioral therapy puts forth one version of this. Freud also values rationality, although he believes we need to be careful about efforts to subjugate appetite, or, using his language, drive. Such efforts are likely to result in the drives or their derivatives resisting restraint in ways that produce the irrationality of neurosis. But in such cautions Freud is offering a re-working of a familiar framework, not proposing something that Plato would not recognize. At least, not as I have so far described it.

Matters become more complicated when one starts to examine more closely how Plato understood reason. Rationality for him is not a product of the mind's processes, nor does it reside in the mind. For Plato, "our becoming rational ought not most perspicuously to be described as something that takes place in us, but rather better as our connecting up to the larger order in which we are placed" (Taylor, 1989, p. 123). Reason involves turning the soul toward the real order of being so that it can be seen. To understand something is for the soul to participate in the Idea which gives that thing its being. As a consequence, one can't be rational and be wrong, for being rational is seeing the order of being, seeing the ideas that give intelligibility to the objects we encounter. This is not just the way to truth. Our seeing the order of being also reveals to us what is good and beautiful. These too are seen, not constructed.

By contrast, modern ideas about rationality do frame it as a process that takes place inside the mind. Descartes is a key figure in the development of the modern conception. Unlike Plato, he argued for a radical disjunction between the realm of ideas and the material world. The latter is not given its sense and being through participation in ideas. The material world does not express anything. It is mere extension and to be understood mechanistically. Ideas, on the other hand, have nothing to do with the material world—they exist only in the mind. The mind is known primarily in its activity of constructing a picture of the world around it. The rationality of mind consists in its capacity to construct that picture accurately, with certainty founded on evidence. Rational activity can lead to incorrect conclusions, for it is not a direct seeing of the order of being, but a process of constructing that order by following the proper method. People can err in applying the method, leave out steps, or utilize the wrong data and come up with conclusions that are at variance with how things really are. An accurately constructed picture of the material world reveals how it functions, enabling effective action that successfully achieves freely chosen ends.

For Descartes the body, too, is part of the material realm. The body and the passions that are rooted in it are not to be ruled by a rational vision of the true cosmic order. Rather, the body is to be used instrumentally by a technical rationality which understands how it works. The aim of understanding how the world works in order to act effectively within it becomes more than a recommended method for successful action. Descartes inaugurates a new ideal for how to live well. The sense of living life well comes not from acknowledging a fundamental good which inspires us and to which we answer. Rather, the agent's sense of dignity comes from having control over one's own body, one's passions, and the natural world through a well-founded knowledge of how these material phenomena work mechanistically. On Descartes' view, the mind is fundamentally reflexive. It is reflection on its own operations, operations that consist of the careful assessment of a world stripped of any intrinsic meaning. Done properly, this assessment guarantees the self-sufficient certainty of knowledge.

According to Taylor, Descartes begins one important version of the modern inward turn. For Descartes, the human agent does not search for a meaning that is expressed in the world, but monitors its own inner processes of reasoning to ensure that an accurate representation of the world has been constructed. The mind is immaterial, and its task is to objectify fundamentally meaningless material that can be mastered if one uses the proper method. Cartesian subjects are fundamentally disengaged from the world and their embodiment within it in order to be able to act effectively.

There are clearly intimations here of the therapeutic vision of flourishing as rational self-mastery that I described in the previous chapter. Descartes' version of this is hardly identical with any particular version of it in modern psychotherapy. But the ideal of disengagement for the sake of effective action in service of one's individually chosen aims echoes throughout modern psychology and psychotherapy. One can frame self-efficacy as a psychological trait that operates across social and cultural contexts (Bandura, 1997). Certainly, part of what it means to act in any context is to hope that one's actions will be effective. But the modern ideal that Taylor traces back to Descartes and that is present in some therapies is more than a desire for an action to succeed. It is a conception of what it is to live well that is built around the maximization of efficacy rooted in a picture of people as acting upon a domain of matter with no intrinsic meaning, in order to achieve freely chosen ends. Descartes' philosophy presages the therapeutic stance of detached observation of one's emotional processes as the basis for decisions about whether to endorse them, to liberate them from prohibition, or to discover how to manage or change them. Such a stance toward the self is present in any number of therapeutic practices and concepts (cognitive restructuring, examining the evidence for feared outcomes, the psychoanalytic observing ego, etc.).

It is important to see that Cartesian disengagement is not quite the same as that of ancient Stoic thought. One can see this in their contrasting views on emotion. For the Stoics, passions are wrong opinions, such as mistaken

beliefs that wealth, honor, the esteem of others, or social position are important. People make themselves subject to unnecessary suffering through such
errors. They may become enraged or melancholy because they believe that
one of these "goods" was taken away from them. But the Stoic sage sees that
such things do not really matter and can thereby rise above the petty fears,
envies, and angers that are experienced by those who misunderstand what is
truly worthwhile. The Stoic sage is free of such passions and instead exhibits
apatheia, equanimity. Stoic insight into what truly matters enables one to step
back from excessive attachment to trivial matters that one cannot change and
focus upon that which one can influence—one's own opinions about what
matters and the intentional actions that flow from them.

For Descartes, however, the passions are not wrong opinions that are the
result of false assessments of what is truly valuable. Instead, the passions are
an extra energy that can be imparted to a course of action. This can make
action more successful if the added emotional energy is directed by the oversight of reason. The effort to succeed at reaching any goal one chooses is not
Stoic equanimity. Further, on the Cartesian view, even violent passions may
be an advantage if they are put in the service of rationally chosen aims. The
task for rationally directed action is not so much to see what matters and what
doesn't, but to see what objects and forces are present in a situation in order
to manage it better, to act effectively in it, and perhaps to use the energy of
the passions to lend greater power to one's actions. This is an ethic of rational
control, of disengagement from a meaningless material world in order to see
how to influence it for one's own ends. It is not the Stoic recommendation to
step back from a false picture of what is worthwhile in order to clearly see
what is genuinely significant.

Descartes conceives of persons as agents who use effective means to pursue ends of their own choosing. Descartes' Christian faith set a frame for his
conception of proper choices regarding a good life with others. But his picture of mind intimates the purely instrumental stance toward self and world
that will take on starker forms in later modern thought, where means can be
rationally discerned but ends appear to have no rational foundation. Much
of the modern therapeutic ethos shares this picture of people. Consequently,
therapeutic aims are usually framed as an effort to restore patients' freedom
to pursue ends of their own choosing, and as refraining from the promotion of alternative goods. Robinson (2010) notes this in his discussion of
some differences between Stoic thought and cognitive-behavioral therapy:
"It is not a trivial matter to observe that, unlike Stoicism and most classical philosophies, CBT lacks any clear account of the ideal toward which it
aims" (p. 137). Therapists generally subscribe to the modern idea that one
settles on aims for living well through personal, even arbitrary, choice. And
since ends can't be rationally established but are subjectively chosen by each

individual, respect for the individual's freedom of choice is paramount. In the previous chapter, I discussed the centrality of this idea for therapeutic ethics under the headings of autonomy and particularity. It is also at the heart of modern liberal views that play an important role in the thinking of therapists. Freud (1919/1955a) gives pointed expression to this idea in his warning that psychoanalytic treatment ought not to move beyond analysis to "synthesis," toward shaping the patient according to an ideal or philosophy that the analyst subscribes to. To do so is "only to use violence, even though it is overlaid with the most honorable motives" (p. 165).

Taylor sees in Locke's theory of mind a further development of Descartes' disengaged self. Locke developed a model of thinking as the rule-governed re-working of what is given to us through passive processes of sensory reception and association. What sensation and association give to us is fine as far as it goes, but the elementary ideas so delivered to us are synthesized into distorted general ideas through the influence of custom, bad education, and the passions. In order to overcome these distortions, we need to take the false ideas we have been taught, disassemble them back into their elementary forms, and then re-combine them by reliable rules of mathematics, deduction, and probable evidence. There are two reasons why it is important for people to think things out for themselves. First, independent rule-governed thinking is more likely to arrive at correct results that are not distorted by the corrupting overlay of tradition and authority. Second, the project to arrive at reliable knowledge through one's own efforts is necessary in order to maintain independence, to escape manipulation and domination by others. The ideal of independent, critical thinking suggests that there is a link between truth and freedom.

Locke added a non-teleological model of motivation to this picture of the self-responsible reconstruction of ideas. Why do we seek what we seek? What makes something appear to be worthwhile or desirable? It is not that we see that an object of desire is in fact good, worthwhile, or desirable in itself. We do not act "for the sake of" something beyond us. Rather, there is an uneasiness inside us that pushes us toward an object. The object toward which we are driven has become a desired object because it has been associated with a decrease of unease in the past. This process might appear to make us the pawns of past associations over which we have no control. However, like the view of the world foisted on us by our culture, the linking of unease with objects that have relieved unease in the past can be disassembled and examined according to canons of evidence. I may have found myself focused on certain objects due to their past association with a decrease in tension, but I can stand back from such associations and consider whether it makes sense to pursue a particular object. Analogous to the way that education and custom have given us false ideas, they have also given us bad habits. Through careful analysis we can challenge the standard views of what is worthwhile, suspend our surrender to the passively established link between certain objects and the relief of unease, and establish new habits in order to bring about greater pleasure or happiness.

Taylor emphasizes that nothing that we find in this sort of reflection belongs to or constitutes us—it is simply material that we can reshape. On Locke's view, what we most fundamentally are *is* just this capacity to reshape. Taylor says that Locke's view of the mind gives us a "punctual" self that has no content beyond its capacity to observe and remake itself. What I observe within myself are not givens that I discover I am, but constructions I can reconstruct. The power to disengage from culture, tradition, and one's own inclinations results in a concept of the person as a disembodied being existing outside of socio-cultural context, as a pure act of examination and instrumental re-working of a material world that has no meaning in itself and that provides no guidance or direction for living. Such a self is "punctual" in the sense that it is a point of consciousness that is distinguished from its embodiment, and can be imagined to be detachable from it. The idea of the detached punctual self has lent plausibility both to modern science fiction stories that depict minds being transported into other bodies or machines, and to psychotherapies that conceive of persons as capable of re-engineering themselves.

Inwardness as Self-Exploration and Personal Particularity

While the detached stance has played an important role in the natural scientific study of how the world works, it has significant limitations for understanding human experience. Taylor notes that there are some human phenomena that are better understood through a deeper engagement or immersion in them, not through detachment. As an example, he points to the explication of our emotional life. Consider the following scenario. I have some vague sense of dislike toward a man I met at a social gathering, but I didn't think much about it at the time. Later, a friend refers to this man and I remember not liking him, but can't specify exactly what is prompting the feeling, or even whether there is something more specific to it than "dislike." So I start to talk about this person with my friend, and the feeling comes back again. I discover in letting myself feel this dislike more fully that it is prompted by the sense that the other didn't listen when I spoke, but always steered the conversation back to something he wanted to talk about. I felt unseen, ignored, as though I were not worthy of his attention. Further, the person talked about things as though he assumed everyone agreed with him, liberally introducing what he said with "of course," or "as we all know." He made pronouncements, not conversation. And I discover that tangled up in my dislike of the person was a wish to argue with him, to assert the independence of my views.

In this example, it is not detachment from my feelings that helps to explicate them, but a fuller immersion in them, letting them guide my articulation. This immersive self-understanding constitutes a radical alternative to the disengaged, punctual self of Descartes and Locke. It too involves a sort of inwardness and reflexivity that is quintessentially modern. And it too has an early modern progenitor—Montaigne. Montaigne's self-reflection didn't seek fundamental truths beneath the flux of experience. Nor was he interested in the rational assessment of what he found within as part of a project to remake himself, to achieve mastery over his thinking and habits. He simply wanted to ascertain and describe what he saw. His reflections on the details of his personal experience were not intended to be part of the development of self toward what is better morally, nor toward what is more rational and effective. In fact, Montaigne held that the demands of self-perfection could be tyrannical and needed to be tempered. The exploration of self here was done more for the sake of self-acceptance and self-discovery than for self-mastery.

> Montaigne is an originator of the search for each person's originality; and this is not just a different quest but in a sense antithetical to the Cartesian … The Cartesian calls for a radical disengagement from ordinary experience; Montaigne requires a deeper engagement in our particularity. These two facets of individuality have been at odds up to this day.
>
> (Taylor, 1989, p. 182)

While Montaigne's version of personal self-reflection is a striking and singular example, widespread forms of self-examination can be found throughout the early modern period. Many of these initially took religious form, being supported by both Puritan and Jesuit spiritualities. Taylor cites social historians who have explored the rise of journal writing out of Puritan practices of inner spiritual scrutiny. This attention to and documentation of personal experience was later continued in secular forms, laying the groundwork for the eighteenth-century English novel.

These two facets of modern individuality are easily linked to elements of the four ethical ideals of therapy outlined in the previous chapter. Certainly therapeutic rational self-mastery appears to be a descendent of the disengaged, punctual self theorized by Descartes and Locke. Montaigne's inward turn to acknowledge whatever is found in the stream of experience, without placing excessive moral demands upon what is found, has many exemplars in psychoanalytic and humanistic therapies. The therapeutic idea that we should value what is particular to who we are and protect it from the impositions of family, society, and moral demands is very much in keeping with Montaigne's views, even if contemporary versions take on forms that he would not recognize.

The pictures of flourishing on offer in the psychotherapies have roots in a modern ethos whose origins go back to early modern thinkers. These cultural roots are overlooked by practicing therapists, therapy theorists, and researchers when they get caught up in the details of practice and technique, the rationales for various orientations, and questions regarding therapeutic efficacy. The latter concerns can obscure the broader aims of therapy that partake of a particular culture's views of what constitutes a well-lived life. Taylor's history makes plain that such views are not the result of a simple scientific examination of "how people really work." They partake of a modern Western ethical tradition that proposes specific ideas about human well-being.

Disengagement, Social Discipline, and the Modern Buffered Self

Linking therapeutic ethics to modern Western culture requires more than finding connections between therapy and the ideas of a few philosophers. In explicating the two modern forms of inwardness I have so far summarized Taylor's overview of three early modern thinkers' ideas about mind and self. But a culture is more than ideas. It includes a widespread set of practices that instantiate such ideas in daily life and experience. By "practices" Taylor means "more or less any stable configuration of shared activity, whose shape is defined by a certain pattern of dos and don'ts" (Taylor, 1989, p. 204). Explicit ethical ideas articulate, support, or "bring to some conscious expression the underlying rationale of the patterns" (ibid.).

The personal stance of disengagement was recommended by Descartes and Locke for epistemological reasons, but it was also an ethical stance. That is, it became an ideal for mature autonomous people who were determined to think for themselves rather than be passively enthralled by the taken-for-granted views of their culture or tradition. The ideal of detachment and re-examination of the culturally accepted also appeared in early modern thinking about traditional social arrangements. Various projects to foster rational control over social practices began in the late sixteenth and early seventeenth centuries. There was a new emphasis upon discipline and rigor in military and civil administration, and in regulating social practices in the arenas of commerce, labor, health, morals, and religion. These are the changes in modern social practice that have been a central focus of much of Foucault's work (Taylor references Foucault's *Discipline and punish*, 1975/1977). The ideal of rational mastery motivated not only the project of individual detachment from unthinking engagement in life in order to remake thinking and habits. This ideal was also operative in a modern project of social objectification, a re-working of practices and institutions for the sake of more effective societal control.

Those social practices and institutions in turn shaped patterns of individual decision-making and personal ideals for how to live well. Taylor emphasizes that the influence between social structures and popular ideals operates in both directions. He differs from theorists like Marx and Weber who see social and economic structures as determinative of how we live, unilaterally creating demands and ideals (or ideologies) that determine our views about how to live well. Taylor does not believe that social institutions and structures create a sort of "iron cage" (in Weber's language) from which we cannot escape. Widely held ideals and social structures shape each other, help to create, sustain, and change each other. One is not the originary source of the other.

If social conditions do not unilaterally determine ethics, they neverthe-less have a powerful influence. Taylor (2007) discusses the ways that modern changes in social structure contributed to changes in the ways that people managed their emotions. He references Elias' (1939/1978) history of increasing bodily fastidiousness and control over emotional expression as social structures were transformed from the medieval to the early modern period. Elias notes that the medieval knight or lord was fundamentally a warrior whose power and prestige depended upon physical might. As such, his capacity to lead and succeed in battle was of prime importance. There was no need to curtail emotional expression—in fact, the martialing of intense rage might be an asset in battle and demonstrate in other contexts that he was not to be trifled with. Nor were ready acts of aggression restricted to knights. The relatively uninhibited expression of "belligerence, hatred, and joy in tormenting others" (Elias, 1939/1978, p. 166) was also present in the life of townspeople. Open and casual acts of violence were common and unremarkable. They were even part of festivities. "In Paris during the sixteenth century it was one of the festive pleasures of Midsummer Day to burn alive one or two dozen cats" (p. 171).

Elias notes that the easy expression of aggression and violence was not a matter of people being continually angry, fiercely scowling, and constantly challenging others to fight. "On the contrary, a moment ago they were joking, now they mock each other, one word leads to another, and suddenly from the midst of laughter they find themselves in the fiercest feud" (p. 168). What he describes is an emotional life that was given free rein to be volatile. With regard to bodily intimacies, what mattered in pre-modern Europe was the social status of others who were present. A knight might well be naked or use a chamber pot in front of a servant or someone of lesser rank, but would not do so in the presence of someone of higher rank.

Social structures slowly changed in modernity as power centers grew larger, there were fewer sovereign lords, and those who had previously ruled independently became dependent upon maintaining their position within a large royal court. Early modern European court life required a different sort of attunement to rank, a courtier's sensibility. That is, court life required the careful assessment of what was owed to whom in a much more intricate labyrinth of gradations of power and status that were arrayed beneath the king. Now it was best to guard one's feelings, to be circumspect about how openly expressive one was, and to be careful not to engage in open displays of emotional expression or bodily functions without understanding the risks and benefits in a far more complex social world. Descartes' disengaged self as an epistemological ideal here matched up with a socially necessary disengagement from, and restricted expression of, emotion and bodily functions.

Elias' work sheds light on how some of our fundamental ideas about psychological health are closely linked to particular social structures of modernity. As an example, consider theories about the role of emotion regulation and mentalization in borderline pathology (see Bateman and Fonagy, 2004, p. 85f). Some capacity for mentalization and rudimentary emotional regulation is necessary for participation in any human society. But emotional regulation is not all or nothing. Our understanding of whether someone's degree of emotional regulation is healthy or pathological can be shaped by expectations that derive from the demands of our particular social organization. Such expectations were clearly different in the pre-modern Europe Elias describes.[1]

The greater restraint in emotional expression and the Cartesian dichotomy between the mental and the material supported other changes in modern lived experience. As modern social life developed there was an increase in the lived sense of a thick boundary separating self and world. For pre-moderns, the boundary between the mental/emotional inside and the material world outside was both theorized and experienced as porous. Pre-modern Europeans lived with a sense of themselves as subject to and influenced by charged objects (charms, potions, relics of the saints, etc.). The world was experienced as full of good and evil spirits that resided in special places and objects, spirits who can protect or do harm. There was not a sharp distinction between meaningless matter and meaningful mind. For example, the medieval view of melancholy was that it resided *in* black bile, and not, as we moderns might re-interpret the theory, that bile causes melancholy. For the earlier view, an emotional quality resided in a physical substance, not just in psychological experience. In modernity, the boundary between the physical and the psychological is understood to be impervious, with a meaningful phenomenon like melancholy being a mental event that can only be understood as caused by material substances (neurotransmitters) that have no psychological meaning in themselves.

The pre-modern view of magic was that it also crossed this boundary between the material and the mental. Love potions or spells were understood to influence personal experience through powers that reside in special materials or speech acts. In the course of modern history, we have moved to living as bounded selves that are buffered in such a way that it is a work of imagination to entertain the possibility of being subject to magical forces and spirits. For the modern disengaged self that stands back from the world in order to understand its workings and thereby act effectively within it, the idea of a substance or spell having an occult effect upon one is an intrusion upon one's autonomy, it is an intolerable "imprisoning of the self in uncanny external forces" (Taylor, 1989, p. 192).

Taylor speculates that the European witchcraft craze occurred when it did because of the instability of the new sense of self in this period (approximately the fifteenth to the mid-seventeenth centuries). A new sense of self as bounded and self-possessed existed in tension with an older notion of our vulnerability to occult forces. The latter, such as the influence of witchcraft, was a threat to this new self. Earlier attitudes toward witchcraft were more skeptical and occult practices were not experienced as a profound threat, for the ideal of a buffered self that would be threatened by them did not yet exist. And, in fact, it was not medieval but early modern Europe that put witches on trial and burned them.

Freud can serve as a useful illustration of the modern buffered self and its connection to therapeutic ethics. He makes many comments in his writings on his well-bounded self, of being impervious to the experience of spiritual forces that were commonly accepted as part of pre-modern life. In *The Psychopathology of Everyday Life*, Freud (1901/1960) notes that he cannot pronounce on the possibility of things like prophetic dreams or supernatural forces for he has had no experience of such things. His tone suggests gentle mocking of those who claim to have had such experiences.

> To my regret I must confess that I am one of those unworthy people in whose presence spirits suspend their activity and the supernatural vanishes away, so that I have never been in a position to experience anything myself which might arouse a belief in the miraculous.
>
> (p. 261)

Of course, Freud linked his uncompromising adherence to science with a resolute atheism and skepticism regarding the supernatural. But one can see in many of his comments on this and similar subjects that Freud is not simply referring to his system of beliefs, but to his way of experiencing the world. In his paper on the uncanny he notes his personal insensitivity to this phenomenon. He links uncanny experiences to animism, including "the attribution to various outside persons and things of carefully graded magical powers, or mana" (Freud, 1919/1955c, p. 240). He argues that we all go through a version of animistic thinking in childhood. But those who have matured leave such beliefs behind, and, with them, the vulnerability to experience the uncanny.

Perhaps the clearest expression of Freud's buffered self is his discussion of the oceanic feeling in *Civilization and Its Discontents* (Freud, 1930/1961a). As in his discussion of the uncanny, he begins by saying that he "cannot discover this 'oceanic' feeling in myself" (p. 65). He then goes on to say that while the self or ego does shade off into the id as one looks further inward, toward the outside world the boundary is quite sharp, at least for the normal adult who is not (his one exception) "at the height of being in love" (p. 66). One sees here a link between the affirmation of inwardness and the resolute insistence on a sharp boundary between within and without. Freud also argues that this sort of boundary is an achievement, that it is not present for the infant or in "primitive" animistic peoples.

It may be that this sense of having strong boundaries also played a part in his indifference to music (see Jones, 1957, p. 408), which, as Adam Phillips points out, was "something of a feat in the Vienna of his time" (2014, p. 18). To be open to music is to be open to influence from something that gets inside and stirs an emotional response, and that can cross the boundary between inside and out without asking permission. Certainly other forms of art (visual and verbal) can be powerfully affecting. But because the viewers can turn their gaze where they will with a painting, or because readers can break off the reading of a poem as they wish, there remains an element of control that is less easily available for music.[2] As sound, music pervades and penetrates, surrounds and gets inside, whether invited in or not. Perhaps Freud was not simply indifferent to music, but protectively walled off against what he perceived as a non-rational intrusion.

What might appear to be an exception may actually reinforce the picture of Freud's buffered self. He does accept the possibility of telepathy in a number of writings (for example, 1925/1961b, 1933/1964, 1941/1955b), although he notes in one paper (again!) that this is not part of his personal experience, that he is devoid of an occult sense (1941/1955b, p. 193). However, his account of telepathy does not dissolve the boundary between self and other, but assumes it and attempts to explain how communication across this boundary is possible. He calls telepathy thought-transfer, and suggests there may be a process of transduction where thoughts are transferred into a physical medium, which has some effect upon the receiving person and is then somehow transferred back into thought. He draws an analogy to the telephone, with the transfer of sound to electrical impulses and back to sound. He does not see telepathy as evidence that selves might be porous. Rather, he wants to find a scientific explanation for what can only appear as a puzzling communication across boundaries that should make such influence impossible. Such communication would not be puzzling for the porous selves of pre-moderns.

It would be understood to be part and parcel of the lived experience of being vulnerable to the impact of all sorts of powerful forces and meaningful signs in the surrounding world.

Freud described himself as buffered. He also believed that a buffered self was what one would expect of any civilized adult. The personal experience and valuation of such boundedness may also have played a part in his conception of psychoanalysis as a practice where analysts' detached objectivity enables them to accurately observe and interpret the manifestations of the patient's unconscious. This view is often contested today, with many analysts arguing that there is a complex entanglement of patient and analyst, each influencing the other and contributing to what appears in session. It seems safe to assume that, to a great extent, Freud did have a buffered self, whether or not this provided any objectivity in his psychoanalytic practice. But more important than his simply being so, he felt it was right to be so, that this was what non-neurotic rationality and maturity looked like. The buffered self was a sort of ideal for Freud that shaped his pictures of psychopathology, maturity, and analytic practice. This may also help to explain why he was always careful when discussing occult or spiritual matters to be sure to remind his readers of his personal lack of experience of them. It is as though it were important for him to say: "I am not one of those people who feel themselves to be subject to inexplicable spiritual forces or to have a mystical attunement to the world. I am thoroughly walled off from such things, and proud of it." Freud was always suspect of his patients' emphatic denials. Denials suggest an effort to shore up a preferred picture of oneself, often driven by moral strictures that lead to deceiving oneself about uncomfortable personal truths. However accurate Freud's claims about his boundedness may have been, the repetition of the claim may also speak to his need to live up to an ideal of being buffered that functioned as a sort of ethical imperative rooted in his understanding of what it meant to live life well.

However, Freud would not have felt the need to proclaim how thoroughly buffered he was if this was the general condition of all selves in modernity. Freud is right that a well-bounded self, like many psychological configurations, is not given at birth. The degree to which it is achieved varies from person to person. Further, the modern emphasis on a sharp boundary between self and world exists in tension with other ways of thinking about the self that are native to modernity. For example, the oceanic feeling of oneness or attunement to the world that a modern might experience, and that Freud claimed to have no experience of, is not quite the same as the porous self of pre-modernity. It is likely to have links to other modern ideals deriving from Romanticism. I examine Taylor's exposition of these ideals later in this chapter.

The Affirmation of Ordinary Life and the Therapeutic Ethic of Intimate Emotional Bonds

The inward turn available to moderns has roots in two versions of reflective self-examination present at the beginning of the modern era: the disengaged self-observation and self-mastery of Descartes and Locke, and the careful attention to and respect for personal particularity of Montaigne. But there are other important contributors to the modern sense of inwardness. A new emphasis upon the importance of one's emotional life grew out of what Taylor describes as the affirmation of ordinary life.

To illustrate what he means by this change Taylor again makes a contrast with pre-modern views. Aristotle makes plain in his writings on ethics and politics that there is a difference between life and the good life. Life requires attention to bodily needs, the management of a household economy, involvement in family, sex, and procreation, and availability to defend one's community. The good life goes beyond these mundane concerns to theoretical contemplation and citizen participation in the polity. Taylor sees in modernity a broad critique of this elevation of contemplation and political life above the day-to-day pursuits of work and family ("ordinary life"). Theoretical contemplation was attacked in the early modern period for lacking the practical value of the new empirical sciences that promised technological benefits. And political life was criticized as the arena for grasping at glory and power. The latter critique was also expressed by ancient Stoics and medieval Christians. But their complaint about political vainglory was that it turned people away from philosophical contemplation or the love of God. For moderns, another basis for this critique arose: the pursuit of honor and glory is a distraction from the sober productive benefits of work and family life.

How did this elevation of ordinary life come about? Taylor points to its beginnings in the Reformation. Medieval Western Christianity was seen by the Reformers as elevating some ways of living the faith above others. There were those consecrated to God in special vocations (monks, nuns, and priests) and those for whom the spiritual life was less central, the laity who benefited from the spiritual efforts of the more fully devoted. The Reformation revised and rejected this view in various ways, affirming the laity as full participants in Christian life. Rather than the special vocations of Catholicism the reformers promoted the idea of a calling. People are called by God to a particular type of work, and no work is lesser or greater provided that it is done in service to the Lord. A leveling of social status began here that went through a number of developments in later modernity.

Further, this demotion of the higher status assigned to a life specially dedicated to prayer and spiritual works was combined with a suspicion of the asceticism that often went with monastic and priestly vocations. Asceticism was critiqued by the Reformers as a prideful refusal to enjoy God's gifts. The material goods that are the fruits of labor and the enjoyments of married life are ultimately benefits bestowed by God, and should be enjoyed as such. What matters for Christian living is not a special form of work, monastic dedication to prayer, or presiding over sacramental rites. Rather, ordinary life, done worshipfully, was seen as sanctified in Reformation theology. This esteem for human productivity in ordinary work took on non-religious connotations in later centuries, heightened by the rise of capitalism. Critics of capitalism like Marx also maintained this focus on human productive capacity. Further, the elevation of the spiritual value of married life over the celibacy of priests and nuns was also given secular form in subsequent centuries in the ideal of a companionate marriage built upon strong bonds of sentiment. But Taylor sees the roots of these later developments in changes initiated at the Reformation.

The value given to work and marriage brings to mind a saying that is often attributed to Freud: the aim of treatment is to be able to love and to work. Freud's view, that to aim higher than this is to court neurosis (even if a few may be capable of something higher), provides a distant psychological echo of what the Reformers understood in religious terms. Such a picture of what constitutes human flourishing would seem alien or paltry both to the aristocratic warrior who sought glory in battle and to the medieval nun who dedicated her life to God. A critic of modernity like Nietzsche might also see in this picture of human well-being the pitiful goals of the last men. But "to love and to work" generally makes sense to us moderns as reasonable aims. So much so that we may not even notice that there is a particular ethic here. It just seems like common sense, common sense being one form taken by the largely uncontested ethic of a culture.

Illustrating the affirmation of ordinary life and tracing its further developments, Taylor emphasizes the role of Deism, the rise of new art forms, and the ideal of the companionate marriage.

Deism

Taylor examines the transformation of the early modern religious affirmation of ordinary life into its later, secular version. He sees the rationalized Christianity of Deism as an important bridge between them. Locke provides an early exposition of Deism in his notion that the order of nature reveals God's beneficence and wisdom. Our disengaged autonomous reason enables us to see this order and thereby to discern and participate in God's purposes. However, Locke's views still contain elements of the traditional picture of human depravity, but now given a naturalistic spin as an innate tendency to be self-serving. Though our reason may enable us to see the lineaments of God's plan in the natural world, our natural egocentric tendencies make us unable to follow it except through the threat of damnation. According to Locke, our very egocentrism and hedonism, our natural desire to experience happiness and avoid pain, is used by God through the threat of punishment in the after-life to help us turn that selfishness toward the good. Our self-love becomes an instrument that leads us to do what is right, to do as God commands.

There were those who were unsatisfied with this picture of human depravity, whether it took the theological form of fallen nature, or Locke's naturalized variant. The objection was to a picture of people as inherently alienated from God, as sharing so little in his goodness that they either require his undeserved grace or must be threatened with damnation. A countervailing trend within Deism viewed people as intrinsically attuned to God. Shaftesbury proposed that people are not fundamentally corrupted by sin, but have an inclination toward a love of the good. The older ethic based on a rational order designed by God was transformed into an ethic of affective attunement to God that naturally leads us to participate in God's benevolence toward his creation. We move toward the good not by disengaging from ourselves and the world around us to examine them rationally and discern God's will, but by engaging more deeply with the love of the good implanted in us by God and that is part of our nature. Our inner nature came to be seen as a moral source that revealed the good and motivated us to pursue it.[3]

Further developments in Deism initiated a new perspective on emotion, where "sentiment" replaces "passion" as the key term. For the ancients, the passions are opinions about what matters. The Stoics saw those opinions as leading us astray, generating desires for that which is ephemeral and beyond our control, like fame, wealth, and the esteem of others. For Descartes, passions are not opinions but a bodily energy that can be put in the service of a course of action decided upon rationally. In the eighteenth century "sentiment" (not passion) came to have a normative value. Sentiments can tell us what is good. We have natural sentiments of affection and sympathy for others that are central to a good life. Attunement to this inner nature can guide us in living well and support the social bonds that are necessary to live with others in community. These are not reasoned conclusions about the good, but a felt connection to and expression of the good. We are not alienated from a good "out there" but can find it within us as part of our very being. This too is an affirmation of ordinary life, not just of the mundane activities of work and family, but of day-to-day emotional experience. This new understanding of emotional life was an important forerunner of later Romantic views.

The Importance of the Particular in the Novel and Painting

The rise of the modern novel further illustrates the rise of middle classes who valued the mundane world of work and family over heroic action and aristocratic virtues. In the novels of Dafoe, Richardson, and Fielding the subjects are middle class people dealing with entrepreneurial virtues and issues of love and marriage. And the characters are particular—their lives are described in the kind of detail that renders them specific. They are not broadly sketched representatives of their class or region. They are not archetypal or "everyman" characters dealing with general issues of life. Nor are they epic figures whose heroic deeds place them outside the realm of daily existence. The general themes that are addressed are presented through the minutely observed details of the ordinary lives of particular people.[4]

Something similar occurs in painting in the modern period. One can see this by comparing a Rembrandt self-portrait with a medieval painting of Madonna and child. It is not simply that Rembrandt considered himself to be a worthy subject of painting. He also seemed to be trying in at least some of the self-portraits to portray what was distinctive about his features and his character. The medieval Madonna on the other hand is an archetypal subject, and is worthy of painting because of a fundamental spiritual significance that transcends the particulars of who the actual mother of Jesus may have been. It didn't matter for medieval painters or their audience that Mary was portrayed with the dress and in the settings of the painter's own day, not those of first-century Palestine. An archetype exists across time and recurs in particular times and places without its fundamental meaning changing. For moderns, however, persons are individuals who can be understood only through particulars, be those the particulars portrayed in paintings like Rembrandt's self-portraits, or in the details of upbringing, relationships, and personal choices that make up the plot of a novel or the content of a diary.

This focus on the particulars of persons is central to therapeutic practice, whether it takes the form of attention to the details of free associations, of patients' descriptions of their upbringing, or of their cognitive appraisals of particular events in their lives. Archetypes are explored in Jungian analysis for their relevance to the specific issues faced by a given patient, not in order to identify universal themes that could apply to anyone. Therapeutic conversation is not general discussion of abstract ideas but careful examination of personal particulars, for therapy shares the widespread modern value assigned to individual particularity.

The Companionate Marriage

The Reformers' elevation of family life above the ascetic life of monks and nuns laid the groundwork for the late seventeenth century's new view of marriage as built upon affectionate companionship of husband and wife and careful attention to the development of the children. The ideal of companionate marriage required a decline in the influence of the extended family, and so choosing a spouse based upon one's feelings began to push aside arranged marriages. There was an assertion of personal autonomy here. This was not the epistemological autonomy of thinkers like Descartes and Locke who called for a critical distance from tradition and authority in order to think things out for oneself. This was personal autonomy, and required the removal of intimate family life from the scrutiny and control of village and clan. The hallway, a new feature in the design of homes, expressed this need for privacy, if initially only among the more well-to-do. Earlier homes were built with one room leading directly into the next. With the new feature of hallways, a couple could escape to a private space in their home while others (servants, for example) moved about the house without intrusion.

Affection and sentiment are an important part of this life within the companionate marriage. Love and affection for spouse and children came to be seen as central to what made a good marriage and family. Taylor stresses that Europeans didn't start loving their families in the eighteenth century. But they did give greater importance to such love, seeing it as more essential to a good life than earlier Europeans. Taylor cites historical research on early nineteenth-century America that also illustrates the new value accorded to family bonds. It is at this period that heaven comes to be viewed not just as the reward for those who are saved. It is now also characterized as a reunion with loved ones who have died. Affectional family bonds are now seen as so important that one of the gifts of salvation is to have them restored in the afterlife.

It is difficult to overestimate the relevance of these modern ideas about family life for much of contemporary psychotherapy. The subject matter of therapy sessions is often focused upon such things as wishes for feeling understood in a companionate marriage, parental guilt over estrangement from children, anger at indifference or emotional neglect of parents, and making peace with a single life that appears to lack these highly valued family goods. Many therapeutic orientations (not just psychoanalytic ones) theorize the roots of psychological problems in various failures or distortions of the family ideal of mutual support and attunement, or in disappointments and resentments that arise in the competition for limited emotional resources in the family. The cultural influence upon such ideas is clear. Can sibling rivalry for a mother's affections have the same meaning or psychological impact in an earlier European culture, where the expectation of affectionate parenting is not given the emphasis it is today? It is possible that people raised in such families would also be less likely to develop the subtle attunement to their own and others' emotional life that is one of the hallmarks of healthy mental functioning laid out in the *Psychodynamic Diagnostic Manual*, for such attunement was not held up as an ideal. But would it make sense to claim that people in pre-modern Europe who lacked this emotional sensitivity were "unhealthy"?

The Voice of Nature: Pleasure, Desire, and Attunement to a Complex Inner Life

Taylor describes the development in the eighteenth and nineteenth centuries of a sense that sentiment has moral significance, that feeling is an integral part of living well. To feel deeply is now worthy of approbation, a praiseworthy quality of character. It is right, beautiful, ennobling, and admirable, even when the life of feeling is tinged with sadness or a sense of the tragic. This greater esteem for a deep affective life also played a part in a changed view of the natural world. The formal French garden was put aside for something wilder, presumably closer to untouched nature. Gardens were still constructed, but the aim was not formal symmetry but the evocation of feelings, feelings of awe before nature's wildness. New ways of being in nature arose, with a value assigned to the tranquility of quiet contemplation on a country walk or to feelings of "melancholy in some lonely woodland spot" (Taylor, 1989, p. 297). The affective connection to nature continued the Deist critique of the Cartesian picture of nature as mechanically interacting meaningless material that people could observe and manipulate from a disengaged stance. People were now seen as having an affinity with nature that was evident in their emotional responsiveness to it.

These inner feelings, awakened by nature and present in personal bonds of affection, have become an important ethical good for moderns, alongside and sometimes in conflict with other ideas about living well through disengaged reason and technical control. The conflict between these ideals is further complicated by the fact that each of them is given greater weight in different domains. This is certainly true with regard to psychotherapy. In the domain of public justification, what matters is the technical, data-driven approach to understanding therapy, the provision of evidence that something works to effect a measurable change. Even humanistic and psychoanalytic therapists point proudly to evidence of their treatments' effectiveness in rigorously designed studies. At the same time, there remain some for whom research on effectiveness is a secondary enterprise that doesn't really capture what therapy is fundamentally about. Some therapists remain committed to the value of a personal transformation in therapy that isn't captured in studies of effectiveness, that can't be easily publicly validated. This commitment has roots in these earlier modern ideas about an inner depth worth exploring for the sake of expanded human possibilities, regardless of whether it directly nets measurable benefits (for an example of this debate about therapy, see the exchange between Hoffman, 2009, 2012, and Safran, 2012).

Early modern ideas about rational mastery and the exploration of particularity have received new formulations and transformations during and since the eighteenth century, reformulations that make them even more clearly part of the lineage of contemporary therapeutic views about human flourishing.

One of these reformulations centers upon a changed valuation of the sensual. The Enlightenment gave a new spin to the affirmation of ordinary life. For the Reformers, the significance of family life and marital love was still expressed in religious terms. These are God's gifts which we should gratefully enjoy. Deists saw evidence of God's goodness in the fact that he designed us so that we enjoy the pleasures of life. With the Enlightenment, the religious frame drops out, and pleasure itself became a measure of the good. There was an exaltation of the sensual, with Enlightenment thinkers like Diderot writing passionately about the misguided traditional devaluation of and restrictions upon sexual pleasure, a view that is very much in tune with Freud's. Indeed, efforts to create a hierarchy of low, sensual pleasures and so-called "higher" or refined pursuits untainted by the biological were looked upon with suspicion. This was a rejection not just of what was perceived to be destructive in Christian morality, but of ancient pre-Christian views as well. Aristotle, for example, ranked theoretical contemplation above civic duty, the latter above labor and family, and all of them above simple pleasure.

Taylor describes how this new sense of the goodness of ordinary pleasure lent support to another modern value, the relief of suffering. The idea that it is unnatural to restrict pleasure was linked to the idea that it is unnatural to inflict unnecessary pain. Cruelty became the object of moral condemnation in criminal justice, family life, and in the treatment of animals. This new rationale for the restraint of violence both reinforced and changed the previous reasons for self-control described by Elias. Now one must practice restraint not simply in order to survive in a centralized court, or to function in growing government bureaucracies and large commercial enterprises. Now restraint of violent impulse was enjoined because cruelty was seen as counter to the fundamental good of bodily pleasure. There was also an assumption among some Enlightenment thinkers that in being freed from traditional prohibitions on sensual pleasure we might come to see that we are all alike in seeking our happiness, and that the happiness of all was our natural concern. On this view, our natural sentiments would incline us to see a harmony of our own good with the good of others.

Although a very optimistic picture of human life is being painted here, it also involves the intensification of a problem that seemed to follow from Cartesian disengagement. Descartes' picture of rationality as the detached observation of how the world works in order to carry out one's freely chosen purposes lends support to a strong sense of instrumental efficacy, but it offers no help in deciding which purposes are worth pursuing. The Enlightenment idea that we naturally seek the good creates a further difficulty: whatever good we find ourselves pursuing is written into us by nature, and therefore not even chosen by us. We cannot help but seek what we are made to seek by our very nature.

Some Enlightenment figures offered an alternative to this picture of people as driven to pursue inherent, naturally determined goods. They argued that the insight into the innocence and goodness of nature was transformative, that it could operate as an inspiring moral source. There was a sense that accepting ordinary desires as worthy and good would release us from the stifling constrictions of traditional ethics, empowering us to live life more fully.

The value of living with vitality, freed of moralistic inhibitions is a common theme in therapeutic literature. This ethical ideal could also be characterized as a form of self-acceptance, which is an implicit message of many psychotherapies. The idea is that there is wisdom in accepting our ordinary desires and forgoing seemingly heroic moralistic efforts to rise above them or master them. This is presented not simply as a scientific fact about people, that they will inevitably pursue ordinary natural bodily desires. There is a further claim: there is wisdom in the acceptance of this fact. Seeing this fact provides the motivational impetus for the pursuit of an ideal.

This ideal takes on new significance in what Taylor calls the expressivist response to the Enlightenment. Taylor points to Rousseau as opening a critique of the Enlightenment idea that we can undo the evils of custom and tradition through a scientific grasp of natural human desire. According to Rousseau, we can't just think our way out of the distortions that have been imposed upon the original impulses of our nature. The problem isn't ignorance of our true nature, but the way we are swayed by opinion in our desire for the esteem of others. The way forward lies in freedom from craving others' approval so that each of us may turn to the inner voice of conscience. Rousseau denies that our inner impulses are simply a set of natural desires that are common to all, desires that everyone can't help but acknowledge and live by if freed from distorting moral strictures. Rather, self-exploration becomes the means by which one discovers a voice within that is particular to oneself, a voice that frees one from seeking the approval of others. The good is now the fruit of a self-determining freedom. Inwardness accesses something particular to oneself, and attending to that is what ensures autonomy and reveals what matters most in living one's life.

The concept of autonomy takes a different form in Kant. Kant's focus on our nature as rational beings links the inner voice of conscience to our rational activity. Unlike the rest of the natural world, the laws of nature do not determine what we do. We can have a rational grasp of those laws, formulate them, and choose to follow them because we see that they are rational. Freedom, rationality, and morality are integrally linked. Morality is not founded on the natural goodness of our inclinations, but on our capacity to formulate laws and maxims whose validity is given by reason and hence is universally applicable. Kant takes a step away from the modern affirmation of ordinary desires and wishes. Instead he emphasizes our agency as reasoning beings, an agency that does not simply pursue what it has been made to seek by its inherent desires, but can assess whether a course of action is rational and worthy of assent.

Kant attributes a new importance to the disengaged, rational stance. It no longer simply brings with it the greater epistemic power valued by Descartes and Locke, or the greater mastery of the material world sought by a technologically oriented science. For Kant, the capacity for reasoned moral choice is what makes us worthy of respect. Since this capacity is central to human worth and dignity, it is essential to living a worthwhile life. Reasoned moral choice is humanity's highest achievement. What makes people both moral and admirable is not following their natural and innocent desires (even if this has a positive outcome), nor obeying laws given by their culture, the state, or even God, but doing what is right because they rationally apprehend what the law requires.

Kant articulates one of the central goods of modernity, the importance of thinking things out for oneself, now not simply because this will get one closer to the truth, or help one to avoid the distortions imposed by tradition and culture, but because the exercise of this capacity is that which makes people worthy of respect. To live fully as a human being is to think things out for oneself. Clearly, this is explicitly promoted in cognitive-behavioral therapy. But Freud (1917/1963, p. 434) also sees it as one of the fruits of analysis—the undoing of repression allows patients to make deliberate decisions about matters that had previously been beyond their grasp, tangled up in neurotic confusion. It also provides another reason for therapists to refrain from telling patients how they ought to live their lives. Nevertheless, an ethical good *is* being promoted here, the value of thinking things out for oneself, of being fully autonomous. Kant grounds this in our nature as rational beings in a way that is certainly not central to all therapeutic philosophies. But his is one version of the modern emphasis upon autonomy as independent critical thinking that recurs in different forms across many therapies.

I want to turn now to Taylor's exposition of a further development of Rousseau's ideas about a personal inner voice. What matters in this further development is not epistemic benefits, the fostering of natural inclination, or autonomy, but an expansion of the meaning and value of finding a unique and original way of living.

Expressivism: Particularity and the True Self

Rousseau offered a new significance to the inward turn. It was not simply a matter of looking within to discover natural moral truths that we all share, but of listening to a personal voice of conscience that revealed one's particular way of seeking the good, freed from concern with the opinions of others. Romantic writers after Rousseau developed these ideas further, emphasizing our role in developing this inner voice through how we give it expression. Since our access to important truths about life comes through our attunement to nature within, we need to develop a capacity for attunement to this inner moral source. Careful articulation of what we discern can enhance and give power to what we find. To bring to expression what we discover within is not simply to name something we perceive independently of the expression. Articulation breathes life into inner personal meanings, helps to bring them into existence. This means that expression plays a role in shaping and defining who we are.

The idea of helping to bring something into being by giving it expression rose to prominence in the eighteenth and early nineteenth centuries. It applied to processes of self-definition, to changed conceptions of art, and to the relationship between the two. No longer was art understood simply as portraying the world. The artist was understood to be creative in a new sense of the word that was akin to the older Biblical sense of God as creator. The artist's vision doesn't just show us the world in a new light, but helps to bring the world into being in a new way. Taylor notes how the Romantic conception of the symbol illustrates this new power of artistic expression. There is an interpenetration of the symbol and the symbolized, of the work of art and its subject matter. Taylor reviews Coleridge's idea that the symbol does not simply designate an object, but helps to constitute what it is about. For Coleridge, the material of a work of art should be so joined to what is expressed in it that meaning and material cannot be disentangled. What is said or shown in a poem or painting should be so fully part of the language of the poem or the way the paints are mixed, applied, or juxtaposed that one can only say or show this "meaning" by use of these materials. The art work does not simply portray or describe an independent object that one could indicate by other means. What appears in the symbol depends upon the symbol in order to appear, even in order to be. Further, the creative expression of self and art was seen as one of the key forms of resistance to the deadening and desiccating effects of the alternative form of inwardness as rational disengagement. The latter's emphasis on self- and world-mastery was critiqued by the Romantics as engendering alienation from living as one truly is, as a betrayal of the self that shares a vital connection with the nature around and within us.

Taylor argues that this notion of giving shape to oneself through the expression of an inner voice became the basis for a far-reaching individualism. The individualism that arose in the late eighteenth century went beyond the obvious fact that people were different from one another. Rather, these differences came to be seen as having a value that should be fostered, "they entail that each one of us has an original path which we ought to tread; they lay the obligation on each of us to live up to our originality" (Taylor, 1989, p. 375). There were traditional roots for this idea in Pauline ideas about the variety of gifts that Christians bring to their participation in the Church. The Puritan idea of each person having their own calling anticipates some elements of individualism. But with later developments there is not simply a variety of callings (baker, deacon, teacher, farmer). Rather, there is something uniquely me that I am called to be true to, to develop, in order to live my life to the full. Taylor emphasizes that the distinctiveness of this idea of personal originality is often overlooked by us, for it is so much a part of our modern culture that we don't recognize that it is a relatively new way of framing what is essential to living well "and would have been incomprehensible in earlier times" (Taylor, 1989, p. 376).

Psychotherapy, as a modern social practice, is replete with this emphasis on the uniqueness of each person and the importance of remaining true to the particular person one is. This is obvious in the theories of many psychotherapies. Humanistic psychotherapists are dedicated to helping people to live more authentic lives. "Authenticity refers to a person's ability to be mindful and emotionally literate in relation to his or her thoughts and feelings and to behave in ways that are consistent with those thoughts and feelings" (Cooper and Joseph, 2016, p. 31). Winnicott (1963, chapter 12) is well known for his theory of a true self that must be protected from impingements so that spontaneity and creativity may flourish, a personal spontaneity and creativity he explicitly links to the arts and culture, as the Romantics did (see also Bollas, 2002, and Loewald, 2000, on the link between analysis and creativity). Contemporary ethical views that descend from Romantic expressivist sources are pervasive in therapeutic ideas about flourishing.

Some analysts work from a different conception of personal uniqueness. Fink (2017) emphasizes that the analyzed patient is someone who follows their own bent, but he doesn't subscribe to the notion that this involves getting in touch with one's "true self." Fink retains the element of originality or particularity, while renouncing the idea that this is a personal possession. In fact, analysis is a sort of self-dispossession. But what comes out of this process is a life lived according to its own satisfactions, no longer in conformity with or rebellion against the impositions of others and in that sense "one's own," or "subjectified."

This is not to deny that therapists have also pointed to ideals for living well that can function as norms. When Kleinians (Segal, 1981) point to a developmental trajectory from the paranoid/schizoid position to the depressive position, they are suggesting that there are better and worse ways of living one's particularity. Cognitive-behavioral theory points to an ideal of rationality that it would be better for everyone to adopt. Freud's developmental progression to genital sexuality implies a normative ideal. But in all these cases, the normative claims exist in tension with the aim of being the particular person one is, unencumbered by externally imposed ideals. For example, Freud's genital ideal exists alongside his repeated admonitions against forcing people to adhere to one form of sexuality. As he writes in *Civilization and Its Discontents*: "The requirement ... that there shall be a single kind of sexual life for everyone [is] the source of serious injustice" (1930/1961a, p. 104).

Post-Romantic Transformations: Darkness Within and the Decline of Self and Meaning

In the nineteenth century there were a number of changes to the Romantic idea that each person has a unique inner voice that provides a connection to the natural world and to important moral truths. The development of natural science in this period led to a view of the universe as a vast and indifferent field of interacting matter and energy. A conception of nature as potentially alien, as an amoral source of power, displaced the Romantic idea of nature as a benign life force.

Art came to be seen as having a meaning that was purely aesthetic rather than moral. The rise of realism in the visual arts and the novel led to a starker picture of the natural world, both around us and within us. Nature was no longer seen so positively as our home, for its forces could be wild and unforgiving (as portrayed in the paintings of Courbet and Manet). The sentiments of characters in novels began to be laid bare more critically, no longer described as a mode of access to moral truth, but as often self-serving and self-deceptive (like Emma Bovary's distorted sense of her romantic feelings). The older Romantic ideal promoted our kinship with nature and its lessons for living in harmony with all of humanity. Nineteenth-century realism recommended the courage to face the stark indifference of the universe, abandoning the naïve consoling hope of feeling at home in it. Nevertheless, something positive was still spun out of this more bracing vision. We may now feel ourselves to be estranged from the world, but we have grown up, gained the dignity of a courageous view of things as they are, no longer clinging to childish fantasies of having a meaningful place in the world or a reliable moral compass within.

Further transformations in the significance accorded to art appeared in Baudelaire and Schopenhauer. The Romantic picture of a beneficent communion with nature is abandoned. Baudelaire believed that art should turn against nature. He opened a new line of thinking that led to the idea that art provided its spiritual benefit through being self-enclosed, justified by nothing outside itself. For Schopenhauer nature is the realm of will, of "wild, blind, uncontrolled striving, incapable of satisfaction, driving us on, against all principles, law and morality" (Taylor, 1989, p. 442). For the early Nietzsche, nature in this Schopenhauerian sense is still an important enlivening source, as it was for the Romantics. But this is not because it is the path to moral goodness. Rather, without a connection to the powerful force of nature we risk losing vitality, becoming flattened and tamed to such a degree that we live a cramped, narrow, and deadened life.

Taylor notes several descendants of these views in later modern thought: Fauvism, Surrealism, D. H. Lawrence, and Freud, who explicitly acknowledged his debt to Nietzsche and Schopenhauer. Taylor sees in Freud a variation on these themes recognizing the importance of contact with wild inner depths. To lose such contact is to lose access to an important source of power, of libidinal and aggressive energies; it is to risk becoming one of those well-behaved weaklings that Freud warned against. But Freud also was an admirer of the disengaged reason descended from Descartes and Locke. He believed in the value of examination of these inner depths, both as a scientific student of them, and as part of the treatment offered to patients. One way to characterize that treatment is that it frees patients from their blindly repeated symptoms by helping them to see through the disguises of defense to the libidinal and aggressive forces they have turned against. And one of the reasons they have turned against them is for the sake of moral injunctions against sexual and aggressive inclinations. So, like Nietzsche, he seeks to undo the damage stemming from projects of moral goodness in order to access a more achievable good: energic vitality. Freud differs from Nietzsche in that he leaves more room for the possibility of a prudential reasoned oversight of that energy (the ego must manage id, superego, and external reality).

Taylor's story of changing modern ideas about who people are and how they might best live is not one of straightforward temporal succession. New views did not entirely replace those that preceded them. For example, the trends exemplified by realism in the arts, the scientific picture of an indifferent and fundamentally meaningless universe, and the even starker picture of nature as reservoir of wild, amoral forces did not sweep previous views aside but existed in tension with them. The Enlightenment hope that a disengaged analysis of the material, personal, and social worlds would be the key to great benefits to humanity remained a viable way to frame human flourishing in the late nineteenth century, and today. The possibility of human improvement through the discovery of one's unique path, realized through an emotional connection to inner depths and outer nature that is brought to personal or artistic expression—this view of human well-being has also had continuing proponents. And older Judeo-Christian views have continued, often influenced by trends that arose only in modernity (as one can see in Kierkegaard and Dostoyevsky). What results is not the triumph of "a" modern ethic, but a situation of unresolved ethical disagreements. As I will discuss in the next chapter, this is also the fate of divergent therapeutic ethics.

Twentieth-century modernism brought about further permutations in ideas about human flourishing. While the inward turn was still present in the sense that subjectivity remained a focus, the self was dethroned. In keeping with earlier Romantic views, there were numerous efforts to show that subjectivity cannot be encompassed by rational or scientific analysis. Phenomenological and existential philosophers explored various ways that lived experience eluded scientific explication. However, what was revealed in twentieth-century descriptions of lived experience was often not the Romantic self characterized by an inner unity that provided the means for the reconciliation of reason and sensibility. What some found in such explorations was a fragmented stream of experience, where a cohesive self, identity, and unity were elusive.

The self was problematized in a sidelining of meaning as well. Some rejected the idea that there are personal inner depths to explore in order to uncover hidden meanings which nourish the development of one's true self. Taylor points to D. H. Lawrence as one writer who sought a liberation from depth, from the freight of meanings. He also sees in Pound's Imagism a call to return to the surface from the depths. For Pound, poets don't discover and express the underlying meanings of the subject matter or object that they are writing about. But neither do they present their subject matter in a cold, flat, or lifeless way. There is an epiphany in poetry, but this is not the revelation of the deeper, truer meaning of the object. One could even go so far as to say that the poem doesn't *express* anything. Rather, the poem effects an epiphany by setting up a space in which certain energies can appear, energies that affect the reader, but that do not yield a meaning one can cognitively grasp and take away from the poem. Energies after all aren't expressed meanings. They nevertheless have their effects.

Lacanian analysis adopts a stance toward the speech of the patient that resonates with these non-expressivist poetics. Fink makes plain that his aim is to change the libidinal economy of the patient, to bring about an energic shift, not to search for meaning. Dreams and slips of the tongue are not telltale signs pointing in a disguised fashion to their underlying true meaning, a meaning that the analyst can discern. They are more fundamentally signs of the breakdown of meanings by which the analysand's ego (via the symbolic Other) has been constructed. The analyst's job is not to offer new meanings, but to point to what is there in the analysand's speech that exceeds or overturns intended meanings. The aim is to break open the tight bonds of self-understanding to which the patient clings in order to free energies the patient has been unsuccessfully trying to subdue with meaning.

Taylor explores more recent twentieth-century developments in views of the self, personal expression, and identity. For example, his discussion of an ethic of authenticity (1991) locates contemporary concerns about being true to oneself in the earlier modern history noted above. He addresses both the criticisms of this ethic (for example, denouncing it as a culture of narcissism) and the efforts to defend it. At this stage of the story, however, therapy no longer appears as an offshoot of earlier modern roots but is part of the "trunk and branches" of modern culture. Therapeutic ideas and practices directly express many of the conflicting ethical views of contemporary Western culture.

Ethical Aims in Socio-Historical Context

Taylor's history of the modern identity covers a complex interconnecting web of ideas and social practices. He looks at the inward turn of modernity, the affirmation of ordinary life, and new understandings of nature as they were articulated in philosophy, theology, political theory, and aesthetics. He points to social practices that were shaped by and influenced these ideas: the Reformation conception of each person's calling; the idea of self-remaking through rigorous self-examination; the value placed upon intimate family bonds and a companionate marriage; the new restraints on bodily functions and emotional expression in the context of social and economic changes; the demand to think for oneself rather than simply accept the opinions of authorities or the assumptions of one's tradition; the attention to the details of everyday experience in personal journals and the novel; the new value assigned to bodily enjoyment and sexual pleasure, which also underlay the new critique of violence and cruelty; the idea of art as expressing important truths unavailable in other forms; the re-design of gardens and homes so that one might be attuned to nature and establish privacy for intimate relations; the value placed on finding one's own way to live.

In linking these practices and ethical views to therapy I am arguing that therapy can be better understood by placing it in this same historical context, seeing therapy too as a social practice shaped by modern ethical ideals. Insofar as they are expressive of this particular culture's ideals, therapeutic aims are not built solely upon objective facts about people. Rational self-mastery, facing unflattering personal truths, liberation from social expectations, and the development of an appreciation for the complexity of one's emotional life are all ideals for living well. These therapeutic conceptions of well-being are neither universally endorsed nor the outcome of scientific research. That does not mean that they are insubstantial fantasies or a pleasant window dressing for the serious findings of science, for people inevitably shape their lives by some notion of the good. Given their deep roots in modern Western culture, therapeutic ethics deserve the respect that is owed to the ethics of any culture. Respect does not mean blind acceptance. Even the most cherished ideals of a culture may be worthy of critique. Indeed, because modern ethics are not monolithic but diverse and conflicted, a culture of critique is central to modernity itself. Further, critics of modernity may find fundamental flaws in its understanding of ethics (MacIntyre, 1984). However, Taylor's history makes clear that whatever their limitations, these ideals are not whimsical preferences but have arisen out of hard-fought debates and repeated efforts to find better ways to live through new social practices. Therapeutic variations on these modern ethical themes deserve at least initial respectful consideration.

Taylor argues that moderns often feel the attraction of competing fundamental intuitions regarding what makes life worthwhile. He is unconvinced by the wholesale dismissal of a major ethical trend of modernity, even if particular versions of a trend fail to be convincing. For example, consider the continuing disagreements regarding whether we should give greater emphasis to the disengaged scientific stance toward self and world, or to a bond of belonging to the natural world and human community built upon each person's attunement to their unique experience. Despite the tension between these two views, one does not cancel out the other. Taylor is unconvinced by one-sided attempts to use one to invalidate the other, and is doubtful that any of us is entirely unmoved by the opposing view. Proponents of technical rationality warn against the irrational and scientifically unsupported views of those who proclaim the value of Romantic ideals. And those influenced by Romantic views make sweeping claims that technical rationality is all about the domination and control of nature and other people. Yet the scientifically inclined also believe in a personal fulfilment that echoes post-Romantic ideals, and the critics of technical rationality are often happy to have scientific expertise on their side in addressing important social issues.

This unresolved tension is also present in therapeutic conflicts. Behavioral therapists are proud of the scientific bona fides of their treatment, pointing to research that demonstrates its efficacy. Yet when seeking their own therapy, many manage to find their way to therapists of humanistic and psychodynamic orientation (Norcross, 2005; Norcross et al., 2009; Norcross et al., 1988). Likewise, the Montaigne-like psychoanalytic call to honest acceptance of whatever appears in the stream of experience does not preclude the need for scientific justification, from Freud's claims that psychoanalysis is the product of scientific research carried out in the consulting room, to contemporary efforts to demonstrate the effectiveness of psychodynamic treatments (Shedler, 2010).

Taylor claims that we moderns often experience the pull of competing views of a good life, that we live with "cross pressures" (2007, chapter 16) that leave us vulnerable to change and instability in our sense of where we can find a full or flourishing life. Because of these pulls in different directions, efforts to definitively declare one view triumphant over the others can sound hollow, defensive, or disingenuous. A declaration of victory in these debates not only risks injustice to competing views, it can appear to be rhetorical grandstanding rather than a fully owned stance. What is needed is a willingness to engage with other perspectives, while recognizing that some of us begin such engagement already feeling an attraction to more than one perspective.

The unfinished nature of our ethical thought and practice is evident in its historical unfolding. Historical context helps to highlight how these views of who we are and who we can be take place in relation to alternative views—challenging, modifying, repudiating, or strengthening them. In being drawn to a vision of well-being we are engaged in a conversation with those around us, those who came before, and those we imagine are to come after us. This conversation can have a spirit of open and welcoming engagement, or of fierce and spirited debate. However, there is also the risk that one party will try to silence others through social-institutional constraints. To do justice to this ongoing and complex conversation means not just avoiding exclusionary tactics, but recognizing that we are always already situated in the socio-historical context of this conversation. Even the historical study of that context does not take place outside the conversation but is located within it. The question for the student of that history is, "How am I entering into the conversation in my very efforts to describe or explain it?"

With regard to psychotherapy, ongoing discussion about ethics deserves attention in its own right, alongside questions regarding theoretical justifications and evidence for the efficacy of therapeutic practice. As I noted earlier in this chapter, Taylor's overview of modern ideas about living well attempts to articulate what made those visions appealing or inspiring. In developing and enacting therapeutic ethics we are also trying to realize a form of life that inspires us. Such ideas have motivational force. To enter into conversation about alternative ethics is to try to understand how someone could be inspired by a different sort of good, or not be motivated to pursue a good we esteem. What will quickly bring such conversations to an end is to claim to have seen through the other's ethical aims, to be able to explain *away* someone's attachment to an ethic. Debate between conflicting ethics may legitimately involve efforts to explain *to* another how an ethic may be serving purposes beyond its express aims, or that its adherents are not seeing the full implications of their position. But if this is to be a genuine conversation, any explanations offered will be made as part of an appeal to the other, not as a dismissal of the other's views because they do not conform to one's own. What I am proposing is that fruitful elucidation and argument for an ethic is best attained through mutual engagement. This entails an interest in what the other is drawn to, and why, as much as an intention to demonstrate the limitations of the other's ethic and the advantages of one's own. I turn to these dialogical possibilities for ethical debate in the next chapter.

Notes

1 Theorists of mentalization have recently begun to explore this link between culture, mentalizing, and emotional regulation. See Luyten et al. (2019).
2 However, some painters strive to destabilize the objectifying and controlling gaze of the viewer, as Merleau-Ponty (1964/1964) notes of Cezanne.
3 The term "moral source" points to a motivational feature of our ethical life: we do not simply reason toward and assent to what is good, but feel drawn to the good, empowered by our vision of it or contact with it, to pursue it and enact it. See Taylor's exposition in chapter 4 of *Sources of the Self* (1989).
4 Taylor bases his discussion of the link between the novel and the modern ethos upon Watt's (1957/2001) more detailed exposition.

4   From the Ethics of Therapy to Ethical Dialogue

I have been exploring the idea that the psychotherapies are more than means to an end, more than technical interventions for the treatment of mental disorders. Each therapy also promotes particular ends through its distinctive ideas about what constitutes human well-being. In Chapter 1 I summarized a companion volume, *The Ethical Visions of Psychotherapy*. In this summary I noted that even symptom-focused therapies promote broader virtues and aims, like courage and autonomy, and that different schools of therapy can be differentiated in light of their different views about human flourishing. Building on these ideas in Chapter 2, I offered a provisional categorization of distinct therapeutic aims: rational self-mastery, honest self-exploration, particularity liberated from social expectation, and the attunement to a complex inner life that is formed in relationships with others. In Chapter 3, I examined the cultural roots of therapeutic views of living well in the context of Taylor's history of the modern identity. This socio-historical context for therapeutic aims helps to reveal their ethical nature, the ongoing nature of disputes about different pictures of flourishing, and the ways that such pictures can serve agendas that go far beyond the treatment of disorders. I ended Chapter 3 suggesting the value of dialogue between diverse therapeutic ethics. In this chapter, I will offer some preliminary reflections on the nature of and prospects for such a dialogue.

Conflicting Ideas About Flourishing

Research on the efficacy of the psychotherapies is unlikely to be of much assistance in assessing the relative merits of contrasting therapeutic ethics. For a variety of reasons, cognitive-behavioral therapies have been more extensively researched in clinical trials than therapies of other orientations, thereby more often receiving the stamp of approval as empirically supported or evidence-based. This is despite the fact that most comparative research shows little difference in efficacy between treatments of different therapeutic orientations. Current evidence-based evaluations of therapy, while claiming to be simply scientific assessments of efficacy, have resulted in the promotion of specific pictures of well-being without any consideration of alternative ethical views. It is good that we can research whether therapy A or therapy B is more effective at reducing the symptoms of a particular disorder (a difference that is not usually due to difference in therapeutic orientation). But such research is of no help in assessing whether to endorse the picture of flourishing associated with therapy A or therapy B.

What do we do with competing ideas about living well? Can scientific research resolve the differences? Are there facts of human well-being that can help us to decide between different therapeutic orientations? If there are ethical facts, we cannot arrive at them by examining ethics from outside of ethics in a way that would allow us to make an objective comparative assessment of conflicting ethical views. Any comparison, critique, or positive judgment upon ethics will itself be made from an ethical position. In Taylor's terms, we don't formulate strong evaluations[1] out of neutral facts, but find ourselves already inducted into certain views about a good life. Ethical critique starts from ethical commitments.

In the last chapter, I examined how the psychotherapies are rooted in already available views about living well that are present in the modern West. Those views are not univocal or static within Western culture, and the psychotherapies do not simply parrot them. Psychotherapists have also contributed to developing, changing, and challenging modern ethics. But the pictures of flourishing enacted in the therapies do not arise from having stepped outside of the cultural matrix that gave birth to them in order to look with an unprejudiced eye upon the facts of human well-being. Rather, therapists are participants in an ongoing conversation about what it means to live well.

It is only within such a conversation that questions about flourishing can have any significance. The effort to ignore preliminary intuitions about living well in order to get a scientific, culture-neutral perspective on what matters results in a technical language that can't address ethical issues. Attempts have been made within psychology and other human sciences to come up with scientific bases for validating ethical ideals. Work on the evolutionary origins of morality is one example. The limitations of such studies for adjudicating among competing ethics is sometimes evident to people who work in the field. But not always. For example, Taylor (1989, pp. 406–407) points to inconsistencies in E. O. Wilson's (1978) conclusions about the evolutionary origins of our emotional responses and ethical practices. According to Wilson, ethics is a biological inheritance shaped by the history of its adaptive advantages. However, Wilson also claims that ethics can be reshaped through a clear-sighted scientific understanding of that history. He argues that the selfishness and tribalism that is natural to us can be changed or re-engineered. The problem with this theory comes when we ask questions about how it is to be re-engineered. To what ends? If our ends are already set for us by evolutionary history, as he has claimed, then how can we change or undo the selfishness and tribalism that is bred in our bones (or genes)? And if our knowledge of this history gives us a freedom from its determining influence, then how influential is it? More importantly, on what basis do we make choices about which revisions to make to our genetically inherited ethics? Presumably, we would have to rely on something other than what was set for us by natural selection or we're right back where we started.

The situation is similar if what is discovered in our evolutionary history is not selfishness and tribalism but prosocial tendencies to empathy, reciprocity, or fairness. Such "building blocks" of morality, as de Waal (2006) calls them, are clearly part of our evolutionary heritage. But what we mean by ethics includes not just being inclined to do something empathic or fair, but having a sense that it is right or good to do so. The idea that an action is right opens the possibility for questions about what constitutes its rightness that can become the basis for reflection, reconsideration, or even challenge to prosocial actions that one finds oneself inclined to do. I can ask myself when it may be wrong to do the empathic thing I feel like doing, or question whether it is pity rather than empathy that motivates me. I can ask under what circumstances I should extend generosity more widely than I am naturally inclined, beyond my circle of family and friends, for example. Such reflections cannot be made simply on the basis that my species is generally inclined to act prosocially, for these reflections put such inclinations in question. De Waal's (p. 77) argument that we humans can and should extend an ethic of care beyond our own species is an example of the extension of ethics beyond the form given by adaptive advantages.

Naturalistic approaches that seek a scientific foundation for ethics often end up defeating themselves on their own terms, then surreptitiously reintroducing an evaluative language that is not itself derived from scientific findings. Skinner's excitement about the benefits to humanity that will come from the scientific control of behavior exhibits similar contradictions (see my discussion in Smith, K. R., 1983, and the more extensive discussion of the limitations of behaviorist psychology in Taylor, 1964).

The theories that undergird therapeutic practices are not just theories about people but proposals for who we might be, not just models *of* people, but models for people to *live by*. Although this runs counter to the picture of therapy as applied psychological science, it is not a radically new idea. Mitchell takes it up on more than one occasion. In *Influence and Autonomy in Psychoanalysis* (1997) he states it quite explicitly.

> Psychoanalysis has become a method for generating a certain kind of meaning, for fostering certain forms of experience and living. There

are many, many forms of human experience, and contemporary psychoanalysis promotes only one of them, a particularly Western, late 20th century form.

(p. 24)

My only disagreement would be with the idea that psychoanalysis promotes only one form of experience endemic to Western modernity. There are a number of conflicting ethical views within the modern West. Mitchell's own overviews of analytic history show that different analytic schools promote different forms of living.

A fundamental question arises regarding the fact that different types of therapy promote different forms of living and experience: why choose one over the other? Greenberg and Mitchell (1983) take up this question in the last chapter of their book. Summarizing their conceptions of the drive and relational models of psychoanalysis, they note that they "constitute two incompatible visions of life" (p. 406). They state that the conflict between them is not capable of resolution through empirical evidence. Instead, deciding between them is a matter of personal choice. "Does the therapy speak to you? Does it seem to account for your deepest needs, longings, fears? In your clinical work does it provide a convincing account of your patients which corresponds with your own experience of them?" (p. 407). They argue that subjective factors of one's personal and professional history will shape the choice one makes. It's not clear from what they say whether they think there can be reasoned bases for preferring one therapeutic orientation over another, although "providing a convincing account" of patients suggests there can be. They liken the move from one therapeutic model to another to conversion. They do not appear to be thinking of religious conversion, but of the shift from one scientific paradigm to another. At least some scientific paradigms are left behind precisely because a new paradigm better accounts for the data. Galileo's concept of inertia has displaced Aristotle's theory of the motion of objects by accounting for phenomena of motion that Aristotle's theory could not. It's not clear that the move from the drive to the relational model (or more broadly, from any one therapeutic orientation to another) can muster that kind of support. Greenberg and Mitchell don't seem to think that it can either (they say that the conflict can't be resolved by empirical evidence). If the choice between therapeutic paradigms is neither arbitrary nor subject to empirical resolution, then what kind of support is there for adopting one therapeutic vision over another?

Greenberg and Mitchell's question about whether a therapeutic theory "speaks to you" points to something important. The idea appears to be that this is a personal choice rooted in basic intuitions. We're not simply in the realm of determining what is the case about who people are, but of raising possibilities for who we might be. So one might ask of the drive and relational models not which is a better account of who people are, but according to which form of human experience is each calling us to live. One could then say that the drive model is offering a form of life where people have either consciously chosen what to do with their impulses and drives, increasing their autonomy (as in Paul Gray), or have been freed from the constrictions of social demands so that they may go wherever their satisfaction takes them (as in Bruce Fink). By contrast, the relational model offers a form of living where people are attuned to how they have positioned themselves in a complex interpersonal world, ready to explore and act within a field of mutual influence and interdependence that is inescapable.

What does it mean to argue for a vision of well-being? And does this bear any relation to demonstrating that one therapeutic model of pathology and treatment has better scientific support? If the therapies offer ideas about living well that go beyond the theories of psychopathology that underlie their methods of treatment, what are the implications for the relationship between therapeutic science and therapeutic ethics? Therapeutic ethics, the pictures of human flourishing on offer in the therapies, may well have some roots in or links to relatively well-founded psychological science. But in most cases those links are distant, for therapeutic theories and practices have developed the basic science and applied it in contexts far afield from the original scientific findings. For example, it is one thing to document the damaging effects upon attachment bonds brought about by the neglect and abuse of children. It is another thing to claim that attachment theory is *the* essential framework for therapeutic work with people diagnosed as borderline. It is certainly a plausible framework, but therapeutic orientations that are not built upon it (like dialectical-behavioral therapy) are also viable. Often the scientific support for an orientation will lend some weight of plausibility. But such support does not prove that only that approach to treatment is valid. If science has a role to play in argumentation about the value of different therapeutic orientations, it is unlikely to resolve all the debates. The ethical aims that are embodied in different orientations require evaluation in ethical terms.

Ethical Reasoning

Merleau-Ponty (1945/2012) has shown that fundamental perceptual orientations like up and down or near and far only exist in a world structured through bodily engagement. For a disembodied view from nowhere, there is no up and down, near and far, left and right, only measurable distances and angles of orientation. Such measurements and angles do not give near and far—nearness is relative to me and my situation, my purposes and capacities. In one sense, the coffee cup on the desk in front of me is near. But in another sense it is not. I placed it where I would have to reach for it ("far") so that I wouldn't accidentally knock it over. The distance in centimeters between me and the cup does not determine whether the cup is near or far. Near and far are relative to a point of view and to particular purposes, unlike measurements, which can be applied "absolutely," without reference to contexts of human significance.[2]

Likewise, to begin to understand what ethics is, let alone to be engaged in ethical practice or reflection, one needs to be in a world that is already pre-formed by certain lines of ethical orientation. This is true whether one is explicitly deliberating about ethics or acting in the light of an implicit ethical understanding. An ethical world is one that is already given as shaped by ethical orientations like good and bad, worthless and worthwhile, dignified and clownish, shameful and praiseworthy, courageous and cowardly, inspiring and banal, constrained and free. Examined developmentally, these distinctions can be seen to arise out of a background of more basic orientations like bodily safety and danger, pain and pleasure, or hunger and satiety. But the entrance into language and culture adds an entirely new level of evaluation, in which our basic bodily sense about what is better and worse is shaped by a rich variety of symbolic forms. And beyond the cultural shaping of bodily givens, linguistic and symbolic forms make it possible for there to be questions about how to appraise the worth of a wide range of actions, events, and social practices. Language even makes it possible to challenge the very language by which we make ethical evaluations. For example, consider the long history of critical examination of the evaluative connotations given to the contrast between "masculine" and "feminine," or between "autonomous" and "dependent" (not to mention the relationship between these two sets of contrasting terms). Language gives us these distinctions and the specific connotations of value assigned to them. It also gives us the means to argue about their nature and significance. By language I do not mean simply individual words like "masculine" and "feminine," but the broad web of the entire language and accompanying social practices which give these words their particular sense and significance.

Just as there is no up and down or near and far without embodied, situated existence, so there are no fundamental ethical orientations for those who do not already exist in a world shaped by some ethical perspective of better and worse. Taylor's critique of Wilson's efforts to explain ethics from outside of ethics (as the result of evolutionary adaptation) reveals the contradictions inherent in trying to find a non-ethical source for ethics. One could say of such a project that "you can't get there from here"; that is, you can't get to ethics from a study of how some of our ethical intuitions may have been shaped by adaptive advantages. Whatever adaptive advantages might explain the origin of some of our prosocial ethical inclinations, one can always ask whether they make sense in our current context, whether they should be blindly followed, whether they can be modified, or whether we should even try to subvert them. In a linguistic-cultural world, "man" does not live by adaptive advantages alone (even if those advantages have played a part in the survival of the species).

There can be objective grounds for judgments of better and worse in non-ethical contexts. This car is better than that one because it has better traction. That food is bad for you because it contributes to heart disease. These kinds of evaluation can be supported or contested by reference to agreed-upon independent criteria. But what about a claim that it is better to be kind than cruel, or the challenge to such a claim, as one can find in Nietzsche? Or, to use an example from therapeutic ethics, can one find independent objective criteria to decide whether reasoned self-mastery is more or less valuable than a nuanced appreciation of the complexities of one's wishes and motives? Are there independent criteria here?

Taylor (1989, 1995a) argues that rather than supporting our ethical views with independent criteria, argumentation about ethical matters uses one ethical view to challenge another. Someone who had no ethical sense, who simply assessed action in terms of whether it helped or hindered the attainment of their weakly valued goals, would have no way to make the strong evaluations that are central to ethics. The criteria for assessing whether something helps one to attain a goal can't be used to evaluate the worth of that goal. There can be independent criteria to support or challenge a statement like: "These investments are good ones because they will increase wealth." But no examination of the stock market, or of the health of the economy, or of particular companies will answer questions regarding whether wealth is a worthwhile goal, how important it is, or how to weigh this goal against competing goals.

Is it legitimate to assess ethics pragmatically, as the means to another end? Someone could claim that following ethical rules is useful for achieving practical goals, perhaps because following the rules will earn others' approval and their positive disposition toward one's aims. However, people who try to be ethical for such practical reasons will not be engaged in ethics, but simply using ethics as a means to achieve their non-ethical ends. Such is the example in Kant (1785/1997) of the shopkeeper who treats his customers fairly because it is good for business, not because it is the right thing to do.

Utilitarian ethics, which assesses the rightness or wrongness of actions in terms of their consequences, would offer a different take on Kant's shopkeeper. Mill (1979/1861) argues that the rightness of an action is determined not by the motives or intentions of the doer, but by the good it does, the happiness it brings. "He who saves a fellow creature from drowning does what is morally right, whether his motive be duty or the hope of being paid for his troubles" (p. 18). Nevertheless, utilitarians also argue that there is a utility value in people who make virtuous strong evaluations, in this case, that the good of others is more important than money. Such people are more likely to consistently bring good to others. They are more likely to act in the service of utilitarianism's fundamental aim, the greatest happiness of the greatest number of people. "The utilitarian standard ... enjoins and requires the cultivation of the love of virtue up to the greatest strength possible, as being above all things important to the general happiness" (p. 37).

A framework of strong evaluation supports reasoning about ethics. It is not enough to desire some outcome (weak evaluation). Ethical evaluation includes assessment of whether the desired outcome is appropriate, justified, or legitimate (strong evaluation). Justification can be based upon fundamental rules or principles. For example, a particular action (or law, or public policy) may be found to violate someone's rights to life and liberty, to free speech, etc. Taylor points out, however, that such principles are themselves dependent upon broader, partly implicit notions of what is important or valuable. To claim that others should be granted rights to life, liberty, or freedom of speech is to assert that we should be guided by these principles in our personal interactions and social structures. But why should such rights be accorded to people? What makes people worthy of them? What constitutes the appeal of a form of society that would recognize them? Answering these questions is not a matter of assessing the ethical status of an action or practice in light of an articulated principle. We are instead articulating our fundamental intuitions regarding what makes people important, valuable, and worthy of being treated with the respect embodied in such rights. These intuitions involve seeing a good that we are moved by, intuitions which give us an ethical world. Without such intuitions, ethics cannot get started.

This is not to suggest that in articulating our intuitions we are simply describing an inerrant seeing of the good that directly gives us ethical truth. My seeing that an action or way of life is good, and is good for a particular reason, can be wrong. But the way to a more perceptive ethical sight comes through a critique of my current ethical perceptions, not from stepping outside of ethical intuitions altogether. One cannot abstract from ethics as a means to improve ethics. There is no non-ethical way to prove that an ethical intuition is correct or incorrect.

Further, an appeal to principles may provide only weak support in ethical debate. An appeal to someone's ethical intuitions can be more persuasive. But for this appeal to make any headway, the person must share at least some ethical intuitions with the person making the appeal. Someone who had no ethical intuitions, or a set that had no overlap with one's own, could not be convinced of an alternative perspective. For example, if someone claimed that there is nothing wrong with killing innocent people in order to provide advantages to oneself, there is little prospect of making any headway in arguing for a right to life. But this isn't in fact how people reason ethically. Even in a case like the United States' willingness to kill civilians in its foreign wars (Tirman, 2011, estimates six to seven million in Korea, Vietnam, and Iraq alone), these actions are not justified by the bald claim that it is acceptable to kill the innocent in order to secure advantages for one's own people. Rather, the victims are pictured as propagating some evil, or of not really being "like us," or their deaths are framed as an unfortunate and unavoidable consequence of the pursuit of some greater good ("we wish we could do it otherwise, but there is bound to be collateral damage"). Such rationales, as self-serving and distorted as they may be, still acknowledge the validity of the idea that it is wrong to kill simply for one's own advantage. Without that acknowledgment, other arguments that would challenge the characterization of the other as evil, unlike us, and thus unworthy of concern would have no traction. Which is not to say that it is easy to persuade—there can be many reasons to deceive oneself in the face of sound ethical arguments. But that does not make the argument unsound. More to the point here, outside of some shared ethical intuitions no argument can get going at all. "The most reliable moral view is not one that would be grounded quite outside our intuitions but one that is grounded on our strongest intuitions, where these have successfully met the challenge of proposed transitions away from them" (Taylor, 1989, p. 75).

Taylor points to the biographical nature of such transitions. When someone moves from one ethical position to another, it is because they see that the new position is an improvement, is more convincing, or clarifies a previously unacknowledged but perhaps dimly felt sense about the matter. For example, a young woman comes to see that idealizing the commodified beauty portrayed in popular culture is part of the subjugation of women, and she begins to question her previous passion for the latest styles in hair, make-up, and clothes. After further reflection, reading, and discussion with friends perhaps she modifies her views again, finds some legitimacy to the appreciation of beauty, but nevertheless remains attentive to how common standards of beauty can be linked to an exploitative demand that keeps women in a subordinate social position. She may later come to a yet different view, but if she does so it will be for similar reasons. That is, each shift will be experienced as a gain upon her previous position in that it addresses something that had been previously overlooked, or is more encompassing of her fundamental intuitions, or clarifies a contradiction or confusion in her previous view.

Such revisions all take place within an ethical world. They start from and reconsider certain ethical assumptions. And they are never finished. The best that can be said about an ethical position is that it is an improvement on a prior position. It's the best sense someone has at present about what is good, how it is right to live, or what makes this or that aim worth pursuing.

Taylor refers to this as a person's "best account" (1989, pp. 58f). Any given best account can be improved upon, but that improvement will come through moving on to another better account.

If this is how an ethical sense develops and improves, this does not mean that the current view is always better than prior ones. I could be wrong now and my older position might have been better. But the only way I would come to realize that my prior take was actually better would be if I came to see that the move to my current position was confused, or self-deceptive, or motivated by factors that only obscure matters. Perhaps I begin to sense that I came to take on my current views because I fell under the spell of a charismatic figure who persuaded me by appealing to a blind fear that I now see as shameful. But the way out of the spell is to acknowledge that this fear was operative within me—moving forward in this case takes the shape of accounting for more of who I am, for what I was motivated by that distorted my ethical views.

Our ethical debates sometimes appeal to principles. But just as often they take the form of appealing to people to examine a contradiction within their views, or to spell out the implications of an assumption, or to acknowledge that they do care about something that they have been overlooking. There is an invitation to articulate something implicit that has not been given its due. The appeal is not to acknowledge a principle that has broad consensus, but to acknowledge something in one's fundamental sense of what is good or right that lies dormant, or has been ignored for motivated reasons.

Sandel (2014) gives an example of such ethical reasoning in his discussion of the way that Lyndon Johnson campaigned for civil rights in the South in 1960. Johnson would speak to white southern audiences not by appealing to principles of justice or equal rights. He appealed to their fundamental, emotionally lived sense of right and wrong. He would ask how they would feel if their child was sick and they had to take her to a distant hospital to get care, or they couldn't buy her a soda at the drug store on a hot day. "To bring his listeners around, Johnson relies on their self-interpretive agency. He urges them to consider the particular things they care about, the things that define their daily lives, and to judge accordingly" (p. 240).

Movement forward in ethics takes the form of transition from a previously held view that is retrospectively seen as failing, inadequate, or incomplete. In a particular person's life such transitions often take biographical form, a story of how and why they moved from one view to another. "I used to believe that X would make my life more fulfilled and now I see I was misguided." Or: "How could I have lived before without this important good in my life?" Spelling out such transitions can require a complex narrative, where someone notes the appeal of the former view, how they came to see its limitations, and how the current view is more viable, complete, freeing, or life-enhancing. For the purposes of simply living through this transition, a less elaborate articulation may suffice. However, such narratives not only help to explain such transitions, they help to sustain them, for the transition is partly constituted by a story of advance. So the explication of what happened, how the transition came about, helps to develop it, to strengthen it, and to enact the new ethical perception.

This is apparent in cultural transitions regarding ethical views. Here the narratives take the form not of personal biography but of historical explanations that shade off into ethical justifications. We saw examples of this in the previous chapter. Early modern thinkers saw themselves as having come to recognize the value of thinking things out for themselves by moving beyond what they saw as a willingness to blindly follow tradition in the medieval period. Romantic era intellectuals critiqued the Enlightenment for its overvaluation of rationality and saw themselves as retaining what was worthwhile about reason while adding an affectively mediated attunement with nature that enriched and deepened life. Romanticism has been critiqued in turn for the way that the moral value of feeling has been used to support irrationalism, or blind allegiance to a personal or national identity. In such transitions, each movement or era understands itself in the light of its advance upon what went before. Debates take the form of questioning whether the transition really constituted an advance, or brought with it some other ill, perhaps one even worse than what was left behind.

Ethical Transitions in Therapy

Unlike the debates that occur in broad cultural change, therapeutic practice does not usually involve efforts to directly persuade patients to adopt a new ethical stance. Rather, therapists point to something that patients have left out of their stories about themselves, or an anomaly in how they tell their stories, or an invitation to look at their dilemmas from another point of view. For example, a cognitive-behavioral therapist may inquire of self-critical patients whether they would be so depressed if they assessed their limitations and mistakes against a less exacting standard, perhaps pointing out that they don't hold their friends to the same standard and yet don't think less of them.

The invitation to reconsider something in therapy may not be directed to particular problems or assumptions. In punctuating patients' speech, Lacanian analysts are pointing to something that has appeared in their speech that they have overlooked, something that puts what they have been saying in a different light. It may be unclear what a specific slip of the tongue has to do with broader aspects of the patient's problems. But the aim here isn't to solve problems. It's to open up a space for the unconscious, to loosen one's grip on an already constituted frame of self-understanding, a loosening that, over time, can lead to fundamental shifts in the patient's libidinal economy that the patient will experience as a gain, even if this gain does not come in a form that is explicitly articulated. When a relational analyst like Mitchell (1997) shares with a patient his sense of a repeated relationship pattern, this is partly an offer of information about the patient. But seeing this pattern is intended to open the possibility for a different pattern. Indeed, the very way this information is offered can be an instantiation of a different interpersonal pattern that allows a less damaging or constricted way of engaging with others.

These are ethical gains, shifts toward greater flourishing, however flourishing may be conceptualized in the particular therapy involved. These gains usually do not entail a change in a principle for living that becomes part of a formal philosophy for how to handle life's challenges. Sometimes they do. This may be the case with how some therapies are sometimes presented, or with how some people take up the gains they have made in therapy. But this can be done in a way that betrays the spirit of the therapy, even with therapies that lend themselves to being formulated in terms of general principles. There is plenty of material in cognitive-behavioral therapy that patients can extract as ready-made principles or maxims ("to avoid what provokes anxiety only increases anxiety"; "black and white thinking is distorted thinking"; etc.). However, experienced therapists know that progress comes not from memorizing certain principles and applying them by rote. Rather, such principles are guidelines for the development of skills for tackling certain kinds of problems, skills that require practice and need to be sensitively adapted to the particular situation at hand.

Formulation of principles is even further afield from the mode of action of many of the psychodynamic and humanistic therapies. Even when therapeutic practice seems to implicitly point to a principle ("beware of structuring your life around seeking the good of others," or "be alert to the nuances of your psychic life that you may be motivated to deny," etc.), it is not offered as a rule for living or a guidepost for making choices. Rather than principles, people are more likely to come out of therapy with a new ethical orientation, a different set of sensitivities about what may be good for them. Perhaps after analysis patients may recognize their capacity for self-deception and understand that they will never have a complete grasp upon their motives. This realization may be more lived than formulated. It may be humbling to accept these limits to self-knowledge. But it may also be liberating, dissipating a prior shame that was generated by the expectation of complete self-possession and self-control. This new realization may function in the background, exerting a pull to be willing to reconsider assumptions about identity, motive, and intention. But it is not likely to become a maxim for general application (to turn it into a maxim may even undermine the gain it represents).

So, unlike some of the more explicit rationales given for broad cultural changes in ethics, the changes that occur in therapy often entail changes in perspective that are less fully articulated. This feature of ethical change in therapy is related to the fundamental ethical reticence endemic to therapy. Therapists of various stripes are disinclined to explicitly promote an ethical vision, even one that is central to their therapeutic practice. There is an acute sensitivity among therapists to the ways that ideas about how to live well can operate as oppressive and constricting demands, and one of the central ethical offerings of therapy is to aid patients to not be so enamored of a vision of flourishing that it becomes a burden. As a consequence, many of the narratives about shifts in ethical perspective that result from therapy will have a tentative quality to them. Some therapists and patients will trumpet the gains available through therapy, but many will be much more circumspect. One of the gains of therapy may well be a sense that no gains are final, that therapy sends people on their way rather than brings them to a destination.

Further, ethical perspectives are quite often just that: perspectives, not conclusions. That is, ethics often take the form of an orienting framework rather than a set of specific ideas or ideals. When there are ideas, their application to particular situations calls for a capacity for deliberative assessment that is not given by the idea alone. For example, a patient comes to see in therapy that her depressing tendency to demand moral perfection of herself has been related to horror at the thought that she might sometimes want to further her own agenda, regardless of whether others might benefit. Over time, something shifts in the moral demand, and her condemnation of "selfishness," as she calls it, eases. While this positions her differently in the future, it still leaves her uncertain as to how to apply this new orientation to particular situations. She will have judgment calls to make regarding how to act upon her new acceptance of a self-oriented agenda in a given context.

When patients do come out of therapy with stories to tell about how they have changed perspectives on what matters in their lives, these are less likely to be stories about therapy than stories about their lives.

> I used to think and live my life under the rubric of implicit views of who I was, of what was wrong with me, of who I was supposed to be for other people, and of what I had to do to be happy. Some of that has changed. Much of it no longer seems so important. I can see why I used to worry about all that, and such thoughts are not entirely foreign to me now, but they don't rule my life or so constantly occupy my mind—I've moved on to other things.

Often all that can be said about therapy is a few positive things about the therapist "who really listened to me," or about a vague idea ("I learned how to challenge some assumptions I was making").

Arguing for the Ethics of a Therapy: Practice and Narrative

Unlike patients, therapists often have a lot to say about therapy, about what they believe is beneficial about it, how it helps people, and with what sorts of difficulties. Arguing for particular therapeutic aims and their implicit conceptions of well-being is not a simple matter, however.

Distinct therapeutic practices that introduce people to different ways of living, acting, and thinking about themselves have the means to become self-validating. When someone enters into a therapeutic engagement they are allowing themselves to be shaped by that therapy's practices. How they are changed can then be pointed to as evidence of the correctness of that therapy. Fink (2017, p. 325) is delighted at the "abnormality" of analyzed people. But is this abnormality something that was always true of them and that they have simply been freed to live? Or does Lacanian analysis bring about this abnormality through the manner in which analysands are continually thrown back upon themselves, unable to find an analyst with whom they can identify, turned away from their preferred self-understanding, in search of a satisfaction that is idiosyncratically their own? When patients learn to observe their thinking patterns, to examine them for the ways that they distort facts and generate depressed mood or anxiety, they learn to become masters of their own psychological houses, able to alter their symptoms. Does this prove that the cognitive theory is correct? Or does this not represent the offer of a way to live in the light of certain notions about reason and emotion? To the extent that patients accept the offer, they have taken on a new way of living with their depression or anxiety that provides certain benefits as they have come to value self-mastery and to discover ways to make it possible. The fact that there are accompanying symptom changes does not prove that the underlying ethic is superior to other therapeutic ethics. For one thing, very different therapies aiming at different forms of flourishing can have equivalent symptomatic success. Further, the idea that symptom change should be the fundamental measure of success already assumes something about which benefits matter most (it favors one ethic over others).

Therapeutic theories are not independent of what they are theories of. Therapeutic practices shape subjectivity in the light of a theory of that subjectivity. Unlike natural scientific theories which can be assessed for the extent to which they accurately account for an independent object, therapeutic theories and practices help to create what the theory is about. Galileo's discovery of the laws of motion didn't change the velocity of falling objects. But a theory that people have repressed wishes and motives that appear in disguised form in dreams, symptoms, and slips of the tongue can change how people live their lives. They begin to pay attention to their dreams, to doubt that they can take their conscious intentions at face value, to look for possible sexual or aggressive meanings in what had previously gone unnoticed, and now come not just to understand but to live their lives as people who are inevitably motivated by sex and aggression. This is akin to a process of enculturation. In therapy, people are brought to live differently via practices that help to create what their theories claim to be the case. Theories of who people are also shape people to be (live, experience) in accord with that theory. This is one of the meanings of Taylor's idea that we are self-interpreting animals (1985a). Who we are is partly constituted by who we understand ourselves to be.

This is not to suggest that therapy simply makes itself true, simply indoctrinates or creates persons in its image, as if there is nothing to the person in therapy beyond what is imparted via therapy. It is clear that therapy can fail. People drop out of therapy. Some people come to therapy with a particular idea of what they are looking for, with regard to the type of therapy or its outcome. Some people do better in one type of therapy than another, or with one therapist than another. Therapists find themselves changing what they do in response to how the patient responds. Patients are not blank slates upon which anything can be written, not raw material that can be shaped in any fashion. As Kirschner (2012) notes, therapists do not "make up" their patients. This is of course just as true for the enculturation that takes place in child-rearing. Parents have to be responsive to the children they have as they try to help them to be better. And some children are especially resistant to some aspects of enculturation, just as some patients are resistant to certain forms of therapy. The response to these resistances can be frustration or despair: "this child is impossible—he's making me crazy," or "this patient isn't analyzable." But the inclination to refuse what is on offer can also prompt parents and therapists to change what they do. Therapists adapt their approaches to new situations, sometimes even change fundamental notions of how to do therapeutic work. For example, many of the transformations in analytic theory and practice (the shifts from drive theory to ego psychology, or to object relations, self psychology, and relational analysis) have had something to do with encounters with people who did not do well with previous approaches.

However, changes in therapeutic theory and practice have also been prompted by the changing aims of therapy. Analysts of different schools make different aims central to their theory and practice. They have different ideas about which potential benefits of analysis are most valuable. Behavioral, rational-emotive, and cognitive-behavioral therapies were developed in part out of frustration with analytic work that did not aim directly at measurable outcomes but was perceived as meandering through a patient's psychological mindscape, offering interpretations of dubious scientific warrant. Their aims, by contrast, were efficient and effective means to achieve objective ends. According to their perspective on flourishing, a pragmatic approach to solving concrete problems was held to be far more valuable than the kind of lengthy personal exploration that might somewhat mysteriously yield symptomatic change.

Therapeutic practices change in response to what is encountered in therapeutic work. There are facts about people that therapy has to attend to. But those facts are to a significant extent also constituted by people's understanding of themselves, of what is amiss with them, what is possible for them, or who it would be good to be. Each therapy in turn has some effect upon the person in therapy that provides support for that therapy's fundamental assumptions regarding who people are and who it is good to be. This transformation is not wrought through indoctrination, but through practices that direct the patient's attention to certain aspects of their experience and behavior in ways that re-write the significance of that experience and behavior so that it becomes something different and open to changes that were not previously possible.

If therapeutic practices change people in ways that tend to confirm therapeutic theories, this does not mean that there can be no argument for one therapy over another, or that each therapy is an entirely self-enclosed system of theory and practice. There are ways to argue for a therapeutic orientation. Such arguments are more likely to take the form of persuasive narratives than objective data. This is not an accident, or an unfortunate limitation of an undeveloped science. Because therapy is at least in part about ethics, about how to live more fully, it will often take the form of a story, of the transition from one perspective, one personal positioning, to another. Clinical stories are not best understood as limited, subjectively contaminated data. Scientific data can give us relatively objective reasons to believe that one thing caused another. A clinical story is meant to reveal something about people and therapy that we wouldn't otherwise see. Clinical case descriptions help to bring something to life, to show us ways of doing therapy, but also ways of seeing certain kinds of human problems and ways of aiming for something better that can only be shown by narrative means.

There is a legitimate scientific concern that such narratives create the truth they would reveal, that they do not provide us with a "clean" perception of what is going on in therapy, but are shaping the depiction of what happened in such a way as to support a particular theory. While this does create the possibility of distortions that favor therapists' preferred views, such narratives are also the product of therapists' efforts to articulate something they are seeing in their patients or in therapeutic process. They may be seeing wrong. But the fact that therapists construct narratives from particular perspectives doesn't make them self-enclosed or immune to criticism. Readers of case studies and clinical narratives have the means to assess whether they make sense from some other point of view, are missing information that might reshape the conclusions, resonate with anything they have seen themselves, or illuminate problems they have encountered. An assessment of this sort isn't like an assessment of whether therapy A or therapy B results in a lower score on the Beck Depression Inventory. It's more like the assessment of a work of narrative history or of whether a recent novel captures the zeitgeist of contemporary work, dating, or family life. Such interpretive assessments rely upon standards even if they don't result in final decisions and are open to further re-assessment and interpretation.

To critique clinical narratives for creating the truth they would reveal is to miss the ethical point of such narratives. They are calling fellow therapists to a new perspective on particular difficulties and on ways to help patients move past them. Of course the narrative helps to create what it is about. That is what narratives do. Not just fictional narratives, but historical, political, spiritual, and therapeutic narratives. Narrative is one of the richest forms for the self-interpreting that gives shape to human life. Clinical narratives are trying to shape us to be better therapists, to draw us toward seeing a therapeutic situation in a new light, to attune us to a new perspective on how patients get into trouble, and on how therapy can help. This is the case even when what is new here is only slightly new, only a variation on well-known themes. Clinical narratives do straddle the boundary that natural science is rightly loathe to cross between creation and discovery, often making something appear that was only dimly sensed before it was invoked in language that helps both to point to it and, in a sense, bring it into being.[3] Freud's Oedipal theory is a kind of fundamental story that has generated myriad particular clinical stories of Oedipal dynamics. It both helped to reveal a kind of problem people can have and created a framework for gathering together the events of nuclear family life into a narrative that was not widely available before, and in the process making it possible for there to be new forms of intervention and new aims for treatment.

What I mean by clinical narratives are not just case reports written up after the fact. Nor am I referring here simply to the narratives about a patient's life that are constructed in therapy by patient and therapist. These constructed narratives are common in therapy, and sometimes helpful, although also open to myriad defensive or self-deceptive uses. Beyond these narratives, I am also referring to those that are enacted in the moment-to-moment action of therapy. Patient and therapist are looking ahead, aiming to get somewhere, even if this movement is entangled with efforts to avoid going in certain directions or to delay seeing certain possibilities. Both participants do what they do, and say what they say, as part of an effort to figure out where to go and how to get there, "there" being framed differently by different therapists and patients: a decrease in symptoms, the depressive position, increased self-mastery, a greater capacity for mentalization, etc. Sometimes the place to go is simply to be more deeply or fully here and now. But in each case, there is an aim and the action of therapy will be in service of that aim, which means that it will have a narrative arc. Even if the story is one of impasse or stalemate, this too implies that there is a path to travel that has been blocked.

So narrative is woven through therapy, whether in the form of case reports, or told in session by patient and therapist, or lived and enacted in therapeutic practice. Narrative is inevitable, and part of the process of therapy. But it is not necessarily benign. I referred above to the defensive or self-deceptive nature of some narratives. Cognitive and behavioral therapists may point patients to the ways in which their stories are irrational, lack evidentiary support, too "black and white," "catastrophizing," etc. Many therapists are aware of the ways patients construct narratives to favor a preferred and distorted self-understanding. Lacanians point to their ego-generated imaginary character. And many of the available narrative templates are derived from a social and cultural world that offers truncated, flat, or oppressive narrative forms that constrict and stifle possibility. Therapeutic work can often involve loosening the grip that a problematic narrative has had upon a person, re-writing it, telling new stories, or learning to live with anomalies and gaps in a story that is never complete.[4] But in all of these cases there is the creation of experience through the narrative and interpretive form in which it is articulated.

There is a sense then that narrative can constitute what it is about rather than simply point to an independent object. However, this does not make narrative fundamentally suspect, for that which it is about can only appear in narrative. Narrative ought not to be relegated to a second-class epistemic status simply because it is not operating entirely within a designative semantic logic where what we talk about has an existence independent of the language with which we talk about it. The history of innovation in therapy has been partly the result of scientific investigation into therapeutic efficacy and process, child development, attachment theory, and basic science regarding processes of habituation to arousal, etc. But innovation is also the product of new ways of narrating lives, of stories formed around different sorts of crises, confusions, struggles, and oppressions. These are such stories as: being the blind victim of patterns of phobic avoidance that sustains anxiety; being trapped in repeated depressive self-statements about oneself and one's options for living; wishes for impossible triumph in tension with expectations of catastrophic punishment (castration) stemming from the difficulties of negotiating love and loss in the nuclear family; loss of self through impingements, subtle and dramatic; self-betrayal and estrangement; thwarted esteem; or living with the consequences of growing up in a racist or sexist culture that battered one's integrity and prospects for flourishing.

Although narratives cannot be held to the standards of traditional empirical research, they do need to be accountable. They need to point to real events in people's lives that support their plausibility. But a project to sort out the real events from the narrative frame in which they appear is a fool's errand. Can such narratives be supplemented, supported, or challenged by extra-narrative data? Certainly. But the result of such supplements and challenges will be a re-written narrative, not a collection of data. For in sorting out the difficulties of their patients' lives, and of what can be done to help them, therapists are bound to frame this in terms of plot or narrative, of how people with these difficulties can be helped to move from here to there, from pathology to health, from constriction to freedom, from self-estrangement to authenticity, from traumatized isolation to life engagement, that is, toward greater flourishing.

Of course, therapists support their particular therapeutic orientations with more than case studies. Even the typical clinical paper often invokes the history of prior thinking about a problem, references prior research, or points to conundrums or unresolved controversies. This is then sometimes followed by the writer's own theoretical contribution, with clinical examples given as support for an alternative approach. In this context, the case report may play a subordinate, illustrative role for the broader theoretical point. But it would be wrong to conclude that clinical narratives simply say concretely what is elsewhere stated in more abstract terms. Clinical stories do not simply play a supportive role to abstract ideas. Insofar as therapy is a social practice, its concretely enacted details are as important as its theoretical articulation. To spell out certain key principles is essential for communicating what constitutes a particular therapy. To tell clinical stories without extracting from them some general ideas about what the therapy's aims are would be of little use. But to only give general maxims for practice would be equally useless (probably worse). Such maxims and recommendations are often made. They serve a purpose, but they leave too much undecided and offer too little of context and exemplars to know how to apply them to concrete situations. Consider recommendations to utilize Socratic questioning in cognitive-behavioral therapy, or the psychoanalytic idea that one should only interpret something that is already close to the patient's awareness. Without seeing a number of examples and trying it out oneself, seeing how and why it does or doesn't apply, the principle can be almost useless. Complex social practices like therapy need to be described in the form of concrete exemplars, not simply to illustrate them, but in order to begin to understand what they are and what their more formal articulations mean.

However, these theoretical and narrative presentations of therapeutic orientation are usually "in house" affairs. They are part of how a particular therapeutic orientation is sustained, developed, or revised. They appear in papers that are published in journals dedicated to a particular orientation (*Journal of the American Psychoanalytic Association*, *Behavior Therapy*, etc.), or a subgroup within it (*Psychoanalytic Dialogues*). They are part of the ethical reasoning within that orientation. They provide support for or critiques of the practices and theories of their respective orientations, and thereby implicitly promote a variation on the picture of flourishing in that orientation. Outsiders can read such work and may or may not be moved or convinced of the validity of what is presented. But such work isn't typically part of an effort to engage or convince those of a different orientation.

Contrasting Ethics in Dialogue

Conversation between the contrasting ethics of different therapeutic orientations will put fundamental beliefs up for debate. Honest dialogue involves the risk that cherished views will be challenged. A conversation about core beliefs can change the participants in a deep and personal way, for personal identity is partly constituted by views on what matters most (see Taylor, 1989). What's at stake in such conversations are basic ideas that both say something about people (they offer descriptions and explanations) and propose aims for people (they include prescriptions, norms, or aspirations). These two aspects come as a package, each implicitly depending upon the other. For example, when psychoanalysts try to make the case that we have wishes and motivations that are in conflict, a conflict that leads to internal division through a process of repression, they are also arguing for certain goods that elude us because of such conflict. For one analyst the good obstructed may be framed as a more complete and honest self-understanding, for another as autonomy, for a third as erotic vitality set free from socially imposed constraints. Focus on one of these goods over others will entail a correspondingly different formulation of the nature of conflict. A formulation of who people are and how things go awry for them both shapes and is shaped by how one formulates the nature of the benefit, good, or well-being that is aimed at by the therapy.

The challenge to one therapist's views from a therapist of a different orientation is also two-sided. Humanistic therapists may take issue with the focus on psychic division in psychoanalysis, or with the conception of wishes or motives as operating like impersonal forces within the person. They may argue that a more accurate conception of the person includes a natural bent toward a healthy, integrated self. Without this inherent tendency toward growth or authenticity there is no possibility of therapeutic change, for one can't just act upon patients with interventions that push them to grow personally (see the idea of the "client-as-active-self-healer" in Bohart and Tallman, 1999). Here too therapeutic aims and aspirations are linked to corresponding conceptions of what is most fundamental about who people are. The humanistic therapist may claim that the therapist's fundamental role is to listen for and support patients' budding efforts to find themselves, to develop the capacities, interests, and strengths that are unique to them and bring them toward their particular forms of flourishing.

Some behavioral and cognitive-behavioral therapists may object that this is all too abstract and speculative, that what impedes people from attaining their goals are specific patterns of behavior and emotional distress that can be changed with targeted interventions. If people are divided against themselves this is not the result of repression or dissociation, but of mistaken beliefs and reinforced habits that can be more directly addressed. It is the removal of impediments to people pursuing their own path that is of most help to them in becoming who they "authentically are." The humanistic project to help patients discern where their true selves lie runs the risk that the therapist will steer each patient toward a self that the therapist thinks the patient should have. What people need is the freedom from symptomatic, habitual, and irrational impediments to effective action in the world. Once such impediments are removed, people can find their own authenticity, libidinal vitality, freedom from the demands of the social world, or whatever else they may think is important. It is not the therapist's job to point them to a particular version of flourishing, or to take them there.

Nevertheless, this apparent neutrality regarding a good life implicitly points to a more specific good. The explicit claim is that the only relevant therapeutic good is the individual's freedom from well-defined psychological obstacles to acting effectively in the world. Beyond that, each person will choose their own good. But implicit here is the assumption that the person's sense of the good is not implicated in their symptoms and that the unhindered self-directedness of the individual is the only good that matters in therapy.

The situation is no different for those who study psychotherapy in a sociohistorical context. They enter the conversation asking whether particular psychological theories and therapeutic practices are expressive of, influenced by, or serve particular social, cultural, or economic ends. But they will implicitly be offering some theory about people, about how they are created or shaped by broader social forces and practices. Depending upon their conception of those social influences, they will also have some implicit picture of what it is possible for people to aspire to. That is, they may question whether the resolution of psychic conflict, the search for authenticity, or the aim to master symptoms and irrational habits of thinking and behavior are feasible self-standing aims, or serve some other social end. They may put in doubt whether intended therapeutic aims are attainable or even make sense, perhaps claiming that they are only possible in a social world that has been radically re-structured, or even that, in a more just society, flourishing will take an entirely different form. If so, then social-political change aiming at that more just society will be the most important good.

So the debates about the conflicting views of human flourishing present in the therapies will include claims regarding both the nature of persons and the form of flourishing that people can reasonably aim for. But how do such debates proceed, what sorts of argumentation can be offered?

Sometimes the argument involves pointing to some relevant factor that another orientation overlooks. In *The Ethical Visions of Psychotherapy* I raise concerns about the effort to conceptualize the problems people bring to treatment in atomistic terms. For example, I note that specific emotional responses and behaviors often can't be given generic labels that determine which interventions should be utilized. What patients complain of and seek help with can rarely be understood outside of complicated contexts that give them their meaning. Understanding those contexts can require detailed exploration of patients' personal experiences, their culture, their views about what is important to them, what they expect from therapy, how they relate to the therapist, etc. A therapy consisting of the direct application of techniques without attention to these larger contexts is vulnerable to a number of critiques.

Sometimes argument about the ethics of different therapies involves an appeal to something that the adherent of another orientation already subscribes to but isn't acknowledging. A cognitive-behavioral therapist might agree with a psychodynamic therapist that a particular patient's panic disorder is ultimately rooted in shame over loss of control or in relationship patterns of passive dependence. This therapist might even acknowledge that the patient's shame began in childhood relationships, and could be effectively addressed through how it appears in the relationship with the therapist (i.e., in the transference). Nevertheless, the cognitive-behavioral therapist could appeal to the psychodynamic therapist along these lines:

> Does it really not matter to you if a twenty week program of treatment can make it possible for this person to leave the house alone, go to the store, or return to work? Perhaps there will be all sorts of interpersonal issues left to address, but isn't this a worthwhile benefit for the patient?

The cognitive-behavioral therapist bases this appeal on some sense that the psychodynamic therapist also recognizes the value of efficiently bringing about concrete behavioral change, at least some of the time, in some contexts.

In fact, this appeal is often on the mark. For psychodynamic therapists' rejoinder is not likely to be: "No, that's pointless." Instead, they are more likely to respond with something like, "Yes, this would be worthwhile, but … it's just a beginning," or "these symptoms may also improve while doing a type of therapy that engages patients more deeply," or "it misses an opportunity to do work that addresses more fundamental issues." That is, there is an acknowledgement of the value to patients of such treatment rather than a dismissal of it. What is added after the "yes, but" is a pitch for other sorts of benefits, not a denial of this benefit. But now a conversation can be engaged about which benefits matter more, in what contexts, and for what reasons.

The debates on such matters can be difficult to resolve. Cases can be pointed to as part of the argumentation. For example, one patient's agoraphobia-resolving mastery of her panic made it possible for her to return to work, which boosted her self-esteem, and decreased her reliance upon a dependent relationship with her oldest daughter. But another patient made some headway with his agoraphobia, returned to work, and developed a dependent relationship with his supervisor, provoking a number of conflicts that led to his being fired. He was only able to begin to see this interpersonal pattern, let alone start to change it, as a later therapist began to address its appearance in the transference. The value of changes in how patients position themselves in living their lives is often only seen in action, as one spells out the particulars of how a patient moves through therapy to a new position. So such case examples are part of the debate.

But the examples above do not directly address disagreements about the more fundamental aims of the therapies. In an earlier chapter, I offered a tentative listing of distinct views regarding human flourishing that are embodied in different therapies: rational self-mastery, honest self-exploration, particularity liberated from social expectation, and attunement to the complexities of emotion and motivation in relationship with others. What would a discussion about the differences between such fundamental ethical ideals look like? They can take a number of different forms: a well-wrought argument that points to unjustified assumptions or a contradiction in the other's reasoning; an appeal to a good the other is overlooking, perhaps because they are focused on a different good; a case narrative that illustrates how a therapy guided by one conception of flourishing brought about specific benefits. There is no set method here. These will be wide-ranging debates about the merits and limitations of each view of well-being. These engagements will look like the disputes between rival pictures of the good in Taylor's history of modernity that I surveyed in Chapter 3. They will be ongoing affairs, unlikely to be easily resolved. I am certainly not in a position to resolve them. But I do want to give some brief indication of what such a dialogue might look like, whether the participants are therapists of different orientations, or social historians and critics of therapy. Imagine the following exchange as the opening statements in a roundtable discussion.

First speaker (a proponent of rational self-mastery):

Without a capacity to assess the reasonableness of one's habits and beliefs, all other goods are elusive. Reasoned reflection and control over emotional responses are essential to success in most endeavors in life. Without this, peoples' efforts to explore the complexities of their psychological depths, to free themselves from social expectations, or to find their authentic selves will be like swimming in a hurricane. Without this, relationships with others cannot be established or sustained. The person who is terrified of the next panic attack or crushed with depressive despair doesn't have the psychological scope or motivation to pursue any of these aims. Moreover, rational self-mastery can be helpful not just for treating symptoms, but for extricating oneself from alienating demands, for developing a life that truly feels like it is one's own, and for other forms of a fully flourishing life.

Second speaker (responding to the first):

Rational self-mastery is just too empty. If therapy only gathers me together under a more solid 'command and control' so that I may pursue aims that I choose, but is mute about which aims are worth pursuing, is it sufficient? Doesn't this approach risk presenting a picture of existence with each of us in charge of ourselves but afloat in a sea of choice, with no reason to move in one direction rather than another besides emotional pain, fear, or the avoidance of depression and anxiety? Further, is it true that psychological difficulties are best characterized as impediments to moving effectively away from distress toward whatever goal the individual has decided is good? Aren't some difficulties that people bring to therapy related to dilemmas or confusions about what really makes for a decent life, or raise questions about what the person has so far considered to be truly worthwhile?

Consider the executive who fears that his panic attacks may signal weakness in a competitive business environment where he believes he must appear iron-willed and tough at all times. Behind his fear that this 'weakness' will show through and undermine his professional success is another concern. He grew up hearing his father repeatedly tell him that he wouldn't amount to anything. The desperate need to succeed is driven by the project to prove his father wrong. There are important questions here for him to consider. Why does he still feel he needs to convince his father, whom he has long since surpassed in career attainment and financial success? In trying to prove himself has he taken on a project that has been fundamentally alienating, which has kept him from exploring other options for a fulfilling life that might actually bring him some joy and relieve him of the burden of a self-imposed life sentence of self-assertion? Won't his way out of the cycle of panic, where fear of panic creates more panic, require addressing these basic questions about who he feels he must be? It is true that the therapist's job is not to tell him what that different version of himself is. But exploring these questions is likely to involve changes in fundamental ideas about how he should live his life, about what is most important for him to do and be. It is not simply the removal of psychological hindrances to the attainment of ends he has already decided upon.

Third speaker (a political critic of therapy):

What appear to be personal goods like rational self-mastery or authenticity are in fact ideological constructs. Without attention to the wider social context, such aims may unwittingly support other ends, like an economic system with unceasing demands for production and consumption. From this perspective, a goal like the search for authenticity may be seen as a pipe dream that gives people the illusion that they are on their way to greater happiness. Meanwhile, this pleasing fantasy serves to distract from the oppression wrought by the economic system they serve, functioning as a psychological 'opium of the people.'

Fourth Speaker (a proponent of liberated particularity):

The project of rational self-mastery is exactly what Freud, Lacan, and others have shown to be illusory. Unless they are freed from the expectations and demands of the familial and societal world into which they have been born, people will think they are rationally charting their destiny only to be following a path set by others.

Fifth Speaker (questioning the proponent of liberated particularity):

How do I know that the good I am aiming at isn't worth pursuing just because it comes from my family or culture? Are you claiming that there is something particular to me that should outweigh all that I have received and that has shaped my sense of what matters in life? What am I left with in this scenario? On what basis do I decide that something is better than what has been bequeathed to me? I may sense ways in which the ideas about what is worthwhile proposed by my social-cultural world are constricting, unappealing, demanding, or damaging to me and to others. But won't my sense of what's amiss also have some roots in that culture? Am I ever entirely outside of such influences? And don't those influences also give me a basis for critique of the picture of the good I find around me? Further, why is that which is particular to me *the* measure of flourishing? Can I just assume that social constriction upon the freedoms and particularities of individuals is necessarily the central problem to address?

Sixth speaker (a proponent of honest self-exploration):

I do not argue for an ideal of personal honesty as simply good-in-itself, as a free-standing virtue that requires no further justification. Such honesty is essential to living with others. There is a kind of courage here, the courage to face and accept oneself without defensiveness. This is the courage people need in order to be themselves in the context of a complicated social world where there are multiple pressures to betray oneself in order to 'get along.' Honesty supports a robust particularity that has been discerned, accepted, and *owned*. It is not the particularity that results from an impersonal shift in libidinal energies.

Seventh Speaker (with sympathies for humanistic therapy and relational analysis):

Self-mastery. An honest self-perception that provides a more robust self-acceptance. A liberated erotic particularity that leads to following one's own bent outside of social expectations. Selves, mastery, courage, going one's own way. How stereotypically masculine, independent, and isolated. Aren't the best things in life really associated with relationships with others? Isn't the reason to explore, master, or particularize yourself so that you can participate more fully in interpersonal life, and contribute to it as well? At the end of the day, at the end of your therapy or analysis, is it really just your particular satisfaction, your autonomy, your self you want? Is everyone who seeks connections in friendship, romantic relationships, family, or community really overlooking what is most important? If you're honest with yourself, haven't your best moments been with others? Yes, the worst can also happen with others: betrayal, violence, indifference. But this indicates the ways that relationships can go wrong. Betrayal, violence, and indifference are wrong precisely because they damage what is most important: relationships, community, a sense of social connection, and commitment to something beyond oneself.

(Some may further integrate these relational aims with the broader sociopolitical aims noted above.)

I find myself drawn, to one degree or another, to all of these positions. None of them seem to me to have refuted the others. Some who read this will no doubt think that I haven't done a good enough job at showing the strength of one of these positions so that it is evident how it wins out over the others. That's certainly true. These opening statements are far too brief to make a very strong case for any one of them. Others may propose a picture of ethical or political aims that are not captured by any of those I have described. But I would respond that a more robust argument for any of these ethics (or for one I haven't included) would provoke vigorous rejoinders, and the debates would go on.

I say this not to suggest that these debates are pointless. In fact, it is because I think they are so valuable that I believe the debates should be protected. What makes them valuable? And what do they need to be protected from?

One value of the ongoing debate between contrasting therapeutic ethics lies in how it can strengthen each position. Debates between rival ethics can help each side to re-work and refine their ideas about how therapy works, what benefits it can bring, and what its limitations are. At the same time, such debates keep any one position from gaining unchecked dominance. This is important, because there are dangers in ethics. I am referring here not just to the psychological danger explored earlier where ethical aspirations become crushing burdens that constrict freedom or provoke crippling guilt. The danger I am pointing to here is the way that an ethic can become insulated and self-reinforcing, rendering itself impervious to critique when it attains dominance within a culture, or within a therapeutic subculture. An ethical hegemony can set in that puts a stop to growth and development.

Further, in claiming to see where the good lies one can be tempted to assume a right to impose that good on others. Debate can be stifled by the "motivational" aspect of ethics. That is, precisely because the draw toward a perceived good can be so powerful, can be like being in love, it can ride roughshod over competing considerations. People can blind themselves to other goods, or to their participation in that which does real harm. Keeping the debate open is one means to guard against ethics going awry in these ways.

Where does this leave us? We're in this swirl of arguments, allegiances, half-justified convictions, pushing and pulling, often feeling pushed and pulled by more than one position. Many of us long for clarity, certainty, a resolution of the debates. Some of us believe we have that clarity, or can see a path to it. Some feel that it is our obligation to seek an adjudicating decision upon the competing views, for to leave us in such a muddle would be irresponsible. Can't we reason or research our way to the truth about conflicting views of flourishing?

We should continue to debate, to examine the pros and cons of various ethics. I am not sanguine about any final resolution, even if some views are so transformed in the process of debate that their original versions no longer appear believable to any of us. There is a benefit for each picture of flourishing in being tested against alternatives. The benefit here is not that one may win out, although that is theoretically possible. A more feasible benefit is that each can improve by responding to challenges posed by the others.

The possibility for this improvement to occur depends upon a willingness to dialogue, to engage with alternative perspectives, to open oneself to letting the other expand one's vision. Genuine consideration of alternative views of well-being can be difficult, but also rewarding. Challenges can clarify what is at stake between competing visions of flourishing, what the dangers and obstacles are to the achievement of any one of them. In dialogue with one another, if the parties involved are willing to listen and potentially be changed, we can begin to see that each of our assumptions allows us to see certain aspects of flourishing, and distorts or limits our vision regarding others. Richardson and Zeddies (2004) argue for the value of dialogue as "a way that serious convictions and profound openness to their needed revision might peacefully coexist and work together productively" (p. 641).

What is not helpful is an evaluation of all therapies based on a criterion that is endemic to one therapy or social theory, such as efficiency at symptom reduction, greater understanding of the origins of problems in family dynamics, a different way of relating to the therapist in session, a patient's reports of feeling more authentic, a sweeping condemnation of therapy for the ways in which it implicitly supports suspect societal aims, etc. Any and all of these are worthy of consideration, but to claim that one of them is the most important measure of therapy, or the only worthwhile benefit to pursue, is to assume that we know more about how to weigh conflicting views of well-being than we actually do. Keeping the conversation going is not well served by elevating one particular good (rational self-mastery, autonomy, socio-political change, authenticity, particularity, libidinal vitality, relational freedom, etc.) to the status of being the standard against which all goods should be measured, against which all aims are to be evaluated. No voices should be silenced, not simply for the sake of equity to all, but because each of us needs, even for the sake of our own perspective, to hear the others.

In this ongoing conversation and debate there may well be stalemates, points where dialogue breaks down or seems impossible to sustain. The participants may turn away from discussion and return to their respective communities of practice, sure that their aims are worthwhile in a way that the others' are not. Sometimes it is better, for the sake of possible future dialogue, to acknowledge that an impasse has been reached. What would be a disaster, however, would be to turn such an impasse into a reason to shut off future discussion. Or worse yet, to use one's own standards to rule out others' approaches as fundamentally invalid.

A pluralism that is more than live and let live, that involves debate and engagement across contrasting aims, can serve as a check against the distorting influence of blind adherence to one perspective. It is important to keep one view from a position of unchecked dominance, drowning out the voices of the others. This is because our ideas about where the good lies, whether this is given psychological, political, or other form, are so easily bent to self-congratulatory and self-serving interests. Theories about people take part in shaping people to be who they are through the aims and practices they support. In this sense, theories about people are attempts at self-definition. We cannot live without self-definitions, but we can be quite adept at fooling ourselves with them. Taylor recommends that we be wary about projects to finalize our self-understanding, for they can embody self-serving distortions.

> We could only be confident of our conclusions after a course of critical scrutiny which we never achieve in a more than halting and partial way. In our detached moments, we cannot but be suspicious of all self-definitions, even our cherished ones.
>
> (Taylor, 1983, p. 57)

From this point of view, it is a good thing that psychoanalysis no longer has the powerful influence that it had in the 1950's and early 1960's in the United States. It is unfortunate that cognitive-behavioral therapy has been promoted by some to such a position today. The contemporary elevation of cognitive-behavioral therapy is often presented as simply the result of scientific findings that have established its greater effectiveness. My discussion of therapy research in *The Ethical Visions of Psychotherapy* shows that such an argument for the hegemony of this therapy is seriously misleading on scientific grounds, and ignores the implications of promoting one view of flourishing over others without even acknowledging that there is an ethical debate to be had. The absurd outcome of the managerial, profit-driven utilization of cognitive-behavioral therapy described by Dalal (2018), which distorts what is genuinely valuable in cognitive-behavioral therapy, reveals even more clearly why a plurality of therapeutic visions of human flourishing is essential.

Ultimately, the ongoing debate about ethics needs to be protected from a scientific view of persons as simply natural operators within a world of cause and effect who can be aided in the effectiveness of their operations. There is certainly a range of human problems where this perspective has legitimate application. But the majority of problems that people bring to therapy implicate assumptions about what it means to live a full and flourishing life. In this context, to promote being effective at attaining one's goals as the fundamental aim of therapy is to promote one ethical view, a particular perspective on human well-being. It should be on the table for comparison with other ethical views, not used to avoid the debate, or assumed as the obvious measure of flourishing.

Evidence-based practice has tended to value treatments that demonstrate efficacy at reducing symptoms so that patients are free to pursue whatever aims they choose. As valuable as such an aim may be, to assume that this is what therapy should be about is to overlook important questions about diverse ethical views. Responses to the current emphasis on symptomatic improvement have pointed to other therapeutic aims. When humanistic and psychodynamic therapists offer alternative aims for therapy they are not primarily claiming to be more successful at reducing the severity of symptoms. Rather than focus upon symptom reduction, these treatments focus on other aims, like the development of a nuanced appreciation of one's own and others' emotional lives, a liberation from the demands of others, a greater capacity for intimacy and empathy, etc. The claim is that there are things worth doing in therapy besides reducing symptomatology. Whether this is right or not is worthy of debate, but this is not a debate that can be resolved by forcing such treatments to prove they achieve the standards for symptom reduction that constitute the criteria for designation as evidence-based.

Appropriate admiration for what can be achieved through scientific research should not blind us to its limitations. Unlike a decrease in symptoms, some therapeutic aims do not easily lend themselves to straightforward measurement. It is often difficult to be very specific initially about the aims of a humanistic or psychodynamic therapy. Exploratory therapies often operate as extensive searches through patients' difficulties on the way to resolutions that can't be formulated in advance. They involve re-interpretations of experiences that were previously overlooked or taken for granted in a process where the understanding of problems and aims changes over time. When has an Oedipal conflict been resolved, authenticity been fostered, erotic vitality and personal particularity been achieved? There are certainly things that therapists and patients can point to as evidence of coming closer to such aims, such as experiences and interactions that patients report from their life outside of therapy, or different ways of being with the therapist in therapy. Researchers can also develop more objective measures of such aims. But the leeway for interpretation and disagreement will always be greater than with symptom measurements, for these aims are not very concrete, can take a variety of forms, and are not achieved once and for all. Often the aim is not "achieved" so much as discovered by the patient to be a path to travel further, with a positive outcome being a sense that one has found one's footing on the path. People can be fooled, and fool themselves about such aims. It's reassuring to be able to point to concrete measures that give more confidence about results. But concrete measures leave a great deal of what people aspire to in therapy off the table, and they don't address the differences among competing aspirations.

Psychotherapy and Ethics

There are many ways to formulate what psychotherapy is, what effects it has, and what it aims to do. What I hope to have shown is that it makes sense to think about therapy in the context of questions about what matters in life, what we can hope for in living well, hopes that include but also point beyond the aim of changing behaviors, reducing symptoms, or treating disorders. The more far-reaching ethical aims of therapy are not simply an edifying patina painted over effective techniques and interventions. Ethical aims are both woven into the fabric of therapy and constitute an "ecosystem" of meaning in which therapy operates. Ideas about the shape of a flourishing life are part of what it is to be human, be those ideas explicit or implicit, expansive or limited. People can *state* that life is best lived without such ideas, that they are invented fictions people use to console themselves. But it is difficult to *live* without some notions of what makes life worth living. Even the claim that life is at best a cramped and tawdry affair is an appeal to face the truth and avoid the snake oil of promised happiness—that is, it is a recommendation to avoid distorting the truth of our limited possibilities with false hope. This too is an ethic.

The psychotherapies play a part in this larger human conversation about what matters, alongside partners with different frameworks for formulating and addressing ethical views. Whether acknowledged or not, therapeutic orientations participate in debates with a wide range of interlocutors: political thinkers, philosophers, theologians, social historians, anthropologists, etc. One of the mistakes that can be made about therapy is to see it as taking place within a self-enclosed, purely psychological realm, whether that realm is conceptualized psychodynamically, behaviorally, or humanistically. Further, this conversation is not simply an exchange of the explicitly articulated proposals of academics. It is also enacted in day-to-day decisions and actions by people who are trying to live well in the best ways they know. What we do, not just what we say, gives expression to our notions of living well. Sometimes what we do succeeds, more or less, in bringing about a better life. Sometimes our actions are part of an ongoing struggle to find something better in the face of tragic events, oppressive social structures, or psychological knots. Engagement in therapy, as patient or therapist, takes place in the context of intimations of a meaningful life, a life lived in the light of what matters most. Therapists and their patients (and philosophers, political theorists, etc.) disagree about what that better life is—the theoretical debates, impassioned pleas, illuminating stories, and perspicacious research will go on. But to do therapy, to be in therapy, or to understand therapy without considering this ethical context is to overlook something central to a widespread social practice that is part of modern efforts to live well.

Notes

1 For weak evaluation, something is of value simply by virtue of the fact that I desire it. Strong evaluation requires more than desire for an object. Strong evaluation is an assessment of whether something is worth pursuing, and on its basis I may judge my desire as noble, worthy, and rational, or as weak, foolish, alienating, cruel, etc. See Taylor (1985a).

2 One can use "near" and "far" outside the context of purposes: "Those two stars are near each other." But this is just a shorthand way of saying that the distance between them is less than that between most stars. This is scientifically loose and all-too-human talk that refers to inanimate objects with language that strictly applies only to animate beings.

3 I am here characterizing narrative in terms that are consonant with the expressivism discussed in the last chapter.

4 See Meretoja (2018) on non-subsumptive narrative practices that are not violent appropriations of the other or of one's self.

Appendix
Charles Taylor for Therapists: A Brief Introduction

Charles Margrave Taylor (1931–) is a Canadian philosopher born to a Francophone mother and an Anglophone father in Montreal. He was educated at schools in Quebec and Ontario, and received his bachelor's degree in history from McGill University in 1952. He was awarded a Rhodes Scholarship to Oxford University, where he received a Bachelor of Arts (1st class honors) in Philosophy, Politics, and Economics from Balliol College. He was a fellow of All Soul's College at Oxford through 1961, when he received his D. Phil. from Oxford with a thesis supervised by Isaiah Berlin. He has been on the faculty at McGill University in Montreal since 1961 (now emeritus), and has had appointments at a number of universities (among them Oxford, Berkeley, Hebrew University of Jerusalem, Northwestern, J. W. Goethe University in Frankfurt, Stanford, and Yale).

Taylor has written on a number of topics in philosophy: philosophy of language, ethics, history of philosophy, epistemology, political theory, and philosophy of the human sciences. He has also written historical-philosophical studies of modernity, secularism, and religion. He has published more than 20 books and over 400 articles. His work has been translated into 23 languages. His intellectual contributions have been recognized by a number of awards, including the Kyoto Prize, the Templeton Prize, the Kluge Prize, and the Berggruen Prize. Taylor's writings have been the subject of a number of secondary works providing exposition, commentary, and critique (a small sampling includes Abbey, 2000, 2004; Colorado and Klassen, 2014; Garbowski et al., 2009; La Forest and Lara, 1998; Laitinen and Smith, 2002; Leask, 2010; Smith, N. H., 2002; Tully, 1994; Warner et al., 2010).[1]

Why turn to the philosophy of Charles Taylor in order to understand psychotherapy? While he has written in depth about various topics in psychology (1964, 1985a), he has offered only brief reflections on therapy. A few studies of therapy have utilized Taylor's work (for example, Slife et al., 2019; Stern, 2019; Tjeltveit, 1999), but Taylor himself does not discuss particular therapies in any detail, and has nothing to say about psychotherapy research.

What his work does offer for an understanding of psychotherapy is a careful philosophical examination of the human sciences rooted in a detailed framework for understanding the nature of persons. Taylor accepts the standard scientific view that humans are part of the natural world, biological beings with a repertoire of behaviors that are partly the result of objective events in their immediate environment, their life experience, and their evolutionary history. But persons are more than this. Objects and events in the lives of persons have a significance that derives from what matters to them, and much of what matters to them cannot be derived from or reduced to the givens of their biology or the influence of the world around them described in purely objective terms. Significance for human beings includes the complex requirements for flourishing that we share with our fellow animals, like health, safety, and the opportunities to exercise basic capacities for living. But beyond these lie symbolically and culturally shaped meanings that can be just as important, and for the sake of which people are even willing to risk health and safety. The care for self and loved ones that derives from our animal heritage is rewritten by humans as the obligation to bring oneself and others toward forms of living well that are understood in cultural terms. These aims for well-being and flourishing vary from one culture to another and include a wide range of ideals: to be a noble warrior, to show proper respect and piety for ancestors, to not act impulsively but to reason carefully about important decisions, to honor one's family, to be successful in one's work, to live in accord with the tenets of one's religion, to seek social justice, fame, or artistic or scientific excellence. Because these meanings are linguistically and symbolically shaped, the study of their role in people's lives points to the inevitability of an interpretive, non-objectivist understanding of human life. Nobility, familial piety, careful reasoning, honor, success, the devotion to one's faith, justice, or beauty—these all have received various interpretations and emphases, both in how they are formally articulated and in how they are practiced across different cultures, and within a given culture. To understand what it means for someone to live their life partly formed by one or more of these goods requires consideration of the background of language and practice within which these goods arise. This requires an interpretive reading of meanings, not just an objective observation of empirically demarcated events or forces that influence behavior.

Taylor's work in the philosophy of human science is rooted in his philosophical anthropology of persons as self-interpreting animals. He is critical of those forms of modern human science that assume that people are natural phenomena that can be studied the way one would study any other natural phenomenon. An example of the natural scientific approach[2] to human phenomena would be the project to use evolutionary history, neurochemical processes, impinging events ("contingencies"), and the cognitive processing of those events to explain the behaviors, desires, emotions, and beliefs of people. In writings on behaviorism (1964), cognitivism (1985a), and the social sciences (1985b), he argues that a natural science approach ignores or distorts much of what is central to human existence: purpose, intentionality, consciousness, personal significance, and the common meanings embedded in our institutions and social practices.

Natural scientific approaches have an allegiance to a naturalistic metaphysics that requires that objects of study be characterized in terms of non-anthropocentric properties. Anthropocentric properties are those which things have only by virtue of the experience of agents of a certain kind. A mountain can be "majestic" for us, but not for the valley below, nor for the squirrel living in a tree on its slopes. To do a natural scientific study is to exclude properties like majesty, nobility, or cruelty. It is to use only "absolute" properties that are not relative to particular sorts of agents. For Taylor, the flaw in such an approach to understanding people is that they are precisely the agents for whom such properties matter, and matter in ways that shape their lives. People are partly constituted by their self-understandings, and those self-understandings incorporate distinctions of worth like majesty, nobility, kindness, cruelty, the sublime, and the degrading, distinctions which are through and through anthropomorphic or subjective (in the sense that they only appear for subjects like us). The "partly" in the prior sentence is necessary because the role of our self-understanding in constituting who we are does not deny the influence of evolutionary history or contingencies of reinforcement. Nevertheless, a human science that acknowledges our self-interpretive nature recognizes that the impact of natural events derives at least some of its influence from the significance of those events in a human world shaped by social-symbolic-linguistic forms. These forms shape human aims in the light of certain distinctions of worth, distinctions that only exist *through* being given symbolic form (which is why the mountain isn't majestic for a squirrel, who lacks the language to constitute concepts like majesty).

If humans are partly constituted through a self-understanding that includes distinctions of worth (or "strong evaluations"), and if so much is ignored or distorted by natural scientific efforts to explain people, why do such theories seem so plausible to so many? Taylor argues that their plausibility stems partly from the well-deserved prestige of the natural sciences when they are applied to the non-human world (although they can lead to distorted conclusions about non-human behavior as well—see Taylor, 1964). But Taylor sees something else motivating the attraction to such theories. This is the modern attachment to a particular picture of human agency, where we are

> capable of achieving a kind of disengagement from our world by objectifying it. We objectify our situation to the extent that we can overcome

a sense of it as what determines for us our paradigm purposes and ends, and can come to see it and function in it as a neutral environment, within which we can affect the purposes which we determine out of ourselves.

(1985a, p. 4)

The natural scientific view of people is not the result of simply taking the scientific approach to the physical world developed in modern science and applying it to the human world. There is also an ethical pull toward an ideal for how we might live, toward being persons who are capable of creating their own aims and purposes, and using a neutral, meaningless natural world as the medium in which those purposes may be realized. This is an aspiration to a particular conception of living well, where we do not submit to purposes that are thrust upon us by nature, society, or God. Rather, our freedom, dignity, and self-respect flow from being creators of our own ends, from stepping outside of a sense of the world as bestowing meaning upon us, seeing it instead as simply a mechanism of causal interactions in which we can intervene to affect our purposes. Taylor has written extensively on the rise of this view of freedom as reflexive self-making. He also addresses the irony of espousing this ideal on the basis of an objectification that extends beyond the world around us to us, that makes our lives the outcome of impersonal forces.

So Taylor claims that the plausibility of the natural scientific study of people lies not so much in scientific data as in this ethical ideal for how we might live. Taylor's critique of this ideal does not suggest that we can simply dismiss it as wrong. The freedom of the disengaged identity that has objectified the world through scientific analysis is so much a part of modern self-understanding that it cannot be completely jettisoned. Nevertheless, these views have also had a distorting influence that needs to be addressed. "The kind of critique we need is one that can free it of its illusory pretensions to define the totality of our lives as agents, without attempting the futile and ultimately self-destructive task of rejecting it altogether" (1985a, p. 7).

This critique is genealogical, examining how the modern self-understanding came to be and what has constituted its appeal. Genealogical accounts of the modern ethos already exist (many deriving from Nietzsche's work). But Taylor feels they are often "underdemonstrated, indeed, rather impressionistically argued for; and they tend to be hostile and dismissive towards the scientific outlook and the disengaged identity" (1985a, p. 7). Taylor's own work is extensively argued for in detailed examinations of the historical rise of the modern identity, where he acknowledges the legitimate appeal of disengagement, as well as its limitations (1989, 2004, 2007). In these writings he explicates the particular path the modern West has taken to develop the moral, political, and personal instantiations of this disengaged identity. I summarize some of this work in Chapter 3, exploring how the history of modern ideas about human flourishing reveals the historical/cultural context for the ethical aims implicit in contemporary psychotherapies.

It is here that Taylor's work is most relevant to making sense of psychotherapy. Different schools of psychotherapy propose different conceptions of what a human being is, of how people develop psychological problems, and of how to correct those difficulties for the sake of divergent ideas about living well. Therapeutic conceptions of living well have roots in the cultural context of modernity. Yet psychotherapy is often theorized by its proponents and practitioners as a means to correct mental disorders or to change behaviors by utilizing context-less facts about human psychology that are revealed through scientific research. There is little recognition that human psychology (both the discipline and what the discipline studies) is shaped by assumptions that are present in our ways of speaking about persons, narrating our lives, and interacting with each other, many of which are specific to our socio-historical context. Our therapeutic theories and practices are rarely simply the application of general scientific findings but promote particular ideals for flourishing, ideals that require an ethical assessment that cannot be accomplished by natural science.

I give a particular slant to my exploration of the ethical nature of therapeutic aims by taking the philosophy of Charles Taylor as a guiding thread. There are a number of other philosophers whose work would support a similar overall approach, even if some of the specific conclusions might differ. In fact, Taylor has been influenced by many of them: Heidegger, Merleau-Ponty, the late Wittgenstein, Iris Murdoch, Gadamer, Ricouer, Polanyi, and McDowell, among others. I make passing reference to some of them, but do not engage the nuances of Taylor's similarities and differences. I am not taking up Taylor's work to do an exposition of his philosophy, but for the aid it brings to answering some fundamental questions about psychotherapy.

Taylor also has a number of critics and friendly interlocutors who disagree with him on various issues (N. H. Smith, 2002, reviews a number of these debates). Taylor has not decisively answered all of his critics, nor are all of the controversies about therapy I address in this book resolved simply by examining them in the light of his philosophy. But I do think that such an examination sheds important light upon several presently unresolved disputes, deepens the conversation, and opens new possibilities for moving beyond current stalemates.

Notes

1 See the bibliography of Taylor's work and secondary sources at charlestaylor.net/Home.
2 Giorgi's (1970) term "approach" has connotations much like those of the "philosophical anthropology" I am using here.

References

Abbey, R. (2000). *Charles Taylor*. Princeton, NJ: Princeton University Press.

Abbey, R. (Ed.) (2004). *Charles Taylor*. New York, NY: Cambridge University Press.

Bandura, A. (1997). *Self-Efficacy: The Exercise of Control*. New York, NY: W. H. Freeman & Co.

Bateman, A., and Fonagy, P. (2004). *Psychotherapy for Borderline Personality Disorder: Mentalization-Based Treatment*. New York, NY: Oxford University Press.

Beck, A. T., Rush, A. J., Shaw, B. F., and Emery, G. (1979). *Cognitive Therapy of Depression*. New York, NY: Guilford Press.

Bohart, A. C., and Tallman, K. (1999). *How Clients Make Therapy Work: The Process of Active Self-Healing*. Washington, DC: American Psychological Association.

Bollas, C. (1992). *Being a Character: Psychoanalysis and Self Experience*. New York, NY: Routledge.

Bollas, C. (2002). *Free Association*. Cambridge, UK: Icon Books.

Colorado, C. D., and Klassen, J. D. (Eds.) (2014). *Aspiring to Fullness in a Secular Age: Essays on Religion and Theology in the Work of Charles Taylor*. Notre Dame, IN: University of Notre Dame Press.

Cooper, M., and Joseph, S. (2016). Psychological foundations for humanistic psychotherapeutic practice. In: D. J. Cain, K. Keenan, and S. Rubin (Eds.), *Humanistic Psychotherapies: Handbook of Research and Practice* (pp. 11–46). Washington, DC: American Psychological Association.

Cushman, P. (1995). *Constructing the Self, Constructing America: A Cultural History of Psychotherapy*. Reading, MA: Addison-Wesley.

Dalal, F. (2018). *CBT: The Cognitive Behavioral Tsunami*. New York, NY: Routledge.

de Waal, F. (2006). Morally evolved: Primate social instincts, human morality, and the rise and fall of "veneer theory." In: S. Macedo and J. Ober (Eds.), *Primates and Philosophers: How Morality Evolved* (pp. 1–80). Princeton, NJ: Princeton University Press.

Doherty, W. J. (1995). *Soul Searching: Why Psychotherapy Must Promote Moral Responsibility*. New York, NY: Basic Books.

Elias, N. (1994). *The Civilizing Process: Sociogenetic and Psychogenetic Investigations* (Rev. ed.) (E. Jephcott, Trans.). Malden, MA: Blackwell Publishing. (Original work published 1939.)

Ellis, A. (1962). *Reason and Emotion in Psychotherapy.* Seacaucas, NJ: Citadel Press.

Fink, B. (1995). *The Lacanian Subject: Between Language and Jouissance.* Princeton, NJ: Princeton University Press.

Fink, B. (1997). *A Clinical Introduction to Lacanian Psychoanalysis: Theory and Technique.* Cambridge, MA: Harvard University Press.

Fink, B. (2004). *Lacan to the Letter: Reading Écrits Closely.* Minneapolis, MN: University of Minnesota Press.

Fink, B. (2007). *Fundamentals of Psychoanalytic Technique: A Lacanian Approach for Practitioners.* New York, NY: W. W. Norton.

Fink, B. (2014a). *Against Understanding: Commentary and Critique in a Lacanian Key (Vol. 1).* New York, NY: Routledge.

Fink, B. (2014b). *Against Understanding: Commentary and Critique in a Lacanian Key (Vol. 2).* New York, NY: Routledge.

Fink, B. (2016). *Lacan on Love: An Exploration of Lacan's Seminar VIII.* Malden, MA: Polity Press.

Fink, B. (2017). *A Clinical Introduction to Freud: Techniques for Everyday Practice.* New York, NY: Norton.

Foucault, M. (1977). *Discipline and Punish: The Birth of the Prison* (A. Sheridan, Trans.). New York, NY: Vintage. (Original work published 1975.)

Freud, S. (1953). The interpretations of dreams. In: J. Strachey, (Trans. and Ed.), *The Standard Edition of the Complete Psychological Works of Sigmund Freud* (Vol. 5, pp. 339–627). London: Hogarth Press. (Original work published 1900.)

Freud, S. (1955a). Lines of advance in psychoanalytic therapy. In J. Strachey, (Trans. and Ed.), *The Standard Edition of the Complete Psychological Works of Sigmund Freud* (Vol. 17, pp. 157–168). London: Hogarth Press. (Original work published 1919.)

Freud, S. (1955b). Psychoanalysis and telepathy. In: J. Strachey (Trans. and Ed.), *The Standard Edition of the Complete Psychological Works of Sigmund Freud* (Vol. 18, pp. 173–193). London: Hogarth Press. (Original work published 1941.)

Freud, S. (1955c). The uncanny. In: J. Stachey (Ed.), *The Standard Edition of the Complete Psychological Works of Sigmund Freud* (Vol. 17, pp. 217–256). London: Hogarth Press. (Original work published 1919.)

Freud, S. (1959). "Civilized" sexual morality and modern nervous illness. In: J. Strachey (Trans. and Ed.), *The Standard Edition of the Complete Psychological Works of Sigmund Freud* (Vol. 9, pp. 178–204). London: Hogarth Press. (Original work published 1908.)

Freud, S. (1960). The psychopathology of everyday life. In: J. Strachey (Ed.), *The Standard Edition of the Complete Psychological Works of Sigmund Freud* (Vol. 6). London: Hogarth Press. (Original work published 1901.)

Freud, S. (1961a). Civilization and its discontents. In: J. Strachey (Trans. and Ed.), *The Standard Edition of the Complete Psychological Works of Sigmund Freud* (Vol. 21, pp. 57–145). London: Hogarth Press. (Original work published 1930.)

Freud, S. (1961b). Some additional notes on dream-interpretation as a whole. In: J. Strachey (Trans. and Ed.), *The Standard Edition of the Complete Psychological Works of Sigmund Freud* (Vol. 19, pp. 123–138). London: Hogarth Press. (Original work published 1925.)

Freud, S. (1963). Introductory lectures on psychoanalysis. In: J. Strachey (Trans. and Ed.), *The Standard Edition of the Complete Psychological Works of Sigmund Freud* (Vol. 16, pp. 243–463). London: Hogarth Press. (Original work published 1917.)

Freud, S. (1964). New introductory lectures on psychoanalysis. In: J. Strachey (Trans. and Ed.), *The Standard Edition of the Complete Psychological Works of Sigmund Freud* (Vol. 22, pp. 1–182). London: Hogarth Press. (Original work published 1933.)

Garbowski, C., Hudzik, J., and Klos, J. (Eds.) (2009). *Charles Taylor's Vision of Modernity: Reconstructions and Interpretations.* Newcastle Upon Tyne, England: Cambridge Scholars Publishing.

Giorgi, A. (1970). *Psychology as a Human Science: A Phenomenologically Based Approach.* New York, NY: Harper and Row.

Glasofer, D. R., Albano, A. M., Simpson, H. B., and Steinglass, J. E. (2016). Overcoming fear of eating: A case study of a novel use of exposure and response prevention. *Psychotherapy, 53*(2), 223–231. doi:10.1037/pst0000048.

Gray, P. (1994). *The Ego and the Analysis of Defense.* Northvale, NJ: Jason Aronson.

Greenberg, J. R., and Mitchell, S. M. (1983). *Object Relations in Psychoanalytic Theory.* Cambridge, MA: Harvard University Press.

Hoffman, I. Z. (2009). Doublethinking our way to "scientific" legitimacy: The desiccation of human experience. *Journal of the American Psychoanalytic Association, 57*(5), 1043–1069. doi:10.1177/0003065109343925.

Hoffman, I. Z. (2012). Response to Safran: The development of critical psychoanalytic sensibility. *Psychoanalytic Dialogues, 22*(6), 721–731. doi:10.1080/10481885.2012.733653.

Jen, G. (2017). *The Girl at the Baggage Claim: Explaining the East-West Culture Gap.* New York, NY: Vintage Books.

Jones, E. (1957). *The Life and Work of Sigmund Freud* (Vol. 3). New York, NY: Basic Books.

Kant, I. (1997). *Groundwork of the Metaphysics of Morals* (M. Gregor, Trans. and Ed.). New York, NY: Cambridge University Press. (Original work published 1785.)

Kirschner, S. R. (2012). Do therapists really "make up" their patients? *Theory and Psychology, 22*(6), 860–865. doi:10.1177/0959354311434072.

LaForest, G., and Lara, P. (Eds.) (1998). *Charles Taylor et l'interprétation de l'identité modern* [Charles Taylor and the interpretation of the modern identity]. Saint-Nicolas (Québec), Canada: Les Presses de l'Université Laval.

Laitinen, A., and Smith, N. H. (Eds.) (2002). Perspectives on the philosophy of Charles Taylor [Special Issue]. *Acta philosophica fennica, 71.*

Lambert, M. J. (2013). The efficacy and effectiveness of psychotherapy. In: M. J. Lambert (Ed.), *Handbook of Psychotherapy and Behavior Change* (6th ed.). Hoboken, NJ: Wiley.

Lear, J. (2000). *Happiness, Death, and the Remainder of Life.* Cambridge, MA: Harvard University Press.

Lear, J. (2005). *Freud.* New York, NY: Routledge.

Leask, I. (Ed.) (2010). *The Taylor Effect: Responding to A Secular Age.* Newcastle Upon Tyne, England: Cambridge Scholars Publishing.

Lingiardi, V., and McWilliams, N. (2017). *Psychodynamic Diagnostic Manual* (2nd ed.). New York, NY: Guilford Press.

Loewald, H. W. (2000). Psychoanalysis as an art and the fantasy character of the psychoanalytic situation. In: H. W. Loewald (Eds.), *The Essential Loewald: Collected Papers and Monographs*. Hagerstown, MD: University Publishing Group.

Luyten, P., Campbell, C., and Fonagy, P. (2019). Reflections on the contributions of Sidney J. Blatt: The dialectical needs for autonomy, relatedness, and the emergence of epistemic trust. *Psychoanalytic Psychology*, *36*(4), 328–334. doi:10.1037/pap0000243.

MacIntyre, A. (1984). *After Virtue: A Study in Moral Theory* (2nd ed.). Notre Dame, IN: Notre Dame University Press.

McWilliams, N. (2004). *Psychoanalytic Psychotherapy: A Practitioner's Guide*. New York, NY: Guilford Press.

McWilliams, N. (2005). Preserving our humanity as therapists. *Psychotherapy: Theory, Research, Practice, Training*, *42*(2), 139–151. doi:10.1037/0033-3204.42.2.139.

Meretoja, H. (2018). *The Ethics of Storytelling: Narrative Hermeneutics, History, and the Possible*. New York, NY: Oxford University Press.

Merleau-Ponty, M. (1964). Eye and mind. C. Dallery, (Trans.) In: J. M. Edie (Ed.), *The Primacy of Perception* (pp. 159–190). Evanston, IL: Northwestern University Press.

Merleau-Ponty, M. (2012). *Phenomenology of Perception* (D. A. Landes, Trans.). New York, NY: Routledge. (Original work published 1945.)

Mill, J. S. (1979). *Utilitarianism*. Indianapolis, IN: Hackett Publishing. (Original work published 1861.)

Mitchell, S. A. (1988). *Relational Concepts in Psychoanalysis: An Integration*. Cambridge, MA: Harvard University Press.

Mitchell, S. A. (1993). *Hope and Dread in Psychoanalysis*. New York, NY: Basic Books.

Mitchell, S. A. (1997). *Influence and Autonomy in Psychoanalysis*. Hillsdale, NJ: The Analytic Press.

Mitchell, S. A. (2000). *Relationality: From Attachment to Intersubjectivity*. New York, NY: Psychology Press.

Mitchell, S. A. (2002). *Can Love Last? The Fate of Romance over Time*. New York, NY: W. W. Norton.

Mitchell, S. A., and Black, M. J. (1995). *Freud and Beyond: A History of Modern Psychoanalytic Thought*. New York, NY: Basic Books.

Norcross, J. C. (2005). The psychotherapist's own psychotherapy: Educating and developing psychologists. *The American Psychologist*, *60*(8), 840–850. doi:10.1037/0003.0666X.60.8.837.

Norcross, J. C., Bike, D. H., and Evans, K. L. (2009). The therapist's therapist: A replication and extension 20 years later. *Psychotherapy: Theory, Research, Practice, Training*, *46*(1), 32–41. doi:10.1037/a0015140.

Norcross, J. C., Strausser, D. J., and Faltus, F. J. (1988). The therapist's therapist. *American Journal of Psychotherapy*, *42*(1), 53–66.

Phillips, A. (2014). *Becoming Freud: The Making of a Psychoanalyst*. New Haven, CT: Yale University Press.

Richardson, F. C., and Zeddies, T. J. (2004). Psychoanalysis and the good life. *Contemporary Psychoanalysis, 40*(4), 617–657.

Robinson, D. (2010). *The Philosophy of Cognitive Behavioral Therapy: Stoic Philosophy as Rational and Cognitive Therapy*. London: Karnac Books.

Rogers, C. (1951). *Client-Centered Therapy*. Boston, MA: Houghton Mifflin.

Roland, A. (1988). *In Search of Self in India and Japan: Toward a Cross-Cultural Psychology*. Princeton, NJ: Princeton University Press.

Rose, N. (1990). *Governing the Soul: The Shaping of the Private Self*. New York, NY: Routledge.

Safran, J. D. (2012). Doublethinking or dialectical thinking: A critical appreciation of Hoffman's "Doublethinking" critique. *Psychoanalytic Dialogues, 22*(6), 710–720. doi:10.1080/10481885.2012.733655.

Sandel, A. A. (2014). *The Place of Prejudice: A Case for Reasoning within the World*. Cambridge, MA: Harvard University Press.

Segal, H. (1981). *The Work of Hanna Segal: A Kleinian Approach to Clinical Practice*. Lanham, MD: Jason Aronson.

Shedler, J. (2010). The efficacy of psychodynamic psychotherapy. *The American Psychologist, 65*(2), 98–109. doi:10.1037/a0018378.

Slife, B. D., Ghelfi, E. A., and Slife, N. M. (2019). Psychotherapy and the moral realism of Charles Taylor. In: B. D. Slife and S. C. Yanchar (Eds.), *Hermeneutic Moral Realism in Psychology: Theory and Practice* (pp. 71–85). New York, NY: Routledge.

Smith, K. R. (1983). Verbal behavior and authentic speech. *Journal of Phenomenological Psychology, 14*(1–2), 3–20.

Smith, N. H. (2002). *Charles Taylor: Meaning, Morals and Modernity*. Malden, MA: Polity.

Stern, D. B. (2019). *The Infinity of the Unsaid: Unformulated Experience, Language, and the Nonverbal*. New York, NY: Routledge.

Sue, D. W., and Sue, D. (2003). *Counseling the Culturally Diverse: Theory and Practice* (4th ed.). New York, NY: John Wiley & Sons.

Task Force for the Development of Practice Recommendations for the Provision of Humanistic Psychological Services. (2004). Recommended principles and practices for the provision of humanistic psychosocial services: Alternative to mandated treatment guidelines. *The Humanistic Psychologist, 32*, 3–75. doi:10.1 080/08873267.2004.9961745.

Taylor, C. (1964). *The Explanation of Behavior*. New York, NY: The Humanities Press.

Taylor, C. (1983). Use and abuse of theory. In: A. Parel (Ed.), *Ideology, Philosophy, Politics*. Waterloo, Ontario: Wilfrid Laurier University Press.

Taylor, C. (1985a). *Human Agency and Language: Philosophical Papers (Vol. 1)*. Cambridge, MA: Cambridge University Press.

Taylor, C. (1985b). *Philosophy and the Human Sciences: Philosophical Papers (Vol. 2)*. Cambridge, MA: Cambridge University Press.

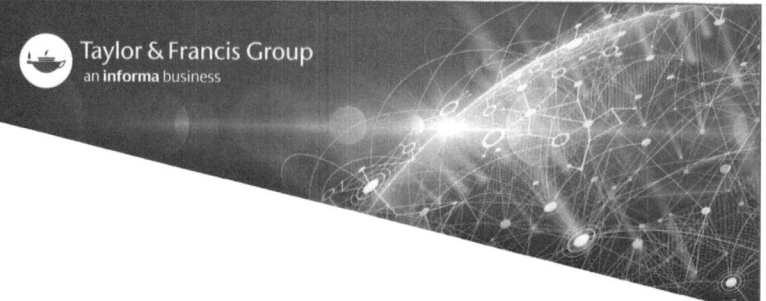
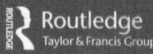
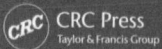

ADVANCED
HYPNOTHERAPY
Hypnodynamic Techniques

JOHN G. WATKINS

ARREED BARABASZ

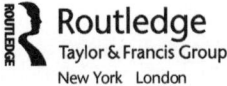

Routledge
Taylor & Francis Group
New York   London

Routledge
Taylor & Francis Group 711
Third Avenue
New York, NY 10017, USA

Routledge
Taylor & Francis Group
2 Park Square
Milton Park, Abingdon
Oxon OX14 4RN

Routledge is an imprint of the Taylor & Francis Group, an informa business

---

Library of Congress Cataloging-in-Publication Data

Watkins, John G. (John Goodrich), 1913-
　　Advanced hypnotherapy : hypnodynamic techniques / John G. Watkins, Arreed Barabasz.
　　　　p. ; cm.
　　Rev. ed. of: Hypnoanalytic techniques / John G. Watkins. c1992.
　　Includes bibliographical references and index.
　　ISBN-13: 978-0-415-95627-7 (alk. paper)
　　ISBN-10: 0-415-95627-7 (alk. paper)
　　　1. Hypnotism--Therapeutic use. I. Barabasz, Arreed F. II. Watkins, John G. (John Goodrich), 1913- Hypnoanalytic techniques. III. Title.
　　[DNLM: 1. Hypnosis. 2. Psychoanalytic Therapy--methods. WM 415 W335a 2007]

RC495.W348 2007
616.89'162--dc22
　　　　　　　　　　　　　　　　　　　　　　　　　　　　　　　　　　　　　　2007019100

Visit the Taylor & Francis Web site at
http://www.taylorandfrancis.com

and the Routledge Web site at
http://www.routledge.com

Dedication

To Doctor Marianne Barabasz for her encouragement,
ongoing love, and understanding and to our patients,
students, teachers, and colleagues, who share with us the
adventure hypnosis brings to the exploration of inner space.

Foreword

Many of the innovative techniques described in this book were devised and developed by Helen Huth Watkins, wife and 30-year colleague of author John G. Watkins. After she died in 2002, a biography of her life (*Emotional Resonance*, J. G. Watkins, 2005) was written at the request of her students, patients, colleagues, and associates, focusing on her "personhood" and her personal life over and beyond her professional contributions and therapeutic skills.

Emotional Resonance covers her life from her birth in Bavaria to her sudden death, including her transition from a simple university counseling psychologist into a world-honored psychotherapist to whom psychiatrists, psychologists, and other mental health practitioners went for their own personal therapy.

Contents

Contents

Acknowledgments

We wish to express very special thanks to the following people and sponsors for their invaluable assistance in the preparation of this volume: Helen Huth Watkins (for cases, comments, and specific hypnoanalytic techniques); Ciara Christensen (for commentary to enhance understanding, for typing and proofreading, and as our "subject" model); McKenzie's Hair Studio (for Ms. Christensen's hair styling and make-up); and "Kat" at Washington State University IT Graphics (for digital enhancement of patients' productions). Thanks also to Archer Photography, Moscow Idaho, for special attention to Ms. Christensen's hypnotic demonstrations with Dr. Arreed Barabasz.

Introduction

To paste a coping skill on the surface of an injured person is to further remove that person emotionally from the "self." The empirical-behavioral tradition, although showing immediate therapeutic results, has done so by ignoring conditions and behaviors that are mediated through subliminal "unconscious" processes, thus severely limiting the scope of its operational area (see pp. 233–268).

This book is for those therapists and clients who desire short-term psychotherapy that leads to understanding the root causes of maladaptive behaviors, and to resolve those unconscious motivations at a fundamental level. In this pursuit, our goals as therapists are aimed at reconstruction of the personality, we seek to create equilibrium, to help our clients to reach a more adaptive, more comfortable, and more meaningful existence while maintaining his or her creative individuality. This book is not for those who are looking for protocols that are aimed at coaching clients to adopt superficial coping behaviors or bandage coping mechanisms that hinder potential for growth.

A *Time* cover article titled "Can Freud Get His Job Back?" (Grossman, 2003) highlighted the resurgence of psychoanalysis by quoting a graduate student in her 30s who went through analysis after a difficult breakup: "It's allowed me to figure out pretty basic things about myself and why certain situations kept coming up." After analysis, she became more productive, less moody, less angry, and less depressed (without antidepressant medication). She went on to comment, "A lot of jokes about analysis talk about blaming your parents, but being in analysis is more about learning to take responsibility for yourself and to take care of the people around you. That kind of control only comes from understanding your past."

A more important underscoring of the resurgence of psychodynamic therapy is the recent publication of the *Psychodynamic diagnostic manual* (PDM) (2006) by the five major psychoanalytic groups: the American Psychoanalytic Association, Division 39 of the American Psychological Association, the International Psychoanalytical Association, the American Academy of Psychoanalysis and Dynamic Psychiatry, and the National Membership Committee on Psychoanalysis in Clinical Social Work. The manual is intended to fill the void in the *Diagnostic statistical manual of mental disorders (DSM IV-TR)* (American Psychiatric Association, 2000) by the latter manual's bias in favor of biological, cognitive-behavioral, and family-systems therapies.

Psychodynamically oriented therapists listen intently when a client speaks of childhood memories, knowing that these experiences may play a crucial role in the current presenting problem. They also recognize that chronic repetitive patterns of interactions within a family and with significant others in the past lead to disturbances in the adult personality more often than overt trauma (Gabbard, 2005, p. 15).

Much of what person-centered and cognitive-behavioral therapists are proficient at applying can be used in the practice of hypnodynamic therapy. This book shows how therapists trained in these limited approaches can approximate reconstructive psychoanalysis without time-consuming, protracted training. The experienced practitioner can learn how to adapt his or her therapeutic knowledge and skills to help patients uncover underlying motivations and blocks to adaption. Therapists will no longer be limited to superficial symptom-removal interventions such as psychoactive medication, supportive humanistic therapy, or cognitive reframings. Practice and experience with what is taught in this book will lead to the appreciation of symptoms as subconscious clues to underlying causes.

We decry approaches that attempt only to categorize clients by similar clusters of symptoms while ignoring their subjective experiences, given that even monozygotic twins with identical genomes develop very distinct personalities (Mauron, 2001). We are far more interested in the individual adaptations and how they differ from other patients as a result of a life story that is uniquely their own. We place the highest value on each patient's dreams, fears, impulses, self-images, hopes, and views of others that constitute the family of self.

Advanced hypnotherapy: Hypnodynamic techniques, is intended to fulfill the promise made in our first book, *Hypnotherapeutic techniques* (2nd ed., A. Barabasz & J. Watkins, 2005). That treatise was largely devoted to elucidating, in detail, nearly 100 different induction techniques. Complete protocols, often sufficient to constitute manualized therapy, were included to facilitate applications to a wide variety of physical and psychological disorders. The orientation of the first volume was on both Ericksonian and directive/supportive approaches to hypnotherapy. We also surveyed the history of hypnosis, hypnotizability, and the recently established neurophysiological underpinnings of hypnotic states.

This second book includes the time-proven classical hypnoanalytic techniques of J.G.W. as well as new hypnotherapeutic techniques, such as digital hypnography and abreaction alternatives. The text shows how hypnosis can be combined with psychoanalysis to make it possible to understand the subjective world of clients. The advanced hypnotherapeutic techniques taught are focused on time-limited hypnoanalysis rather than protracted psychoanalysis. Thus, time-consuming psychoanalysis can be approximated by brief hypnodynamic therapy, which can be applied by those with typical doctoral training backgrounds in counseling psychology, clinical psychology, and psychiatry.

The first book was written from the viewpoint of the learner rather than the professor who doles out information, leaving the reader responsible for mastery. Given the praise bestowed upon that volume for adopting that approach, we again have endeavored to ask ourselves, "If I were a therapist new to this, what would I want to know, what would help me master my own insecurities in the use of hypnodynamic therapy, and what techniques would be necessary to use it skillfully?" To help ensure this perspective, we again drew upon the inspiration provided by the viewpoint of Ciara Christensen, who is now a published PhD student with training in hypnosis, and cognitive-behavioral and humanistic approaches. Ciara read and discussed each chapter with A.F.B. and offered numerous insightful suggestions to improve clarity and readability for those new to hypnoanalysis. We also owe her an enormous debt of gratitude for her professionalism and dedication to weekends of work in typing endless hours of dictation and proofreading. Consistent with our earlier book (Barabasz & Watkins, 2005), Ciara also served as the "subject" model for the photographs in this book. Special thanks are also due to Jamie Scheopflin for her assistance in entering corrections to several chapters in the initial draft.

This book elucidates the use of hypnotherapeutic techniques through giving detailed procedures for adapting such processes as hypnodiagnostic evaluation, Watkins' abreactive techniques, Kluft's fractionated abreaction, Spiegel's split-screen technique, sensory hypnoplasty, hypnography, dreamwork, fantasies, projective hypnoanalysis, dissociative hypnoanalysis, transference, counter-transference, the therapeutic alliance, existential hypnoanalysis, and ego-state therapy. Also included are related techniques rooted in psychoanalysis and hypnosis. Many detailed illustrations of actual interchanges with patients are presented as well as photographs of specific induction procedures and the products of inductions from hypnography. Vignettes clarify specific examples of recommended practices, and six fuller case reports show the interactions in successive sessions and the ultimate outcomes.

Similar to the layout of our previous book, wherever appropriate among the cases presented in this book, the specifics are shown. Pictures and protocols are incorporated to illustrate how those initially trained and experienced in cognitive-behavioral or humanistic therapies can use their backgrounds to interpret patients' clues to unconscious processes. This book is designed to aid therapists to learn how to help their clients resolve the underlying issues involved.

We believe that *Advanced hypnotherapy: Hypnodynamic techniques* will prove useful to all mental health practitioners who have ingested and practiced the hypnotherapeutic techniques taught in our previous book, regardless of their special interest in hypnoanalysis. It is our hope that this book will help move forward the acceptance of clinical hypnosis among the healing professions as the resurgence of psychodynamic therapy continues.

1

Introduction to Hypnoanalytic Techniques

Psychotherapists who have acquired the ability to hypnotize and apply hypnotherapeutic procedures will likely recognize their need to acquire more complex ways of using hypnotic interventions. A few of the more advanced techniques were introduced or hinted at, but not truly described, in Barabasz and Watkins (2005). As promised in the introduction to that book, this one will carry on where the first treatise left off.

This book teaches sophisticated procedures, practiced within the hypnotic modalities, which are aimed at a more fundamental reconstruction of a patient's personality. This is the goal of both hypnoanalysis and psychoanalytic therapy. Hypnoanalysis accepts the psychoanalytic principle that neurotic symptoms are generally, although certainly not exclusively, the consequence of intrapsychic conflict. Our aim as therapists is to eliminate or at least reduce symptoms by emotional as well as cognitive restructuring, not merely by social influence, placebo manipulations, or mere suggestion without actual hypnosis per se (A. Barabasz & Christensen, 2006; see Barabasz and Watkins, 2005, pp. 203–206). When the hypnoanalytic process is successful, it is usually accompanied by "insight."

Accordingly, hypnoanalysis should be regarded as a form or variant of psychoanalysis in its broadest sense. Freud (1953a) explained that any treatment can be considered psychoanalysis if its effectiveness comes from "undoing resistances and interpreting transferences." Given these criteria, hypnoanalysis is definitely "psychoanalysis" in spite of Freud's vacillating history with regard to the use of hypnosis, which began with embracing the modality, then rejecting it, and finally depending on it to manage the pain of his cancer in his final days. Hypnoanalysts are very much concerned with undoing resistances and interpreting transferences. The specific step-by-step techniques to accomplish these goals will be made clear as the chapters in this book unfold.

Hypnosis, when applied according to psychodynamic understandings, is a part of the hypnoanalytic strategy. The therapy becomes "hypnoanalytic" when its hypnotic aspects are so naturally applied by the practitioner as to become secondary to the patient's developing focus on the main objective of achieving reconstructive understandings.

Hypnoanalysts, like psychoanalytic practitioners, attempt to reconstruct and deal with memory material, lift repressions, release bound affects, and integrate previously unconscious and unegotized aspects of the personality. They are also concerned with factors of resistance, transference, and counter-transference as are the psychoanalysts. Similar to Freud (1953a), many hypnoanalysts see dreams as a "royal road to the unconscious" and dream interpretation as a major hypnoanalytic technique. In that sense, their theoretical views of personality structure and neurotic symptom formation closely parallel those of the classic psychoanalysts. The analysis of transference has always been a major psychoanalytic method, along with free association and dream interpretation. Freud simply emphasized its importance.

Free association may ultimately unearth early memory material and ingrained interpretations of early experiences represented as reconstructed memories. Unfortunately, many sessions are required to secure the same data, which within a much shorter time may become apparent through hypnotic hypermnesia, regression, and particularly regressive abreactive techniques. Furthermore, in doing so, there is little if any evidence to support Freud's contention that the ego is bypassed by hypnosis and his notion that consequently such personality changes would be only temporary. As early as 1979, E. R. Hilgard and Loftus showed that memories reconstructed by hypnotic regression can be distorted, but, of course, Freud had already found that through "screening memories," these recollections (more accurately termed reconstructed memory material) secured by free association could also be distorted. There is no evidence whatsoever that hypnosis is any more likely to distort memories than numerous other commonly used therapeutic or detective-like questioning techniques. Furthermore, there is no data extant comparing the validity of hypnotically secured memory material versus those elicited through free association.

Dream interpretation has been a valuable psychoanalytic tool, especially in the hands of gifted and intuitive practitioners such as Wilhelm Stekel (1943c). Hypnoanalysts also employ dream and fantasy analytic procedures (Barrett, 1998). The hypnotic modality provides greater flexibility in the activation, analysis, and interpretation of these creations.

Transference reaction analysis is a very potent psychoanalytic procedure for achieving reconstructive changes in the basic personality. Such reactions appear during an analysis when the patient projects onto the analyst feelings and attitudes that he or she once experienced toward earlier significant figures such as a love for one's mother or hatred toward a dominating father. As these inappropriate reactions are pointed out and explained to the patient by the analyst's interpretations, new insights and growth can be achieved. However, without hypnosis, many weeks and months will typically elapse before such responses develop and become manifest in such a relationship.

More significant is the fact that the patient's regression (Menninger & Holzman, 1973) that brings this about can be far better achieved and appropriately controlled by the use of hypnosis because hypnosis itself is a form of regression in the service of the ego (Gill & Brenman, 1959) or, as Hartmann (1939/1958) termed it, "adaptive regression." A personal communication (August 11, 2002, to A. Barabasz) from Erika Fromm is referred to in Barabasz and Watkins (2005) (pp. 68–70). Fromm explained that a person suffering from a cold might well curl up in bed "just like a child," watching hours of senseless lightweight TV programs, letting him- or herself simply be taken care of by others. This regression helps the person to get well, healthy, and independent once again more quickly. She further likened the activity to taking a vacation in which one engages in entertainment, napping, or reading nondemanding materials. Clearly, these regressions in the service of the ego are nonpathological and healthy. Regressive experiences in the hypnotherapeutic relationship can help to bring about self-healing and facilitation of inner strengths (Frederick, 1999b). In a brief period of time, of course, the patient might be willing to engage in the experience under the guidance of the hypnoanalyst.

This book will also focus on hypnodiagnostic procedures and new, revised, and updated approaches to abreactive techniques. Abreactive techniques, which remedy the early criticisms voiced by Freud and Breuer (1953), are still voiced by some hypnoanalysts. We will also explain the use of hypnography and sensory hypnoplasty as methodologies to derive information about unconscious processes that go beyond verbalizations alone. The reader will learn how to hypnotically facilitate dissociative and projective approaches so that an even greater degree of flexibility is offered to the psychoanalytic practitioner. The latest developments in ego-state therapy beyond those described by J.G.W. and H. H. Watkins (1997) will be presented, with extensions of dissociative techniques that provide yet another dimension in psychoanalytic theory. The theoretical origins of ego-state therapy (Frederick, 2005; Frederick & McNeal, 1999; Emmerson, 2003; J. G. Watkins and H. H. Watkins, 1997) stem from the writings of both Paul Federn (1952a) and Edoardo Weiss (1960). In this book, we approach it from the perspective of concepts concerning the structure and functioning of the self as foreshadowed by Kohut (1971) and Kernberg (1972). However, this book is primarily about treatment techniques, not theory.

Hypnoanalytic techniques should not be regarded as competing with the traditional practices of psychoanalysts or those employing psychoanalytically oriented therapy, but rather as a means of complementing their work. Hypnoanalysis can be viewed as merely an extension and an elaboration of the methods by which Freud and his colleagues undertook to explore the fascinating world of the human mind, one that continually influences our behavior and well-being, but of which we are often so little aware.

The enormous time and cost required for traditional psychoanalysis (three to five times a week for several years) limits its use to a very special and typically affluent population. Hypnoanalysis provides a much more rapid and incisive form of psychoanalysis, while also dealing with deep-underlying conflicts. Hypnoanalysis, as described in this volume, is intended to achieve genuine personality reorganization in a much shorter period of time, thus making the enormous capacity of psychodynamic thinking and psychoanalytic therapy more widely available.

Hypnotherapy is much more than a collection of techniques, because its success involves the very "self" of the doctor (A. Barabasz & Christensen, 2006). Therefore, we have attempted to place our procedures in a broad and philosophical context. That is to say, two practitioners may employ "identical" techniques, yet one achieves far better results than the other. In our chapter on existential hypnoanalysis and the therapeutic self, we explain how to integrate our two books using the concept that all "techniques" in psychological therapy must be practiced within a constructive interpersonal relationship and that in the final analysis, our success or failure may depend more on how we relate with the patient than on what we do to the patient.

We hope that those skilled psychotherapists and analysts who have experience in clinical hypnosis will find this book stimulating, in that a number of new and exciting therapeutic techniques can be added to their practice. As behavioral scientists, we must all continue to explore the inner human condition. Hypnoanalytic techniques offer many sophisticated ways of accomplishing this, both in the clinic as well as in the hypnosis research laboratory.

2
Hypnoanalytic Insight Therapy

Rigorously controlled studies show hypnosis is not only an effective adjunctive intervention but also superior to a number of widely employed treatment procedures when applied directly to influence symptoms as reviewed in Barabasz and Watkins (2005) (also revealed by Lynn, Kirsch, A. Barabasz, Cardeña, & Patterson, 2000). Perhaps it is because of this demonstrated efficacy, combined with cost-efficiency in the face of soaring medical costs (Lang & Rosen, 2002), that its potential for even greater contributions to the sophisticated reconstructive therapies involving insight has not been fully appreciated.

Despite there being many variations of psychoanalysis, all are based on the assumption that neurotic symptoms are the external manifestations of underlying conflicts and lifting the repression of unconscious factors and achieving "insight," will resolve the symptoms. Indeed, the classical psychoanalyst would likely hold that this is true of all neurotic symptoms and that unless insight has been achieved into the underlying dynamic structure of a specific neurosis, no permanent cure can be expected. In the face of now hundreds of studies to the contrary (reviewed by J. G. Watkins, 1992a), this extreme position is no longer tenable.

As discussed in Barabasz and Watkins (2005), many symptomatic conditions respond favorably and permanently to direct hypnotic interventions. Hypnosis has enormous facilitative effects when used in conjunction with standard therapies. For example, two meta-analyses (Kirsch, Montgomery, & Sapirstein, 1995; Kirsch, 1996) showed that the addition of hypnosis substantially enhanced treatment outcomes, so that the average client receiving cognitive-behavioral hypnotherapy showed greater improvement than at least 70% of the clients receiving nonhypnotic treatment. However, there are often neurotic symptoms that do not seem to be permanently relinquished unless unconscious conflicts, at their root, are brought into conscious awareness and reintegrated through that kind of understanding called insight. Therapies that aim at such insight, whether they are person-centered, cognitive, cognitive-behavioral, psychoanalytic, or any of numerous brief psychoanalytic approaches, can often produce lasting results with the addition of hypnotherapeutic interventions.

Intellectual and Experiential Insight

What is intended by the term *insight*? Much that appears to pass for insight in therapeutic interventions turns out to be nothing more than intellectualizations or intellectual understandings limited to only the cognitive (surface-deep) sphere of personality. Thus, reconstructive alteration of the personality is not possible with such superficial approaches. Even a number of analytic therapies go on month after month without showing significant change, despite the fact that the patient has learned to verbalize the dynamic constellation that underpins his or her neurosis. The point is that the patient has achieved nothing more than superficial insight, which has failed to adequately pervade the entire personality. Such examples fuel the arguments against the use of psychoanalytic therapy by those who are insufficiently educated or experienced to appreciate the issue at hand. These situations are responsible for the time-honored joke that "after 7 years of analysis the patient still bangs his head on the floor, but now he knows why." Our goal here is pervasive reconstructive change rather than mere superficial self-understanding.

Many years ago, J.G.W. interpreted to a depressed patient that he unconsciously hated his father. The evidence from his associations and dreams was quite clear on this point, so unmistakable that he immediately agreed: "You're absolutely right, Dr. Watkins. I am depressed because I hate my father. It's really clear now." However, no change in his symptoms occurred until several weeks later, when the patient burst into the office. He stood, wild-eyed and with a horror-struck expression, shouting, "I really *do* hate my father." That was genuine insight, not his first agreement with the interpretation. His initial understanding had only been at the cognitive intellectual level. Nonetheless, it had managed during the ensuing weeks to work its way through to an emotional level, which at long last mobilized feelings as well. A significant reorganization of his entire perceptual network was the result. Finally, the patient really understood. His depression began to clear. He had achieved true insight, and the symptoms never returned.

Reorganization of the patient's understanding is more than verbal or cognitive. Insight as we use it here means a thorough-going understanding including an essential alteration at the emotional level, the perceptual level, the motor level, and even the tissue level. It is a "gut" comprehension that, to be successful, must pervade the patient's entire being in all of these areas: physiological, psychological, and social. It is an alteration in meaning that changes the entire Gestalt of his or her personality. As such, it resolves inner conflicts and thus achieves a permanent impact on the dynamic factors that have maintained the symptoms. Using this definition, insight is a significant and profound experience that genuinely influences the entire lifestyle of the patient. There often remains a presumption that insight is ineffective. This is based on the erroneous, yet pervasive, definition of it as simply an intellectual understanding.

The techniques described in this treatise for achieving insight are intended to teach you how to achieve this greater and more comprehensive objective even though a superficial cognitive understanding is at first attained. The point should always be borne in mind that therapy has not achieved much if you stop at that level. It can, but it is best viewed as a precursor to more permanent changes of feelings and behavior.

Criticisms of Hypnosis by Psychoanalysts

Psychoanalysts have frequently criticized hypnosis because they misconstrue it or assign it to the role of nothing more than symptom suppression through direct suggestion. Anna Freud asserted that, even if some insight may have been achieved, this understanding is "bypassed by the ego" and hence cannot be reintegrative (1946). This criticism has been repeated and believed by numerous analysts ever since. Somehow, it is assumed that when one is hypnotized, the ego is laid aside, that it is not involved in the uncovering process, and that, accordingly, such material as does emerge cannot be absorbed or utilized by the patient for genuine change. The notion is that loss or reduction of symptoms must, thereby, be temporary because no change, or at best only a superficial one, has been made in the basic personality. Therefore, the neurotic conflicts are assumed to reassert themselves, and the symptoms will then return as soon as the influence of the hypnotherapist is no longer present. This position, though unsupported by clinical or empirical findings, has been positively and repeatedly stated in G. Blanck and R. Blanck's (1974) frequently cited volume on ego psychology.

Hypnotic Depth

It would seem obvious to all but the most casual observer that adequate hypnotic depth should be produced before expecting a hypnotizable participant to complete a task difficult enough to elicit pain control for major surgeries (see A. Barabasz & M. Barabasz, 1992). Nonetheless, achieving great depth does not necessarily require a lengthy procedure. Very brief inductions as well as spontaneous trances can often produce deep hypnosis.

One of many interesting examples appeared in a study involving stringent selection of high and low hypnotizable subjects in an experimentally controlled investigation of the effects of alert hypnosis versus the identical suggestion only on EEG event-related potentials (ERPs) (A. Barabasz, 2000). Consistent with numerous studies of hypnosis and ERPs, the data showed that only the hypnotic induction with efforts to insure adequate depth made it possible for high (but not low) hypnotizable individuals to significantly alter their brain activity in response to a hypnotic induction plus a suggestion, in contrast to the identical suggestion without the induction of hypnosis. This finding added further disproof to the sociocognitive notion that suggestion alone can account for all that can be wrought with hypnosis.

Interestingly, and perhaps of the greatest clinical significance to the findings, was that one highly hypnotizable participant produced almost identical responses in both conditions. He altered his event-related potential brain activity, in both the suggestion-only and the hypnotic-induction-plus-suggestion conditions. Simplistically, this would appear to be a statistically nonsignificant exception to the overwhelming findings of the study, but nonetheless it was an exception supporting the sociocognitive position. However, the postexperiment independent inquiry conducted by researchers not otherwise engaged in the investigation revealed the participant's strategy. This subject stated, "When I got the instruction to make like there were earplugs in my ears, I just did what I learned to do when I was a kid."

"Tell me more," replied the inquirer.

"Well, when I got spanked by my dad, I could turn off the pain just like going to another place, so that's what I did with the suggestion, same as the hypnosis part." As discussed in Barabasz and Watkins (2005, p. 85) this could be a classic example of spontaneous hypnosis with apparent dissociation. Alternatively, the suggestion alone constituted the hypnotic induction (Nash, 2005), and the highly hypnotizable subject merely responded with a level of depth sufficient to alter his ERPs.

We recommend that hypnotherapists should always be on the lookout for such behaviors. It is also of importance to understand that a nonhypnotizable participant may provide a greater number of simplistic or easy motor responses to a hypnotic induction after exposure to a hypnotic induction calling for increased depth. In such cases, because the subject is incapable of true hypnotic responding, the evocations for greater depth by the hypnotist provide nothing more than social influence demands for performance on the requested items. Clearly, social influences can produce alterations in a participant's behaviors and production of simple voluntary responses when the subject has little or no hypnotic capacity.

Let us consider the issue of hypnotic depth or trance depth from a different light. Consider hypnotic depth to be a continuum extending from total alert awareness, through hypnoidal relaxation (such as occurs on the analyst's couch), into intermediate states, then to deep (somnambulistic) regions of consciousness (where hypnoanalytic therapy has generally been practiced). The deeply hypnotized individual may achieve what Erickson (1968) termed a "plenary" trance, perhaps something similar to coma. Hypnosis can then be viewed as a dimension of personality, and the question becomes: "Does the most effective therapy occur when the patient is sitting up, wide awake, relaxed, slightly hypnoidal, and reclining on the couch, in an intermediate hypnotic depth or trance state, or only within a profound level of hypnosis?" Furthermore, is the therapy best conducted in one area on this continuum or should there be movement from one dimension to another, first uncovering repressed material on the deep end of the spectrum, and then bringing it back to the more conscious position for ego integration?

From this point of view, hypnoanalytic therapy and psychoanalytic therapy can be perceived as similar uncovering and integrating approaches that owe their difference primarily to the position on the hypnotic depth dimension in which they are commonly practiced. Hypnoanalysis is capable of using the traditional analytic techniques of free association, dream interpretation, and especially analysis of transference, but does so at different points on this depth-of-conscious dimension.

Hypnoanalysts have developed a number of new methods and sophisticated procedures for revealing preconscious and unconscious material, isolating and activating defenses, eliciting dynamic patterns of impulse, bypassing or working through resistances, dealing with transferences, and achieving integrative insight. Therefore, it would seem that practitioners of hypnotherapeutic insight therapy, as well as hypnoanalysis, can employ the same therapeutic techniques as do the more traditional analysts. However, they have in addition another dimension of impact and a number of unique therapy streamlining procedures that can be used to achieve the same result in less time than traditional approaches.

Let us compare this to the military commander who follows the same basic war strategies that have been effective over the years, but who now has available a number of newer weapons, recently developed technologies, and advanced tactics for the achievement of battle objectives. The commander need no longer fight engagements with troops armed only with rifles. Similarly, it is our position that, although much of basic analytic theory (including the developments of the last century in ego psychology and object relations) continues to be valid, psychoanalytic treatment tactics that were developed nearly a hundred years ago can be much improved with the advanced techniques available through hypnoanalysis. It is time that classic psychoanalysts adopt more flexible procedures, including the hypnotic modality.

The relationship between depth of hypnosis and ego participation is shown in Barabasz and Watkins (2005, p. 188, figure 7.1). In psychoanalysis, the patient is induced to relax on the couch and become preoccupied with inner associations. His or her field of external participation is restricted and attention is focused on inner thoughts. This process is time-consuming. But it is precisely what happens when we induce a hypnotic state. The patient can achieve rapid relaxation, the patient's external awareness becomes focused and restricted within his or her own control, and the patient is induced to experience a world consisting only of the therapist and him- or herself. It is when the narrowing of the field of attention (H. Spiegel & D. Spiegel, 2004) is focused on inner processes that we can begin to make progress toward restructuring of the personality.

The majority of a psychoanalyst's patients, upon achieving relaxation on the couch, may well develop a hypnoidal or light hypnotic state. Therefore, psychoanalysis in most cases probably involves, at least, light hypnosis, but it is uncontrolled. The patient is merely left to develop spontaneously whatever state of consciousness he or she may wish to develop, or a level precipitated by the currently salient defense mechanisms, which further delay or complicate the development of true insight regardless of their accuracy. Had the instruction to lie on the couch, relax, and occupy concentration with inner associations been continued further, we would have termed it a hypnotic induction technique, and many patients would have drifted into a medium or even a deep trance. As noted at the beginning of this subsection, some patients develop a deep level of hypnosis upon initiation of the initial suggestion. The difference in hypnoanalysis is that the therapist is keenly aware of the process taking place and uses it to the patient's advantage. The psychoanalyst stops far short of this and simply leaves the patient with a significant degree of ego alertness, but with some ego "relaxation," which Freud (1953b) felt necessary to precipitate preconscious material and unconscious derivatives, making it possible for them to seep through to conscious awareness.

In figure 2.1, the line on the left (e–g) shows the position of the patient in psychoanalysis where most of his or her ego (f–g) is alert and that only a small amount of behavior and experiential potentials stem from unconscious process (e–f). As one proceeds along the continuum of hypnotic depth from left to right, the participation of the ego becomes progressively less, and the emerging of unconscious material increases. In the deep hypnoanalytic position (h–j), there is minimal ego involvement (i–j) as more underlying unconscious and repressed material (h–i) is activated. However, the situation is not at all as it has been traditionally represented in the psychoanalytic literature,

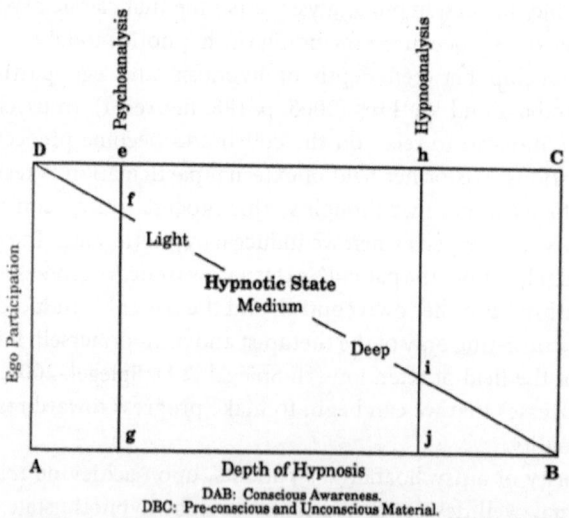

Figure 2.1 In the psychoanalytic position (e–g), a small amount of raw material (e–f) is activated and submitted to a final processing (f–g). In the deep hypnoanalytic position (h–j), a small ego factory (i–j) must confront a huge amount of unconscious raw material (h–i).

in which the ego is presumed to have been bypassed by the use of hypnosis. Lessened, yes; eliminated? No.

If we can agree that the first part of the analytic process is to activate unconscious material and bring it into awareness, then it should be obvious that a much greater amount is accessed and secured in the hypnoanalytic position than in the psychoanalytic one. These data might be compared to the raw material provided for fabrication into an article. The finished product is to be genuine insight, which is the basis upon which one can achieve significant personality restructuring or change, but it must be fashioned into its final form from the original raw material. Only after it is worked through in such a manner can it elicit a significant adaptive personality change. True reintegration cannot take place without this.

To answer the question as to which position on the hypnotic depth continuum shown in Figure 2.1 would be most effective to combine uncovering with reintegration, let us return to our analogy of the factory and the raw material. In the psychoanalytic position (e–g) in Figure 2.1, a small amount of raw material (e–f) is activated and submitted to a final processing (f–g). In the deep hypnoanalytic position (h–j), a small ego factory (i–j) must confront a huge amount of unconscious raw material (h–i). On this theoretical basis, it would seem perfectly reasonable to infer that neither the psychoanalytic position nor the deep hypnoanalytic one could be the most productive area for therapeutic work, but rather somewhere in between may represent an optimal balance of these factors.

The greatest likelihood of therapeutic progress would appear to lie in a psychoanalytic approach conducted within a medium or mid-level of hypnotic depth rather than a deep one. Almost 50 years ago, Conn (1959) emphasized the advantages of working in the mid-level to light states of hypnosis. An equally tenable position would be that we could elicit material during a deep hypnotic state and then bring it back for submission to a more vigorous ego, as represented by the left-hand area of the hypnotic-depth dimension. We opine that hypnoanalytic therapy then may best proceed when it consists of moving back and forth on this continuum. When employing the briefest of the powerful hypnoanalytic procedures, ego-state therapy, A.F.B. suggests that it is essential to ensure full egotization (ego integration) of memory material elicited during deep hypnosis. Abreaction must be brought to full conscious awareness in the context of a supportive soothing re-emergence from deep through light hypnosis.

In both psychoanalytic therapy as well as hypnoanalysis, it would seem valuable to control the level of hypnotic depth and not merely leave it to chance. As discussed earlier, the defense mechanisms (or even momentary whims) of a patient may impel him or her to carry through the analysis at a comfortable and convenient intensity level, rather than one that he or she is capable of achieving. Such patients have histories of flight from therapeutic intervention when the going becomes demanding rather than working to their potential and achieving self-actualizing results. By permitting the ego factory to work at a comfortable level when we submit only small amounts of raw material (such as may be elicited slowly by free association, if at all) to conscious awareness, integrating patients work far below their capabilities. The uncovering and integration of new material proceeds at a lazy and unsystematic pace. Thus, the analysis takes far longer than necessary.

Now, if we uncover unconscious matter at an accelerated tempo, we supply our integrating ego with substantial quantities of raw material. Conscious or light hypnotic state patients will often be strongly resistant to this and will quickly muster the usual defensive postures, such as rationalization or flight from therapeutic interaction. Alternatively, hypnotized patients have the resources at hand to move in an accelerated manner, achieving remarkable therapeutic results. By controlling the variable of trance depth, we have the opportunity to provide sufficient participation of our ego factory so as to maximize desired productivity, thus making possible the most rapid achievement of genuine reintegrating insight.

The "working through" process, repeated by contact between the ego and previously unconscious material, is a key element in psychoanalysis. It is not dispensed with in hypnoanalytic treatment, but it may be speeded up. Repetition of material elicited while in hypnosis is still essential. Such repetition, especially of emotions, as well as cognitions, is particularly effective in the conduct of hypnotic abreactions (see Chapter 5 in the present volume).

Hypnotic Depth at the Intermediate Level

Material elicited and submitted for egotization in the intermediate level of hypnotic depth (Figure 2.1) can and frequently does stimulate considerable anxiety. The confrontation at this point is much more severe for the patient than using either the slow psychoanalytic free-association technique or the deep hypnoanalytic end of the continuum. For example, if the patient cursed his or her father (unconscious raw material) but he (ego) is not present, no actual confrontation takes place, and no therapeutic movement is possible. This would be represented by the extreme right-hand position in the figure discussed earlier. There is no meeting of the incompatible elements. It is like trying to teach a completely unconscious person. Alternatively, if the father is present, but the patient does not express any negative thoughts about him (that is, they are thoroughly repressed), then again there is no confrontation and no therapeutic movement. This is like the position at the extreme left-hand side of the figure. The ego is completely present; hence, defense mechanisms are at the maximum, and the ego is, thereby, not in contact with any of the preconscious or unconscious impulses that drive their behaviors.

Alternatively, if the patient utters an oath against his or her father while he is present in the room (as represented by the intermediate zone level of hypnotic depth dimension), then the sparks will fly. The confrontation takes place. If the contact continues, the unpleasant heat of the anxiety that is developed can be dissipated only by a change in the attitudes and acceptances of either or both of them. A new Gestalt of understanding and relationship must be forged. They can no longer be in conflict with each other or dissociated from one another. Genuine therapeutic change has thus been achieved. The process then is no different in hypnoanalysis than in psychoanalysis, but a greater flexibility of technique and ego participation has been available to facilitate this objective.

The intermediate zones of hypnotic depth involve working through at a high intensity and, thereby, have some potential hazards. If more material is liberated from repression than the ego can assimilate, and if its defenses are incapable of warding off painful contact with such material, then they may be overwhelmed. This conflict can precipitate a flight into a psychotic reaction. It is very rare and quite acute, but it can happen. However, in most cases the patient's defenses arise and thus do not permit it to occur. In some way, the patient's ego will break off contact with the undigestible material, which is now emerging in too great a strength. Sometimes, the patient may spontaneously emerge from hypnosis and seek the extreme left end of the hypnotic depth spectrum (light hypnosis or complete conscious awareness) or, in a very few cases, decathect his or her ego temporarily and enter a profound trance state.

The state may be so profound that the patient may become deaf to your words. Such hypnotic deafness is not absolute. The laboratory-controlled and fully replicated experiential evidence (A. Barabasz, M. Barabasz, Jensen, Calvin, Trevisan, & Warner, 1999; A. Barabasz, 2000; Ray & De Pascalis, 2003) clearly reveals that EEG event-related potentials, as in the earlier studies (A. Barabasz & Lonsdale, 1983; D. Spiegel, Cutcomb, Ren, & Pribram, 1985) of reactions to verbal stimuli, are attenuated, not obliterated. Your voice is dissociated, but contact can be reestablished. Patients are taught in less deep levels of hypnosis that they will hear every word that the therapist is saying when the therapist touches their shoulder. It is, therefore, possible to reestablish contact quickly. Rest assured that this reaction happens very infrequently, and you, as the analyst, can minimize any potentially catastrophic reactions by your normal caring attention to the therapeutic relationship.

Perhaps the most important point is that the ego strength of the patient is never a constant. It is greater sometimes than others, whereas the demands of significant daily relationships can lower it. If the patient maintains alliances with constructive others, particularly you as the therapist, ego strength can be reinforced. It is times like these when even somewhat pathological significant others in the patient's life can be especially destructive to the overall growth. Such destructiveness fuels the patient's needs to maintain control over them.

Hypnotic Depth at the Optimal Level

If you are practicing insight therapy at the intermediate level of hypnotic depth, it is essential that you offer an intensive therapeutic relationship, an alliance involving much "resonance" (J. G. Watkins & H. H. Watkins, 1978). This process involves a partial merging of the ego of the therapist with that of the patient, a temporary identification balanced with appropriate objectivity. This is a partial merging of your ego with that of the patient, a temporary identification with you. Patients are then reassured and can approach the analytic confrontations with a fuller mobilization of their resources because they perceive that they (in a "with-ness") can succeed, where alone they could not.

The analyst who guides his or her patient through the dark labyrinths of unconscious representations is like the good parent who takes the child by the hand and goes with him or her into the dark closet to confront the "Boogie Man." The therapeutic "with-ness" is a temporary and partial merging of the patient's and therapist's egos. The intensity of the hypnotic relationship enhances such togetherness, as the therapist and the patient make a common commitment to the analytic task. This "with-ness" is not counter-transference, which is the projection of the therapist's immature needs onto the patient (Frederick, 2005).

Given various levels of hypnotic depth, we can reveal different facets of impulse and defense during the analytic interview. Because hypnosis is also a form of regression, it can sometimes indicate the contents that may have to be merged during a more classical psychoanalysis session. As one proceeds into deeper and deeper levels of hypnotic involvement, the nature of defenses may be revealed that would only be uncovered at much later stages in classical psychoanalysis. Even if the therapeutic plan were to proceed in more traditional analytic ways, the prescouting value of an overview of the patient's neurosis might aid the psychoanalyst in planning his or her strategy, and facilitate his or her timing of interpretations.

Some analysts (Stekel, 1943c) asserted that the first dream in analysis was like an overview of the entire structure of the patient's neurosis, one whose full meaning would only become clear by the end of the analysis. Similarly, a hypno-diagnostic prestudy can frequently reveal the order in which the various transference reactions would have emerged had the patient free-associated on the psychoanalytic couch. Some analysts may prefer not to use so much control. There has been, even among the older analysts, substantial controversy as to how much the analyst should permit the material to emerge without directivity or to evolve according to a plan based on his or her conceptualization of personality structure (Reich, 1949).

Working through and Hypermedia

Hypermedia can facilitate the reconstruction of memory material, which is experiential and not always veridical. The fact that such reconstructed material may or may not represent true happenings but rather remembrances or screen memories should be explained to your patient at the onset of therapy. Claire Frederick and Maggie Phillips (2004) recommended that a release form be signed by the patient and be kept on file. We think this is controversial, because signing a release form protects the therapist but it impairs the therapeutic relationship, because it implies that the therapist does not fully trust the patient. In hypnotic abreaction, strongly repressed affects can be mobilized so that a re-experiencing, not merely a remembering, takes place. The re-experiencing is critical, in our view, to therapeutic movement and reconstruction of the personality. Hypnotically facilitated release of such bound affects provides a fuller participation by the patient in genuine insight reactions. It thus becomes possible that newer and constructive meanings can initiate real and lasting therapeutic change.

Abreaction and other specific hypnoanalytic techniques will be described in later chapters that explain how to initiate the lifting of repressions, the activation of transferences, the release of bound affects, and the revivification of early experiences.

One tactic might be noted in comparison with classical psychoanalytic technique. During psychoanalysis, the state of consciousness equivalent to the light trance depth is held constant or at least is not directly manipulated by the analyst. The repressions are gradually lifted, and the preconscious and unconscious material is submitted to the patient in gradually increasing doses. In hypnoanalysis, we lift a repression; release a great quantity of unconscious, unegotized material; and then manipulate the trance depth to submit this larger amount of now unrepressed material to increasing impact with the ego. These are simply two different ways of working through the end result of complete egotization, and reintegration may be the same, only the procedures for its accomplishment have varied.

In conclusion, our goals and basic strategies in hypnoanalysis do not differ greatly from those in traditional psychoanalysis. The underlying theoretical concepts are quite similar. However, their employment in conjunction with hypnosis offers the possibility of greatly increased flexibility through the alteration of hypnotic depth and the availability of a much wider variety of techniques.

Summary

Basic hypnotherapy, as discussed in Barabasz and Watkins (2005), involves primarily, although not exclusively, the amelioration of symptoms by direct hypnotic intervention via the establishment of the hypnotic state and the use of appropriate suggestions coupled in some cases with self-hypnotic techniques. Hypnotherapy at this level is a kind of "putting in." Alternatively, and with much greater elegance, hypnoanalysis is a "pulling out." Hypnoanalysis in practice involves the addition of the induction of hypnosis, plus the use of special techniques that hypnosis makes possible. As in psychoanalysis, hypnoanalysis attempts to eliminate symptoms indirectly by the lifting of repressions and the achieving of true insight.

To be effective, insight must be more than intellectual; it must also be experiential, involving affective and motor responses as well as cognitive ones.

Following Freud's renunciation of hypnosis, psychoanalysts for years criticized the process as being "superficial," "bypassing the ego," and not resulting in permanent character/personality change. At one time, these criticisms may have been valid when the hypnotic state was induced solely to potentiate suggestions. Such arguments are no longer tenable. Trance depth is related to the amount of ego participation. In the deeper stages, much preconscious and unconscious material may be uncovered, but there is far less ability to "egotize" this. In the lighter stages of hypnosis, less material can be elicited but with greater ego participation. It appears that the most effective areas for treatment are in the medium zones of trance depth or the weaving back and forth between deeper and lighter states. A.F.B. maintains that the greatest and most rapid changes can often take place when material is reexperienced in a deep abreactive state, but that it is essential that this be brought through to the lighter and fully conscious states in the context of a Rogersian-like, supportive, postabreactive intervention. Just as in psychoanalysis, material lifted from repressions with hypnoanalysis must be worked through to achieve lifelong therapeutic benefits.

3
The Psychodynamics of Hypnotic Induction

As one becomes more and more intensely involved in the study of hypnosis, one is drawn to the view that the response of entering a hypnotic state, perhaps at the uttering of the very first suggestion, deepening, and terminating the condition, is intimately related to the interpersonal communications between the therapist and the patient as well as to the motivational needs of both. The amateur tends to think of hypnosis as simply a state entered by the subject in reaction to certain cues provided by the hypnotist. Such a beginner (although this concept is certainly not limited to those who would view themselves as beginners or amateurs) often shows the greatest interest in reading about and memorizing "techniques," completely ignoring that it is the *meaning* of the interpersonal interaction implied in the so-called technique and not the simple stimulus value of certain words that is of most significance in determining the kind and extent of the hypnotic response rather than hypnotic experience (J. G. Watkins, 1992). Nash (2005) explained that even in the American Psychological Association Division 30 definition of hypnosis (Green, A. Barabasz, Barrett, & Montgomery, 2005), some experts in the field apparently are still stumbling over whether or not the word *hypnosis* must be uttered during the procedure. The notion that the word *hypnosis* is somehow essential does nothing more than perpetuate naïve operationalism, which reflects little upon human nature, hypnosis, or the meaning of the interpersonal hypnotic interaction.

Psychodynamics of Personality

Let us consider the promiscuous Don Juan, the lover renowned in literature and opera. At superficial glance, the fellow seems to be quite a man. After all, he has possessed many women. One might think that he would be very proud of his masculinity. However, it turns out from a psychodynamic viewpoint that quite the opposite prevails. Don Juan is a very insecure male. He doubts his potency, is uncertain of his masculinity, and at an unconscious level, is defending himself against latent feminine or perhaps even homosexual drives. His seductive behavior is necessary, as constant proof to himself that he really is masculine. Each conquest temporarily allays his inner anxiety but does not last long. The issue is unresolved. He is driven to seek a new affair to quell the small inner voice that whispers that he is really not a man. Only from such a psychodynamic point of view can we really understand his behavior, deal with it rationally, and help with an appropriate treatment strategy, which will create or restore in him a sense of confidence that he is truly what he was structurally born to be: a man. Once he has acquired this new understanding, genuine heterosexual love becomes possible. A woman is no longer a possession to control and flaunt. A meaningful relationship with a woman then can replace his promiscuity and need for control.

Yes, psychodynamics represents the psychological subscience that deals with the complexities of unconscious motivational patterns in the determination of behavior. It considers cause-and-effect relationships in psychic life, especially those that are covert. Thus, the origin of behavior may lie far from the actual response, so that neither the subject nor nearby observers suspect its true cause. Like the words in a popular song half a century ago, "You push the first valve down, the music goes round and round, and it comes out here." Psychodynamics is, in a sense, the study of the "round and round."

The participant in hypnosis reacts similarly in an interpersonal relationship with the therapist via the communications received during what is termed the hypnotic induction. He or she enters trance, does not enter trance, or does so, but only lightly. J.G.W. (1954) once attempted to equate the hypnotic state with transference, but later (1963) updated this stance and maintained, rather, that hypnosis was much more than transference (see Barabasz & Watkins, 2005, p. 58). He explained the phenomenon by elucidating the transference needs in the hypnotized individual and counter-transference motivations in the therapist that determined whether a hypnotic state could be induced easily, with difficulty, or not at all, as well as to whether the state produced would be limited to light levels or deep levels. Through the study of psychodynamics, we try to understand the complex of inner and outer motivations, which cause the participant to make a response. Then and only then can we learn to control these more effectively, with the aim of increasing the likelihood that he or she will react with a hypnotic state deep enough for the constructive application of hypnotherapeutic techniques.

Hypnosis as a State of Regression

The interdependence of the hypnotic state on the quality and intensity of the interpersonal relationship between the therapist and the participant was recognized by M. V. Kline (1958). He concluded that there is no constancy of itself in the hypnotic relationship, but there is a constancy to the hypnotic trance state. The trance state was seen as a very basic and fundamental reorientation in perceptual and object relationships. Kline claimed that hypnosis is in no way a unitary "something" or "either-or." Rather, it exists quantitatively to varying degrees and different depths, as well as qualitatively in different forms depending on the nature of the unique relationship between the two parties, before the induction, during the induction, and during nonhypnotic therapeutic interactions. Thus, as discussed in Barabasz & Watkins (2005, p. 58), it can be concluded that the state of hypnosis induced in participant A by therapist B is not the same as that induced in the same person by therapist C, that it is not the same in participants A and D when both were induced by therapist B, and that it is not the same in participant A when induced by therapist B at one time and at another time. The difference in each of these cases is both quantitative and qualitative. The point is that the hypnotic state should not be regarded simply as a unitary state without considering the relationship in which it occurs. Hypnosis is both a state and a relationship. As a state, it has a number of specific characteristics such as lowered criticality, diminished control, the cessation of making plans, less emotional inhibition, and a return to child-like patterns of behavior-regression. Regression by hypnosis is more than a theoretical hypothesis. A. Barabasz et al. (2003) and A. Barabasz and Christensen (2006) conducted experimentally controlled investigations that provided empirical evidence supporting regression.

During sleep, illness, psychosis, and psychoneurosis, we "regress." Hence, we return to earlier and simpler patterns of response. This regression is sometimes forced upon an individual. When he or she is confronted with aggressive environmental demands, such as might be present in a relationship with a significant other, they may overwhelm the ego. The person is unable to cope with them. The ego suffers a devastating annihilation. Psychosis results. However, in most cases, the ego, like a good military commander faced with superior forces, knows enough to withdraw from the scene of battle. It pulls back, shortens its lines of responsibility, and by conserving its energies within a simpler existence prevents its total destruction. In the long term, such behavior may be very destructive, but in the short term, as with most any medical or emotional symptom, the purpose is preservation of the organism. Even in normal sleep, the ego can rest and await the time when, with renewed strength and vigor, it can venture back into the human struggle. Hartmann, as early as 1939, referred to this response as "regression in the service of the ego."

Influences on Hypnotic Regression

When inducing and deepening hypnotic trance, we are concerned with understanding the factors that initiate regressive trends in our patient and how these can be stimulated and controlled. Actually, all methods of trance induction represent some form of initiating regression. Gill and Brenman (1959) classified these under two subheadings: (1) sensorimotor/ideational restriction, or (2) the stimulation of an archaic (hence transference) relationship to the therapist. In other words, we regress when we do not receive adequate stimulation from the environment (A. Barabasz, 1982). We also regress when we are in intimate personal contact with a person who (through transference) represents an early authority figure toward whom we have established immature and primitive patterns of response. The psychodynamic approach to the hypnotic induction will concern itself with both avenues, but it is the second where it can make the greatest contribution to our understanding, therapeutic skills, and effectiveness.

Comparing the induction of a regressive sleep with the induction of regression in hypnosis, let us note that in order to sleep, we first restrict our sensorimotor input. The room is darkened. We lie still. We are made warm by covers and, when possible, protected from undue skin stimuli by comfortable clothing and sheets. Verbal interaction ceases, and we do not want to listen to the sounds or the distractions produced by others. It is in this absence of stimuli that the ego withdraws its energies from the sensory organs and nearly eliminates its communication with the outside world.

Conscious thoughts fade and are gradually replaced by those bits of more archaic mental material referred to as dreams, in which the logic (or rather psycho-logic) proceeds according to the rules that govern unconscious or primary process thinking. The dream becomes like the psychosis, a "legitimate psychosis." The dream is irrational and concretistic, illogical, yet still subject to ego-defense maneuvers. The ego vacillates between the external world, which demands social-reality behavior, and the inner world of primitive drives, which psychoanalysts call the id. At this stage, the state of regression is not unlike that which exists during deep hypnosis. Indeed, the major scales of hypnotizability, including the Stanford Hypnotic Susceptibility Scale (SHSS) Forms A, B, and C (Weitzenhoffer & E. R. Hilgard, 1959, 1962) and the Stanford Hypnotic Clinical Scale (SHCS) (Morgan & J. R. Hilgard, 1975), involve regressive suggestions.

As energies (cathexes) are further withdrawn from the dreamer's ego, mental activity becomes less and less and may finally approach a deep state of coma in which only the continuation of minimal, vital, organic functions indicate that the individual is still alive. Classically, Erickson (1952) described such a hypnotic state as a "plenary trance," which he induced through very prolonged induction procedures in a very limited number of participants. Some 20 years later, Sherman's (1971) doctoral dissertation revealed that profoundly hypnotized individuals reach a stage in which the awareness of "knowledge identity" ceases. Even with the limited EEG technology of that time, he was able to show electroencephalographic changes reflecting a drastic reduction of apparent activity.

Similarly, various stages also seem to appear in a patient regressed chemically through anesthetization of his of her functions, such as in a surgical procedure. Research on restricted environmental stimulation (A. Barabasz, 1980a–d, 1982) has shown that individuals may even experience hallucinatory material and similar mental phenomena as they dream. The hypnotized participant vivifies or perhaps hallucinates inner past or suggested experiences. Sensory restriction when a person remains conscious rather than sleeps has been shown (A. Barabasz & M. Barabasz, 1993) to have lasting effects on the development of the person's hypnotic capacities as he or she develops elaborate defenses involving imaginative involvement (A. Barabasz, 1980d, 1982, 1983, 1984a; A. Barabasz, Gregson, & Mullin, 1984; A. Barabasz & Gregson, 1979; A. Barabasz & M. Barabasz, 1989; Suedfeld, 1980).

We facilitate this regression during hypnotic induction by telling our patient to stare at a fixed point (restricting sources of visual stimulation), or requesting that he or she attend to the relaxation in the muscles, eventually lowering motor activity, calling attention to involuntary actions such as eye closure or hand levitation. These behaviors demonstrate that increasing parts of the body are becoming de-egotized and are longer subject to voluntary control. We suggest falling during a standing, body sway approach (thus disorienting kinesthetic and equilibratory sense contacts with reality). Alternatively, we may ask the participant to become preoccupied with a soothing inner fantasy that stresses comfort, rest, and peace, thus pushing away the outer world. In so doing, the therapist helps the participant tip the balance between cognitive controls and the inner process of more primitive needs. The patient can relax, close the eyes, and regress. By relinquishing direction from conscious mental processes and sources outside the ego, hypnotic suggestions from the therapist become more operative. The hypnotized person is not exactly a child, nor psychotic, nor just dreaming, but does demonstrate behavior that may closely resemble all of these.

Hypnotic productions often look like the reactions of a dissociated individual such as are found in dissociative identity disorder (DID) (multiple personalities). It is not surprising that most DID patients have been studied through hypnoanalytic procedures, because in the hypnotic state, it is so easy to induce the various personalities to appear or disappear. When doing so, the therapist must be critically careful to not produce another new personality entity by suggestion, one that did not exist in the individual before hypnosis. We often forget that the induction procedure is a communication between two parties, and it is the meaning, the essential inner significance of each communicative act, which determines our participant's response, not the fact of administering a technique.

To close the eyes may mean to one participant that he or she is supposed to rest; to another, it may mean he or she is to ignore the outer world; to a third, it may mean that something is about to be "put over" on them without their control; to another, it may mean he or she is to die; to still another, it may mean he or she is to pretend or imagine. Not only may each hypnotic participant interpret the meaning of a hypnotic suggestion differently (particularly those with borderline personality disorders, who misinterpret suggestions far more frequently than normal subjects), but a single participant may interpret the suggestion one way when given by hypnotist A, who is viewed as a helper, and another way when the identical suggestion is administered by hypnotist B, who is regarded as an exploiter. What we tell ourselves makes a critical difference. These two different attitudes may have been determined by differences in the real behavior of the two therapists because inner-personal (transference) attitudes stimulated within the two elicit different physical and psychological characteristics.

The Hypnotic State has Special Meanings to the Patient

All patients are different, and all patients have varied conceptualizations, both consciously and unconsciously, toward hypnosis or its induction. To one patient, to relax, either in a chair or on a couch, is to relinquish defensive postures and to give one's self over to the hypnotic suggestions of another, and this can mean to involve one's self in a state of submission. This can also arise in the patient who is undergoing relaxation on the psychoanalytic couch as well. Both submissive needs and fears can be simultaneously stimulated. Two different patients, both of whom equate being hypnotized with submitting one's self to another, may still react quite differently. One may see it as an enjoyable experience where one is no longer held accountable for one's actions or fantasies and is freed of guilt. The patient can then hold the hypnotherapist responsible for whatever transpires. These patients can sink rapidly into a very deep trance and welcome the hypnotic experience.

To a patient who has spent his or her life struggling for independence, to whom dependence or submission to another constitutes a threat, thus meaning they could be taken advantage of, the induction can become a signal for a "battle of wills." Such a patient intends to show the hypnotherapist that he or she cannot be imposed upon. Unconsciously, such patients may feel fragile and weak. They are consciously striving to be a "rock of Gibraltar," that is, impregnable in the face of an assault that they perceive as dangerous to the integrity of their ego. Thus, the patient is either unhypnotizable or highly resistant, despite the possibility that they may have the natural talent to enter a state of hypnosis.

Recognize this resistance and either bypass it through appropriate technique or overpower it through superior skill and the mobilization of the patient's stronger motivations. Alternatively, this can be analyzed and worked through to reduce its strength. When such resistance is encountered, the wise therapist terminates attempts at induction for the present time and inquires of the patient's views about hypnosis. What has the patient read about it, has he or she seen a demonstration, and what feelings did these demonstrations initiate in him or her? This may be necessary even though the initial debunking of myths about hypnosis may have been quite well covered at an intellectual level prior to beginning hypnosis. At other times, a patient will be resistant to the induction of hypnosis because of the arousal of some new fear (see Emmerson, 2003, pp. 60–76, Resistance Bridge Techniques).

J.G.W. was treating a young woman hypnoanalytically who had typically responded with a medium-deep trance in about 5 minutes, with suggestions involving eye fixation, relaxation, and the dropping of her arm. On one particular day, she was late for her session. She was much disturbed after watching a CNN news program that had been repeating and repeating an account of a sadistic murder in which a girl had been killed while on a tropical island vacation. Her body had been cut into pieces and strewn about!

Instead of her usual response to trance induction, the patient reacted with fidgeting, resistance (manifested by asking questions to delay the induction), and, in general, much anxiety. Only very slowly did she involve herself in the hypnotic regression. Toward the end of the induction procedure, J.G.W. was accustomed to lifting her arm by the wrist and suggesting that when he dropped her hand she would fall into a profoundly deep state. This time, when her wrist was touched, she shrieked and shrank away from him. Further attempts at deepening the trance were abandoned until she had been asked about her fears. It so happens that in this session, she perceived J.G.W. as a potential sadistic murderer. Obviously, she was frightened. Nonetheless, the full airing of this feeling during a light trance state enabled her to achieve a deeper state of hypnosis, which proved to be one that produced a great deal of reconstructed memory material beneficial to her treatment.

Curiously, upon returning to her normal state of alertness after hypnosis, she reported that on the way to J.G.W.'s office she had seen a child's shoe lying beside the walkway and immediately felt frightened, perceiving it as an amputated foot. Had J.G.W. failed to sense her changed emotional reaction and simply proceeded mechanically, there might have been an overwhelming traumatic fear response, perhaps even a permanent termination of treatment. J.G.W. interrupted the induction to inquire into this source of anxiety. Thus, it was possible to resolve the presented matter and induce a productive hypnotic state and also gain knowledge about her own psychodynamic needs that were being projected (transferred) onto J.G.W. during that session. The issue here is not with determining the full meaning of her reaction to the sadistic news event and its significance to her neurosis, but rather with its impact on the process of trance induction. What started as a resistance to J.G.W. and the therapy became a valuable source of new understandings and a basis for progress. The mechanical application of any induction procedure, however initially effective, may lose much of its efficacy if the hypnotherapist fails to be sensitive to the subtle psychodynamic interplay within the patient.

Hypnosis as an Erotic Experience

The hypnotic state is welcomed by some participants as an opportunity in which they are free to enjoy erotic fantasies. During regression, the later-formed psychic structures tend to be eliminated first, hence, the super-ego that is the conscious controls. Then, the ego defenses are also lessened, leaving immature and erotic impulses more free to gain expression in fantasy. This lowering of inhibition is characteristic of both the ingestion of alcohol and hypnosis. Such lowering of criticality with the release of a person's true wishes and fantasies was, perhaps, first noted by Milton Kline (1958).

At times, the desire to enter trance becomes so pleasurable that the patient enters hypnosis at the slightest provocation or may undergo spontaneous hypnotic reactions (H. Spiegel & D. Spiegel, 2004). These responses represent the patient's character traits and can be the result of much practiced experience in dissociating, as is found in highly hypnotizable adults who, as children, were subjected to severe discipline. Josephine Hilgard (1979) noted that is not a matter of some form of learned authoritarian response, but rather that as children these individuals learn to dissociate the pain of spanking by spontaneous hypnosis; for example, when sent to their rooms to think about what naughty kids they were, they would engage in long fantasy involvements (see also A. Barabasz, 1982).

In other cases, it can be pleasurable seduction, similar to the behavior of schizoid individuals who find indulging in fantasy life more pleasant than real existence. Such a tendency in a hypnotic participant is probably not healthy and may be a contraindication for the continued use of hypnosis. What is happening is that the regression is no longer temporary; hence, it is no longer in the "service of the ego," but rather has become a movement toward a permanent, pathological, perhaps psychotic state. Patients who are too easily hypnotized demand our very careful evaluation as to what therapeutic procedures are most appropriate. Clearly, in such cases hypnosis may be contraindicated.

A very small number of patients may interpret the hypnotic induction as some sort of prelude to sexual seduction or as itself a symbolic seduction. Gill and Brenman (1959, p. 140) went so far as to note that "the hysteriform symptoms of rigidity, which may develop in the early stages of hypnosis, often bear a distinct resemblance to the motions in sexual intercourse. If you question hypnotized subjects, they frequently report that they experience a pleasant sensation of fatigue, and some openly admit feelings of sexual excitation." Obviously, this can mobilize either wishes or fears, or both. Whether or not the participant so perceives it depends on the relative balance between the wish to experience such possible reactions and the fear of being seduced. Once such a patient has received adequate reassurance of protection from the fear of seduction, his or her unconscious erotic wishes may serve as a strong motivating agent that facilitates the induction of hypnosis. Being hypnotized and being sexually influenced may have the same meaning for schizophrenic patients and for patients with borderline personality disorder, who are more prone to dissociation.

Death Fears

As Federn (1952a) noted, the fear of death is universal, and few people can master it. The ego simply cannot accept or face its own nonexistence. Death is equated with the loss of self, stillness, immovability, and the end of volition. It is not surprising that certain participants view the induction of hypnosis as dying. We do ask the patient to remain still, close the eyes, and relinquish volition unless the therapeutic situation demands some form of active alert hypnosis. If fears of death are mobilized, resistance to hypnosis will increase. Remarkably, some people are afraid to sleep because they think they may die during their sleep. This fear was most likely initiated in childhood, if the patient was brought up in a Christian background and given bedtime prayers such as "If I should die before I wake, I pray the Lord my soul to take." There are no doubt other similar examples from other cultures and religions, of which the astute therapist should become aware. Fortunately, resistance based on such a fear occurs very infrequently, as most people are not afraid to go to sleep.

The Hypnotic Relationship

As in any interpersonal relationship, but especially in psychotherapy, the patient perceives the other through the eyes of his or her past. Not only the state of hypnosis but also the hypnotic relationship and any interactive communications between doctor and patient have inner and special meanings. Therapists are endowed with characteristics, good or bad, which they experience as inhering in parental and other early authority figures. Furthermore, the same distortion of perception can occur in the therapist, affecting his or her evaluation of the patient by their attitude. This phenomenon is referred to as "transference," and in the therapist, "counter-transference." It operates both in the induction process and throughout treatment. Chapter 11 provides a discussion of these issues in greater depth.

Fantasy and the Induction

Light hypnosis and daydreaming have some close similarities. The schizoid individual constantly revels in such indulgent imaginations. Of course, it is perfectly normal to daydream, and the normal person often indulges in such pleasures. Perhaps one of the more sophisticated approaches to the induction of hypnosis involves the use of fantasy in a guided way. At first, the participant is merely asked to visualize, imagine, or think themselves in a specific scene and then to progressively live within it. It is then possible to move the person time-wise (topographically, not actually temporally) to obtain regression to some earlier age level (A. Barabasz & Christensen, 2006). The fantasy becomes the experienced reality of the moment, just as a dream in sleep is often felt as real.

A participant can become involved in a fantasy experience if this "dream" involves pleasurable stimuli; thus, it precipitates enjoyment that is highly satisfying in some very personal situations. Who among us has not enjoyed daydreams of acquiring success, fame, and vanquishing enemies? Especially potent for the induction of hypnosis can be those fantasized situations that appeal to immature childlike or childhood cravings. For example, skin eroticism has been considered as genetically preceding genital eroticism. Thus, when the therapist helps the patient picture the soothing touch of a soft, grassy slope on which he or she is reclining, or the smooth velvet sensation about one's body when floating on a cloud, the therapist is invoking tactile erotic fantasy reminiscent of the maternal touch in earliest childhood. It is not surprising that the patient is encouraged to regress and may accomplish this end with greater success than more direct induction procedures.

Common unconscious fantasies found in psychoanalysis include the desire to return to the womb, to an early, warm, and environmentally perfect existence or similar, but less obvious, enclosed safe places. The "safe room technique" described by Helen Watkins (see Chapter 11 in this volume and J. G. Watkins, 1992a, p. 249) owes its success to the desire to return to the womb and live in an environmentally perfectly safe existence. The process of birth is a violent detachment from that environment, which once met all of our needs (Rank, 1952). Birth then represents perhaps the greatest trauma of life. We need not argue this point or Rank's conclusion in order to recognize that when the therapist hypnotically talks about a "soft, warm, space with the most beautiful feelings of comfort and peace," he or she is clearly trying to encourage hypnotic regression through revivification of unconscious "somatic memories" related to the period prior to birth.

The practitioner may suggest that in entering hypnosis, the participant will experience great feelings of omnipotence. Thus, the child in the dental chair is asked to close his or her eyes, to picture a television screen, and to imagine watching some cartoon figure, perhaps Mighty Mouse, that little character who is so successful in overpowering the great cat, dog, or other animal representation of parent figures. Reliving the exploits of Superman or Superwoman helps tap into the child's needs for power. The widespread need of children to acquire omnipotence is reflected in the popularity of the Harry Potter books. Various menacing entities (substitute parents) are thwarted by Harry through magic (wizardry). Child readers identify with Harry (Rowling, 2005). The patient's fantasy wish-life is stimulated to aid in getting a regression into hypnosis. Sensations from the dentist's drill or otherwise unpleasant dental probing can become completely dissociated (Smith, A. Barabasz, & M. Barabasz, 1996).

In the initiation of such fantasies, the pictorial descriptive powers of the hypnotist should be fully utilized. This means vivid description, attention to minute details within the images, the allowance of time for involvement, and the willingness to modify the fantasy as directed by the participant. The more we understand the motivational needs of our patient, the more skillful we become in flexibly adapting our induction techniques to different individuals. In some cases, such as the little dental patient, we may expect that his or her need for omnipotence and desire to best his or her elders represent a part of a fantasy life. This is characteristic of almost every child, as well as of the behaviors that we sometimes see in adult borderline personality disorder patients, when they engage in destructive teenager-like rebellions against the very people who have their best interests at heart. Reik (1948) pointed out we must rely on our knowledge derived from interview contacts with the patient and the degree of sensitivity for less-obvious communications to which we have learned to condition our own "third ear."

The Highly Resistant Patient

Contrary to the extravagant claims of some practitioners, the research and clinical practice of most hypnotherapists clearly demonstrate that not all patients can be hypnotized (E. R. Hilgard, 1962, 1992). Even the famous Milton Erickson admitted he was unable to elicit even a single genuine (vs. role-played) hypnotic response, despite a weeklong effort with subjects in Hilgard's Stanford University Laboratory who had been identified as nonhypnotizable using the Stanford Scales (see Barabasz & Watkins, 2005, chapter 4, pp. 89–120) (personal communication to A.F.B. from E. R. Hilgard, 1990; see also E. R. Hilgard, 1979).

Hypnotizability is about as inherited as IQ (E. R. Hilgard, 1979), and unless clever sensory restriction techniques are employed (A. Barabasz, 1982), it is an extremely stable trait over time (E. R. Hilgard, 1965). Nonetheless, skills, experience, and a thorough understanding facilitating close communication with the patient can dramatically increase the number of participants who can respond well to hypnosis even though initially appearing to be highly resistant or lacking in hypnotic talent.

Much of Barabasz & Watkins (2005), was devoted to the conditions that can be set to greatly improve the rate of successful inductions. Nevertheless, every practitioner will be confronted at times with individuals seeking hypnotherapy who appear to be quite refractory to practically every approach and to every hypnotherapist. There are, in fact, some "professional patients" who make the rounds of one therapist after another, ostensibly seeking that one clinician who will be successful, but in reality their unconscious motivation is to prove that no one can hypnotize them. They believe they simply cannot be hypnotized, and as the data from decades of research from Ernest Hilgard's (1979) lab has shown, this may be the case. However, many patients may have hypnotic capacity but unconsciously perceive hypnosis as a battle of wills and want to demonstrate over and over again that they can defeat every practitioner (J. G. Watkins, 1963).

The initial approach of such patients is frequently somewhat as follows: "Doctor, I have been to Doctor A, and he said he couldn't hypnotize me. Then I went to Doctor B, and he couldn't hypnotize me. Doctor C tried but he failed too. But Doctor, I can only be cured if hypnosis is used as part of my treatment. I know you can hypnotize. I have heard of you, and you are recommended." Then they reel off the names of a number of well-known hypnotherapists whom they have already consulted. One often notices that they seem more preoccupied with the renown of the doctors whom they claim failed than their suffering from their reported symptoms. They stoutly maintain that their only motivation is to be "cured" at last.

Such is a common trap designed to ensnare more therapists and enlarge the patient's current collection of symbolic scalps. If one accepts the challenge, one will soon find one's own name added to the list when the patient consults the next practitioner. Perhaps such patients should be rejected at once. And indeed, they often mention clinicians who, after hearing their story, refuse to accept them. As taught in Barabasz & Watkins (2005) chapter on hypnotizability (pp. 89–120), prehypnotic testing and formal hypnotic testing can play an important role in setting the stage for a success where others have failed. Let us recognize that narcissism is not a characteristic lacking among many of us who practice hypnotherapy. It is quite human to wish to succeed where one's respected colleagues have failed. We are ripe for the trap. Accordingly, such patients can usually find more and more therapists who are willing to try.

Let us put cynicism aside. Here we are being confronted with a person who apparently has genuine symptoms and who is seeking our help via the skill that we are reputed to possess. Let us recognize that under all the passive-aggressiveness and need to dominate, there is a struggling human being who unconsciously has pathological feelings of inferiority and is locked into a neurotic obsession to overcome therapists (who are often parent figures in transference). It is difficult for the sincere practitioner to refuse to at least try rather than turn the patient down from the onset.

Let us proceed with the recognition of what is going on and the knowledge that we are being seduced into playing the patient's game. Is there a way that we might get through a patient's defenses, overcome the resistance, and achieve a successful outcome for the patient? Practitioners who have secured some national recognition are more frequently accosted by such individuals, and the more you are known (through publications, national recognition, or even local repute), the more likely you will be approached. The patient's ego is fed by "knocking off" big names in the field. He or she can then brag about their failures to their next victim therapist.

Illustrative of this situation is the following case, for which we provide many techniques and considerations that may be brought up in trying to deal with such an individual. J.G.W. was contacted by a man from a distant city in Canada over a period of several months. The patient stated that he wanted a therapist who was a hypnoanalyst and who would treat him by "regression," which he "knew" was the key to his problems. He had seen quite a host of hypnotherapists and psychoanalysts and reeled off a virtual who's who in the field. Moreover, he had read volumes about all the great masters of analytic therapy including Freud, Jung, Reich, Reik, Kohut, Hartmann, and so on, not to mention practitioners outside of the analytic realm including those of cognitive-behavior therapy, reality therapy, Gestalt therapy, Rogersian therapy, and transactional analysis.

The man was a mild, soft-speaking individual, outwardly friendly and willing to cooperate. After describing his symptoms, which did not appear to be so severe as to affect his work or his normal living activities, he launched into an hour of recounting the failures of all the practitioners he had consulted. They were "not competent" and could not hypnotize him; they were failures. One of them, whom he claimed had hypnotized him, did not have psychoanalytic training, and he "needed hypnoanalysis"; others were too permissive, not authoritarian enough, or simply didn't seem to know what they were doing. He talked incessantly, hardly ever stopping. When asked questions, he would interrupt in the middle of them and launch onto digressions, which avoided answering the question. The greatest of difficulty was in obtaining information about his early childhood, his parents, and his social relationships. He avoided those areas almost completely despite repeated questioning. There was an obsessive avoidance of anything about his personal life, only a continuous recounting of the failures of the hypnotherapists. He was daring J.G.W to try, just try to hypnotize him.

Drawing from our knowledge of Reich's (1949) contributions to character analysis, let us think about what flaws there might be in this patient's defensive armor, what motivations might move him to become so involved in hypnosis rather than to seek other people to meet his need to dominate. He even complained about the chair he was sitting in. A few seconds after being asked to concentrate on his watch, because he claimed he had once been hypnotized that way by a general practitioner (generally a successful tactic), he would shake his head, break off, and declare that "it" isn't working.

Now, this suggests a number of possible tactical options. First, inquire as to what all the others have done so that you can avoid doing the same thing, if you haven't already done so. Such an approach used by you must be different and one for which the patient is not prepared. Normally, of course, it is wise to use a technique that a patient has indicated has worked with another practitioner. This is not the case with such patients. Next, draw from the more rapid techniques discussed in Barabasz & Watkins (2005) and use a quick induction, because if it is slow, the patient will have time to adapt defenses accordingly. Because of the severity of the resistance, one might also consider whether he is defending himself against a possible psychotic break if he should lose control. This would contraindicate the use of hypnosis. However, there were a number of possible positive indicators in his speech and mannerisms, such as bulging eyes, fixed stare, and slight neologisms. If fear is the primary motivation, one's manner will be different than if power needs are the prime and underlying force. J.G.W. judged both were present in this case. The patient, of course, loudly denied having any fear of entering hypnosis.

Economic motives were also possible, in which case the fee might be excessively high to see if he would be willing to invest in the treatment, or excessively low to counteract the claim that "all the doctors want from you is your money." One might even offer that if the treatment is successful, the fee will be substantially reduced. Many of these fee tactics are complicated by the 21st-century emphasis on requiring that therapists provide detailed and legalistic disclosure statements prior to treatment. Such statements, often by law, require carefully outlined fee structures. Nonetheless, the patient's needs must take prominence if we are to act as ethical practitioners. This patient had already spent thousands of dollars traveling around to dozens and dozens of practitioners, yet he claimed he could not afford any long-term treatment such as psychoanalysis. What was essential to him was the "quick fix."

Varying the technique and the therapist's manner seemed to have no differential effect. The patient's response remained the same. He would break off from any concentrated attention in a matter of moments, shake his head, and reiterate, "It isn't working." Sometimes the "opposed-hand levitation" approach (see Barabasz & Watkins, 2005, pp. 162 and 164–165, for details on how to apply this technique) is effective. It was not effective in this case. When J.G.W was most authoritative, the patient claimed that he was not authoritative enough. Using a "rehearsal method," (Barabasz & Watkins, 2005, pp. 171, 174–175) the patient was asked to relive the experience with the general practitioner. He went into regression almost immediately and began sobbing and grimacing, but after a moment he spontaneously emerged, smiled, and denied the reality of the experience, claiming, "I was only demonstrating to you what I did with Dr. M."

This is a remarkable switch in ego states (see Chapter 10 in the present volume and J. G. Watkins & H. H. Watkins, 1997). Sometimes one can appeal to a frightened little-boy need for control ego state, which underlies such passive-aggressiveness. Yet, here a change to a softer manner met with the same stubborn resistance. Under no circumstance was the patient willing to change.

Changes of manner or techniques, analytic probing (for possible sources of conflict and hurt in the patient's life), efforts at sensory underlying needs, and attempts to empathize all met with a stone wall. It was then hoped that confrontation and direct interpretation of resistance might reach the patient. J.G.W. pointed out the patient's strong underlying need to sabotage treatment, the satisfactions received from besting every practitioner, the repetitive searching for an ideal therapist that no one could meet. When you do this, do it in a way that the maladaptive behavior is interpreted, but the self or person of the patient is not rejected or scorned. Accepting the patient does not mean accepting their maladaptive behaviors. Unfortunately, some patients and therapists alike misunderstand this critical difference. Yet even in this case, the fear of entering trance, the fear of losing control, and the need to triumph over the therapist were too great. Only denial and continued resistance appeared. It was essential to establish a trusting relationship, but it was just not available. The patient continued to demand a quick cure by hypnotic regression. He was completely unwilling to spend a long time at it, just enough time to make the attempt and proclaim failure.

Such resistance is based on transference, possibly the need to defeat a parent figure. J.G.W.'s patient would not talk about his parents. He saw it as none of my business. Each time a question about them was asked, within 5 seconds or so he was no longer discussing his parents, but describing in technical jargon some psychoanalytic theory that he had read. He was willing to talk all about therapy, but not to experience it. A logical therapeutic tactic was to continue with repeated questions such as, "Let's talk about you, your unhappiness, and your problems, not what Freud once wrote." However, all these were met with denial and digressions. The patient was a pathological rock of defensive postures.

When it became evident that J.G.W. probably could not help him with any real, underlying problems, it was decided to terminate the consultations. Yet, showing his ambivalence about seeking and then denying treatment, the patient did not want to leave. He took a long time going to the door, and even called later in the day to know if there was a recommendation to yet another hypnotherapist. This later reaction showed a remustering of his defenses, which were obviously evoked to emphasize even further his "victory." J.G.W. declined the invitation to burden others with this case (many of whom he had already contacted) and repeated his firm conviction that he could only be helped when he faced the fact that his need to vanquish therapists was greater than his desire for treatment. He was wished well, and the departure was on a friendly note.

The point we are trying to make here is that we cannot always be successful no matter how we try using every bit of technique, skill, and relationship we can muster. However, in this case, we see a wide variety of approaches that had been found to be effective on numerous other occasions, techniques that when they are tried, usually can open the door for the patient but may not always work. It is a trial-and-error process. They are reviewed here in the case presented above because we often learn more from our failures than our successes, even though it would have been pleasant to have finished this chapter with a brilliant triumph.

Terminating Hypnosis

Given that hypnosis is a form of regression, then its termination means a return to reality, maturity, and the demands of the present. Just as the physicist must be aware of both centrifugal and centripetal forces, so must the effective hypnotherapist consider both the regressive and progressive needs of the participant. In one sense, the termination of each trance is a return to maturity, a rebirth. The regression itself has truly been "in the service of the ego," not a permanent state. Hypnosis, by itself, can have restorative characteristics even when there is no deliberate therapeutic goal in mind (J. G. Watkins, 1963).

Participants need reassurance upon emerging from an emotionally moving hypnotic experience. They fear that maybe they "won't come out of it," despite the fact that this misconception was debunked prior to their first hypnotic experience. Despite the therapist's own personal limitations, he or she stands on the side of the patient's ego, of reality, and of mature adjustment. The therapist's excursions into the hypnotic regression are limited, purposeful, and only for the benefit of the patient and must be concluded at some point. You, as the therapist, will do well to see that the patient understands this quite clearly, whether it is communicated directly or by implication.

Bringing the patient back from the hypnotic state is a process that requires care. Be sure to respect the participant's regressive needs. The therapist must take time and not demand that the patient make an instant response to the dehypnotizing suggestions. If the regression has been deep, that is not a time to use the snapping of fingers and the change to a bright voice of "Wide awake, alert, and refreshed!" Rather, the sudden return of the ego awareness to the deeply hypnotized patient can, in some cases, be traumatic. The patient may not be ready to face the world again quite so immediately, nor to face some of the unconscious material about which he or she was becoming aware. It is essential that we as therapists protect the patient's ego and not submit it to a sudden battery of external or internal stimuli until the patient is ready. Take your time. Progress at the patient's rate of returning to the reality situation of the nonhypnotic state when a deep hypnotic experience has been particularly moving.

The patient sometimes transmits his or her reluctance to leave the comfortable, regressed state. He or she is simply not ready to return to unpleasant realities of life. Some patients simply stay in hypnosis or may temporarily go deeper in spite of efforts to bring them back into a full, normal, alert waking state. The specific dynamics between the therapist and the patient at the time may also play a role, and in spite of hypnotic suggestions for returning to a state of alertness, the patient may go deeper and deeper. Do not panic. Merely convey to the patient an understanding of his or her enjoyment of the present blissful condition and the wish to remain there a bit longer. Either permit the patient to emerge "when you are ready and at your own speed," or in a very kindly manner suggest he or she can return to this pleasurable state "the next time" when he or she can reexperience and understand better the sensations he or she is enjoying at the moment. Under no circumstances should the therapist react as if this was some sort of a challenge, even though it may so represent. If such a "challenge" continues, it may be essential to understand and interpret its meaning to the patient. However, this is seldom necessary. If told to awaken when ready, and then left to him- or herself, the patient usually soon becomes alert.

The issue of a challenge is interesting and depends on the specific dynamics between the therapist and patient that may exist at the present time. A.F.B. was telephoned by a panic-strickened vice principal of a local high school. It seems that a drama teacher had hypnotized one of his students and "could not bring her out of it no matter how hard he tried." I reassured the vice principal, informing him that participants can seldom stay in self-hypnosis for any length of time if left to themselves. As Erika Fromm (2001, personal communication to A.F.B.) noted, even the very best and deepest subjects in our Chicago paradigm study were only able to stay in a state of what they perceived as self-hypnosis for as much as a half hour. The vice principal remained panic-strickened and insisted that the teacher "had already done all things, and that the girl was unresponsive."

I agreed to visit the high school immediately. Upon my arrival, I found a large number of students and teachers gathered around the girl and the drama teacher, who was now sweating profusely. He was red in the face and was blowing at the girl's closed eyes, exclaiming, "Wide awake, alert now!" But she was unresponsive.

I asked the crowd to disperse and also the teacher to leave. The vice principal remained, as I had asked, to observe at some distance. My interaction merely consisted of saying that I was a doctor who had been asked to visit and that "I enjoyed hypnosis as much as you must be doing right now." I also mentioned, in almost a passing tone, that of course everyone knows it is impossible to stay in a state of self-hypnosis for any more than a few minutes. After that, it is nothing more than a form of regular relaxation or an act. I then asked the subject to enjoy those pleasant feelings a bit longer, and "when you are ready, your eyes will know exactly when to open, and you will feel wide awake, alert, calm, reassured that you will never hear about this from anyone in the school administration." Within moments, the girl opened her eyes, smiled, and said, "That was just fine, thank you."

What were the actual dynamics involved here? As it turns out, this 18-year-old girl had been secretly dating the drama teacher. They had had some sort of fight the night before, and she just wanted to show him that "he can't control me." The effect, at least initially, from his alerting procedure was, in all likelihood, a genuine deepening of hypnosis effect given the underlying motivations of which she was now consciously aware.

It is important to establish a full state of ego awareness upon termination of the hypnotic state before letting the patient leave the office, to perhaps drive home. Accordingly, a few minutes should be permitted at the end of the hypnotic period for interactions in the fully conscious state.

We can only aim at increasing our sensitivity, communication, and flexibility in our technique. Psychodynamics is not an exact science. Often there will be times when we are at a total loss to understand what is happening within our participant or why he or she seems so completely unresponsive to our induction attempts. But the counselor or clinician who considers the patient's conscious and unconscious motivations, and who pays close attention to his or her own feelings and their relationship with the patient, will improve their success rate. Attention to those parameters will help you develop a practice of hypnotherapy with increasing effectiveness.

Summary

Psychodynamics deals with the unconscious process that transpires between an original source or stimulus and the final overt behavior or experience. The induction of a hypnotic state is subject to these processes. The "meaning" that hypnosis has to the patient affects his or her resistance, the speed with which hypnosis can be entered, and its depth. The sophisticated hypnoanalyst will take all of these factors into account while inducing hypnosis.

Hypnosis can be considered a state of regression. In that it is a temporary return to earlier patterns of behavior and thought, we see it as regression in service of the ego. Hypnotic regression is unlike regression in psychosis. Psychosis involves fleeing reality frequently and for long periods of time. The ego can voluntarily return out of hypnosis. There is a significant relationship between the depth of hypnosis and the amount of ego participation: The deeper the state, the less the ego is involved. The regressive process of hypnosis in the service of the ego can have a restorative effect itself on the individual.

Hypnosis has a number of special meanings to participants, such as an erotic experience, a death, an interpersonal relationship, or submission to another. It is usually influenced by transference reactions. Individuals may have highly personalized fantasies when entering or experiencing hypnosis, such as returning to the womb or perhaps possessing power. If the hypnoanalyst understands these special meanings, he or she will more likely be able to reduce resistance and have a greater likelihood of success in producing the hypnotic state. It should never be forgotten that the termination of hypnosis may also have very special psychodynamic meanings to patients. Careful observation and care should be taken in re-establishing the full state of normal ego awareness after deep hypnosis.

4

Hypnodiagnosis and Evaluation

Unlike the practice of medicine, diagnosis in psychotherapy should mean more than the attaching of a label to a disease syndrome. Hypnodiagnostic techniques enable us to uncover further information about a patient to permit a more in-depth understanding. This makes it possible to meet the criteria specified in the *Psychodynamic diagnostic manual* (PDM) as well as the *Diagnostic statistical manual of mental disorders* (DSM-IVTR, 2000). This evaluation may precede the application of treatment techniques, but more often it is an ongoing process that continually updates our comprehension of the disorder. We are concerned with ways of evaluating the patient that involve hypnosis. Behaviors included are those elicited during the hypnotic state and its induction, and specialized psychological maneuvers designed to explore the experiential world of our patient. Every single reaction of the patient while in or entering hypnosis has special meaning. The sensitive therapist notes these responses and infers from them significance in the emerging picture of his or her areas of functioning as well as problems.

For example, a slight frown appears on the patient's face during an induction. We might wonder if something is troubling to them. Perhaps we have said or done something that is upsetting, and thus the frown is a manifestation of the patient's resistance. If the induction then proceeds very slowly, or is unsuccessful, the question arises as to just what it was that caused such a reaction. Alternatively, a sudden descent into a deep hypnosis during a fantasy of smooth feeling on the skin may indicate skin eroticism. We have just uncovered a useful clue. Tactile hypnotic suggestions may well be more effective in deepening this state than those that describe lulling sounds. These images may also be related to unconscious conflicts such as are manifested by neurodermatitis or some other skin disorders. At all times, we try to find out what images, what areas of the body, and what needs are most significant to our patient. All of these provide indicants or at least clues as to how we should couch our inductions and therapeutic stratagems.

Negative or affirmative noddings of the head, however slight, can tell us whether we are using effective hypnotic suggestions or not. These may be very subtle. It is virtually impossible for therapists who are tied to fixed protocols and reading from scripts to notice minor shifts in posture, like leaning forward, sitting back stiffly, subtle tensions, relaxations, and nearly inaudible sighs. These all can communicate much to the observing clinician. Reactions to alterations in the voice of the hypnotist, when he or she changes from a strong, forceful manner to a gentle one, may also tell us much about the patient's desires and points of resistance. Perspiring, rubbing of the head, or wringing of the hands may let us know that some inner conflict has been precipitated, even though nothing other than an induction has been attempted. The sources of the disturbance should be determined before further deepening of the hypnotic state. Deepening should be avoided until such understandings have been reached.

Experimental research by E. R. Hilgard and Tart (1966) demonstrated variations in hypnotic trance depth. As explained in Barabasz & Watkins (2005) in the chapter on hypnotizability, they found that asking the subject to report numbers corresponding to the level of depth could be used as an indicant of trance change throughout a hypnotic process. But why does trance depth vary? Variations in trance depth, such as a sudden emerging from hypnosis, or rapid sinking from a constant, light state into a deep one, often occurs as a result of contact with new, conflictual material. Inquiries about the sources and meanings of these reactions are more useful to the hypno-therapeutic process than simple indicants of trance depth. The inquiries can be made directly to the patient without removing the hypnotic state. In fact, it is frequently more fruitful to make such inquiries while a patient is in a light to moderate level of hypnotic responding. Immediately after the patient has returned to the waking state and fully dehypnotized, he or she can also be queried. However, as alluded to earlier, waking states are more likely to give rise to defensive maneuvers, postures, and reactions.

It is particularly important to observe the manner displayed by patients when they are in hypnosis. Some patients are relaxed, passive, and quiet. Frequently, they make a response only upon being initiated to do so by the therapist. Yet others can be very active, talking and acting as if they were almost in a fully conscious condition. The late Helen Watkins (personal communication to A.F.B., 2001) found such an active talking state the most productive in revealing keys to inner conflicts. Some patients display their resistance by a slowing in their responses. Others, through a rapid associating on many topics, reveal they are afraid of losing control. The effective hypno-therapist recognizes these cues and incorporates them into the inductions and hypnotherapeutic process. By recognizing the patient's needs and meeting as many of these as possible, we lower resistance, intensify the therapeutic rela-tionship, and facilitate the treatment process and outcome.

A common question of beginners to the field of hypnotherapy, who may otherwise be highly experienced counselors or clinicians, upon completion of an introductory hypnosis workshop is, "Just what should I do in my first hypnotic session?" Our reply frequently is, "Do within the hypnotic state whatever you have been accustomed to doing without hypnosis. If you are an analyst, have your patients free associate, as they have done before, but hypnotize them first. If you are a person-centered counselor, conduct your treatment sessions as you usually do them. Reflect feelings to the client, use incomplete thoughts, etc., but when he or she is in hypnosis. If you are a cognitive-behavioral therapist, reframe the patient's thinking, but hypnotize them first. If you are a strict behaviorist involved in treating a phobia, "administer under hypnosis the desensitization process your patient will likely already be in" (Wolpe & Lazarus, 1966). Use the hypnotic state to speed the process by employing hypnotic suggestions, so that the next-to-be-visualized item on the hierarchy will be met with greater relaxation, and so on (A. Barabasz, 1977; Woody, 1973). The practicing clinician who has learned to induce hypnosis can make the transition from psychotherapist to hypnotherapist most easily by simply continuing the techniques to which he or she has become accustomed and the ones that reflect his or her years of training and expertise, but do so within the hypnotic modality. Even the intake interview can be conducted after the induction of hypnosis.

Interviewing in Hypnosis

The typical case history can take on greater richness and clues to treatment plans when conducted in the hypnotic context. This is the simplest hypnotic uncovering method. Place the patient into hypnosis before beginning the intake. Ask the usual questions relating to the patient's symptoms, disorder, social history, previous prior treatments, relationships, job, and living situation. Inquiries into childhood, interaction with family members, and early illnesses, as well as adjustment in school and sexual experiences, can follow. It is essentially like any other intake interview, except that the patient is in a state of hypnosis. The interviewer who has been conducting standard nonhypnotic intake interviews for years is usually astonished to find superior recall and a greater richness in detail when hypnosis is used. Reconstructions of memory of events reported in the nonhypnotic state, perhaps in a sentence or two, may well become expanded into several paragraphs, and occasionally they will take on a "reliving" quality when elicited in hypnosis. The recollection, of course, may not be factually accurate. However, what has been reconstructed often provides the keys to therapeutic intervention, keys that might not otherwise have been revealed until many sessions had been conducted. The enhanced ability to uncover material, removed at least to some degree from normal awareness, often provides information that might not otherwise have been uncovered in the early stages of therapy.

The flow of reconstructed memories is facilitated. Not only is the number of recollections substantially increased, but various modifications of questioning technique are also possible within the hypnotic context. For example, one might inquire into the state of mind of a patient at the time when he left his family to volunteer for military service as follows: "You are 18 years old; you feel it is time to prove to your parents; you are a man. You enlisted in the Army. You are saying goodbye to your family. You are talking to your father to let him know how you feel about military service. What are you saying to him?" This is regression, inducing him to experience the 18-year-old period as if it were in the "here-and-now." The present tense is used to reinforce the regression while asking questions.

Including information about the patient's relationships with friends when he or she was a child can be particularly helpful. You could phrase the inquiry as follows: "You are 9 years old and talking to your best friend. Who is your best friend? O.K., you are talking to Sue now, and what is happening?" You can then take the role of Sue and ask the kinds of questions a 9-year-old best friend/companion would ask while interacting with the regressed patient. The patient may then reveal to "Sue" many things she would not discuss with parents or with a stranger. Another way to do this might be to frame the interaction psychodramatically, such as: "Sue, my mother says I gotta clean the house Saturday. How do you think we can get her to let me off, so that we can go over to Sidney's house and use her new makeup kit?" The conversation between "Sue" and the patient might tell the therapist much about the ways in which the patient as a child interacted with and manipulated her parents and other children.

When using hypnosis with very young children seen for therapy because of trauma, A.F.B. found that an imaginary friend or a hand puppet can often serve the same purpose as discussed above. Using the hand puppet to break through might be viewed from an object-relations conceptualization (Winnicott, 1965), which explains that the child's development from a completely narcissistic self-view of the environment to the establishing of object perspectives and relations with others can be facilitated by an intermediate interaction with a transitional object (e.g., a bunny, teddy bear, "security blanket"). The object provides a barrier protecting the child from external contact. But it is a barrier that is real, one that is not hallucinated, and one over which the patient has complete control (Barabasz & Christensen, 2007; Christensen & Barabasz, 2007).

The importance of this intermediate step is especially effective in interactions with psychotic patients (Baker, 1981). In the interview, the patient's child-like regressive states can be contacted and activated when they are provided with such a transitional object, which is like one he or she may have possessed when he or she was a child. There will be an immediate effect in diminishing fear of disclosure. It can represent an internal hurt child that the patient holds in the therapy office, an object the patient can speak to and give reassurance or whatever positive messages are pertinent. A cuddly object, of course, is a representation of part of that inner world and much less threatening than attempting to address that part of the patient's regressed state directly. There is less threat in speaking to the object, rather than directly to the patient.

Such an object gives distance when emotional distance is necessary and when the patient's child state has been reluctant to reveal experiences of a traumatic nature because of the early threats or actual reprisals. Speak to the object, perhaps a teddy bear or bunny; simply tell it that it's O.K. to reveal the pain during a dream that "it" is having. Your goal is to keep the entire procedure within the control of the patient. Once the initial mandatory intake questions are concluded, the follow-ups can be done in an entirely Rogersian nondirective manner, rather than attempting to coerce the patient to reveal things that he or she might otherwise may be unable to talk about.

Case history interviews are simply ways of expanding into a number of different dimensions and are made possible because of the focusing effect of hypnosis and its ability to permit role-taking under circumstances that would elicit rejection if attempted in the conscious state. Many individuals have engaged in sexual or aggressive behavior when under the influence of alcohol, when they have not done so at other times. The altered state of consciousness provided by alcohol offers an excuse for the denial of responsibility. So also may people reveal details of their life, while in hypnosis, which they would normally conceal. By telling it in hypnosis, they can disclaim responsibility and even subsequently deny they said it through actual or claimed hypnotic amnesia. Hypnosis, like many other psychological defenses, provides the opportunity both to reveal and conceal. Using hypnosis in such a defensive manner is normal and should not be confused with the pathological use of such denials and disclaimers by alert individuals about what should be accurate memories of significant events.

What can be elicited in the hypnosis interview may be reconstructed memory material that the patient is not yet ready to confront and understand consciously. The added knowledge, for the time being, must remain the possession of the therapist. However, this comprehension can help the counselor or clinician plan his or her therapeutic tactics more effectively, even if the new understandings cannot be shared at that time with the patient.

While at a university counseling center, a student came to J.G.W., ostensibly in need of advice concerning her educational and vocational future. For 30 minutes, various possibilities were discussed. Almost as an afterthought, I hypnotized her, whereupon she began describing a tangled situation in which she was involved in her hall of residence. She had been "recruited" into a small lesbian clique from which she wanted to extricate herself, but could not seem to find either the courage or the method to achieve this. In hypnosis, this was discussed at length. Various possible options occurred to her in the nondirective hypnotic intervention that might help her leave the group without making any enemies. On emerging from hypnosis, she manifested an apparent amnesia for the discussion about lesbianism. It was as if it never happened, a normal, if not typical, posthypnotic reaction.

During the next few sessions in the counseling center, each interview was conducted at two levels: first in the conscious state about educational and vocational matters and second in hypnosis about her relationships with the lesbian group. Eight sessions later, she terminated counseling, having satisfactorily resolved her problem with the lesbian group. She was able to form new attachments without antagonizing her former friends. At no time did she discuss the expression of her lesbian behaviors or the problems with guilt over having joined the group out of needs for attachment, companionship, and friendship in the conscious state. That entire situation was handled within the hypnotic context. She thanked me for this help and left, either amnesic of the hypnotic discussions, or without a loss of face by having been confronted with them in the nonhypnotic state. The simple interview, at first diagnostic, and later combined with nondirective (person-centered) counseling, was conducted within the hypnotic context, but without any complex hypnotherapeutic interventions. There was a kind of "unspoken hypnotic contract" between the patient and me, and she would have considered it a breach of confidentiality if I had ever brought up references to the lesbian problem when she was not hypnotized. By preserving her right to dissociate confidentially within the hypnotic context, I was able to show respect for her needs while facilitating her willingness to reveal the problem and resolve it successfully. Other examples of the use of hypnosis to facilitate the counseling process, particularly in university counseling center, without the need for deep psychotherapeutic work appear in *Hypnocounseling: An Eclectic Bridge between Milton Erickson and Carl Rogers* by Hugh Gunnison (2004) and J. G. Watkins (1987).

The "In and Out" Technique

As foreshadowed in the case presented above, data obtained in hypnosis may differ somewhat from the replies elicited outside of the hypnotic context. A comparison of the two can sometimes reveal areas of conflict. It is reasonable to assume that the memory material reconstructed in hypnosis may be that which had come under greater defense needs and hence not verbalized in the fully conscious condition. If a patient describes a family situation in hypnosis and then mentions the presence or role of a sister, when previously outside of hypnosis, he or she had discussed the same situation but neglected to point out her impact, one might hypothesize that there is something conflictual about this sister, such that it required repression in conscious recall. As discussed earlier, one of the characteristics of hypnosis is a reduction in criticality, thus permitting previously unacceptable material to be verbalized, material that might otherwise take years to uncover at conscious or merely relaxed levels.

The "in and out" technique allows us to interview simultaneously at two different levels, outside of hypnosis and within the hypnotic context (see fractionation in J. G. Watkins, 1987, pp. 171–172). Let us assume that you are working with a patient who has at least near average or better hypnotizability and there has been adequate hypnotherapeutic experience to establish that the patient will respond to a rapid induction technique. Given those generally met prerequisites, the following posthypnotic suggestions can be administered: "When I tap my pencil on the table like this [pencil is tapped on the table], you will go immediately into hypnosis, a deep, deep hypnotic state, but you will always hear me clearly, no matter how deeply you decide to go. When I tap twice you will at once wake up and become very calm and alert."

The patient is then brought out of hypnosis, and the "in and out" interview might continue in the following manner: "Well, I intended to study for the final exam on Thursday evening. However, a friend of mine came over to discuss a problem with me, and I didn't study. I could have cut him off, but I didn't. By the time he left, I was too tired to study. I flunked the test, and I felt angry at him for ruining my A in that class."

(Pencil is tapped and patient enters hypnosis). "Tell me about that time when you said you received a failing grade in an examination."

"Well, I intended to study for the final exam on Thursday evening. However, a friend of mine came over to discuss a problem with me, and I didn't feel I should cut him off. I was too tired to study by the time he left. I was also angry at him for spoiling my grade in that class. I guess, though, I also felt a little guilty and responsible. I could have told him I had to study and asked him to come over the next day, but somehow I didn't. Maybe a part of me didn't really want to study."

(Pencil tapped twice. Patient emerges from hypnosis). "Tell me about that time when you got a failing grade in an examination."

The patient repeats his first description of the situation again, omitting the part about feeling responsible and guilty at his failure to postpone the meeting with his friend.

What is happening here is that at a conscious level, he blames his friend for the bad grade. Underneath, he recognizes that he was at least partially responsible, but he represses this feeling of personal guilt and fails to take responsibility for his failing the examination, so he reports it only while in hypnosis. By using several of such "in and out" maneuvers, we become more aware of his defenses and resistances and can, therefore, plan our therapeutic strategy.

Beyond its ability to potentiate hypnotic suggestions, perhaps the most important attribute of hypnosis is the facility with which it permits the crossing of experiential time lines. Within the hypnotic modality, reconstruction of memory material is more easily obtained, and reliving experiences activated. Always bear in mind that such reliving experiences do not necessarily represent what actually happened and, in fact, are unlikely to do so. However, veridicality of the reconstructed memory has little, if anything, to do with the goals of therapy. The issue is that what is reconstructed is what is representative of the patient's conflicts. The unresolved living problems may be reinitiated so that renewed attempts at their solution become feasible with the help of the therapist and with the patient's skills of greater maturity and more recent understandings. Satisfaction of unfilled needs and closure of uncompleted Gestalts become possible when the reconstructed memories of these earlier events are reactivated in the here-and-now hypnotherapeutic context.

All of this is precisely what psychoanalysis intends to accomplish via transference reactions. Our point is that hypnosis provides a medium where we need not always wait until the recall and revivification of these earlier events spontaneously arise. Within the intensive hypnotic relationship, we can direct and control the regressive process, or at least we can bring it under more control than would be the case in the fully conscious state. Regressions and transference reactions are expedited in classical psychoanalysis simply because the patient is lying on the couch and is more often than not in a spontaneously induced hypnoidal or light hypnotic state. In hypnoanalysis, we add more therapist involvement to this factor, bringing the strength of a therapist's ego in combination with that of the patient, so that the patient is freed, or at least somewhat more freed, to engage in the reconstruction and revivification of earlier events that would otherwise be so challenging as to precipitate elaborate defensive maneuvers. Hypnosis only adds a new dimension to the uncovering and reintegrating processes. Hypnosis does not change either the goals or the conceptualizations of psychoanalytic therapy.

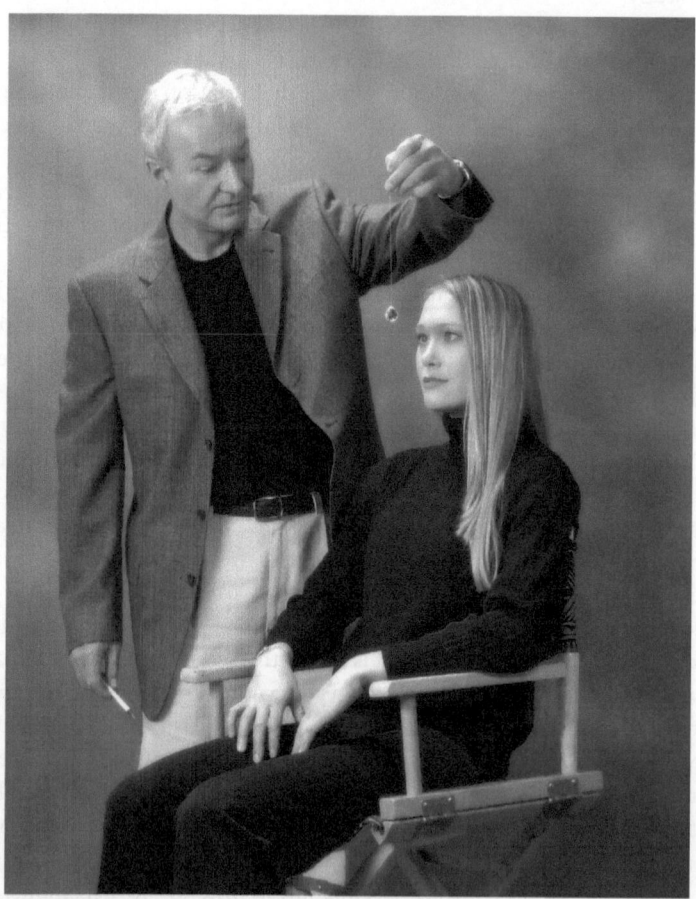

Figure 4.1 Arreed Barabasz and Ciara Christensen demonstrate the "in and out induction."

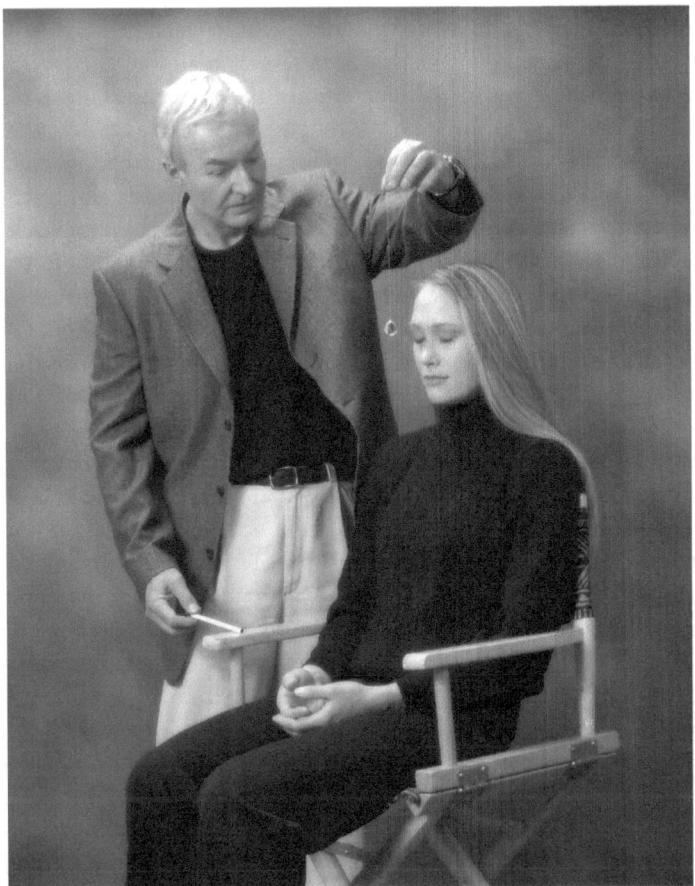

Figure 4.2 Eyes close as the hypnotic state is facilitated.

Just as in psychoanalysis, the hypnoanalytic uncovering of early behaviors and experiences is not generally on an "either-or" basis. Rather, it is more like a continuum in the sense that one can elicit small bits and pieces of reconstructed yesteryear material as verbalized memories and then hopefully move on into more genuine reliving experiences, which involve full emotional, as well as intellectual and behavioral, responses. Regression and hypermnesia are the two basic methods we use for uncovering.

Regression and Hypermnesia

As demonstrated empirically and reviewed by Fligstein, A. Barabasz, M. Barabasz, Trevisan, & Warner (1998), hypnosis facilitates the ability of individuals to recall many situations in far greater detail than would be possible without hypnosis. Under conscious recollection, a patient might describe an instance involving a schoolyard fight with a bully, perhaps when he or she was 6 or 7 years old. The incident may be related in less than a minute. However, when asked to describe the same incident within the hypnotic context, he or she launches into a vivid picturization of the situation, such as the circumstances under which the conflict began, the clothing worn by the opponent, the various blows landed, the outcome, the intervention of friends and teachers, the reactions of parents later at home, and so on. What had been told in less than a minute consciously and unemotionally involves perhaps 10 or more minutes of descriptive details when reconstructed in the hypnotic context. Accuracy of recall is not the issue! The issue is that whatever was encoded about that event is recalled as meaningful to the patient and may hold keys to the resolution of underlying conflicts that remain challenges.

It is important to recognize that the human brain does not have some sort of flawless digital video or audio recorder built in. Many memory traces are simply lost and truly forgotten, but others are repressed and can easily be released through hypnosis. It is extremely important, in our view, that memory reconstruction procedures in hypnosis must be very carefully conducted in as nondirective a manner as possible to facilitate the recall of accurate clues to what the patient has encoded as "memory," rather than manufacturing or fabricating new things by hypnotic suggestion that the patient weaves into what might be presented as recollections. Always bear in mind that patients readily enact unusual roles when asked to do so in hypnosis, and that is not the goal when we are attempting to access repressed material. We wish to identify truly repressed material and not the manufactured guesses of the therapist. Be humble, be open, and avoid making direct suggestions about anything specific that you think may be important. Remain nondirective in your questioning. Reflect what the patient is saying, rather than suggest to the patient what you hypothesize might be important.

The amount of recall elicited will be the product of many factors. The hypnotizability of the patient is critical, as is the depth of trance, yet the relationship with the therapist is paramount. The therapist's skill in working in the hypnotic modality is the key to making all of this work properly and to the patient's maximal benefit. We cannot emphasize enough that reconstructed memories elicited can be reasonably factual, but this is not the important feature. They are filtered through the perceptual and experiential systems of the individual and more likely than not have been altered in one way or another to fit underlying motivations and wishes. The patient is usually more transparent within the hypnotic context. Hypnosis is in no way a truth serum nor is the veridicality of the recalled situation really of much, if any, importance to our goals in therapy. This is also the case in conscious recall as well. A.F.B. was seeing a couple for treatment of sexual dysfunction. In his interview, the man reported, "We hardly ever have sex, perhaps once a week, usually on a weekend." She reported, "We have sex all the time, every weekend!" Indeed, hypnosis has no special ability to create new filters or alter recollections any more than any other form of recall.

What has been said about hypermnesia applies to regression, and even more so. By regression, we mean more than superior reconstruction of memory material. By the term *regression,* we imply a more genuine reexperiencing at the primary process level. The experience, when genuine, is accompanied by emotional, perceptual, as well as behavioral components as they were presumed to have occurred at that time when they first happened. Experimentally controlled research provides empirical evidence to show that this is neither fabrication nor mere role-playing. A. Barabasz and Christensen (2006) demonstrated that tailored hypnotic inductions involving topographic regression to primary process at the age of 5 showed that adults so regressed responded to a set of abstract figure pairs with responses that coincided closer to 5-year-olds than adults. The blind manner in which the experiment was designed, and the nature of the entirely abstract figure pair stimuli, was such that no alternative explanation to the findings could be offered. The regression to primary process was genuine at even the perceptual level.

As we will discuss in greater detail later, regression does not involve the holistic recapitulation of veridical reality, but rather is a reenactment of the person's "memory-experience" of reality. It is a subjective reality; it may or may not be an objective reality. However, symptoms are based on a patient's subjective reality, so the material uncovered has therapeutic validity. The patient experiences them as if they were occurring in the here-and-now. A women regressed to age 3 actually plays with her dolls. The adult who has recovered from earlier speech defects now stutters when regressed. The patient speaks in the first person and in the present tense when regressed: "I am afraid Mommy is going to hit me. Go away, Mommy, don't hit me."

Changes in the physical structure of the individual are obviously a result of maturation and may limit or alter primary process childhood responses obtained by hypnotic regression. For example, Orne (1951) reported "incomplete regression" in his experiment using regressed handwriting samples that were found to be different from those of the regressed adult subject but "not identical to the genuine childhood samples done at age 6." Of course, they couldn't be. Orne failed to consider the simple maturational increase in the size of the patient's hands as he or she reached adulthood. Regression is a mental process and not a physical one. The patient doesn't actually become physically smaller. Yet, within such changes, the truly regressed individual appears to revivify and repeat earlier patterns of behavior and experience.

As discussed by A. Barabasz and Christensen (2006, 2007), to be therapeutically valuable, regression need not be complete regression. It is a misconception to require that regression must be complete to be successful. The notion of completeness is also at variance with even earlier concepts of age regression where Kris, noting his statements of 1936 and 1949 (1952, p. 188), explained that "the ego regulates its own capacity to regression [degree of regression] such that the organizing functions of the ego include the function of voluntary and temporary withdrawal of cathexis." Later, Schilder and Kauders (1956, p. 96) observed that all regressions are only partial, "whereas a considerably portion of the personality maintains its normal relations with the outside world." The psychoanalytic conceptualizations of attenuation of contact with reality in hypnosis are consistently reported by a wide range of controlled laboratory experiments using EEG event-related potentials, which demonstrate the reality of the hypnotic state (A. Barabasz & Lonsdale, 1983; A. Barabasz, M. Barabasz, Jensen, Calvin, Trevisan, & Warner, 1999; A. Barabasz, 2000; D. Spiegel, Cutcomb, Ren, & Pribram, 1985; D. Spiegel, Bierre, & Rootenberg, 1989).

Regression brings a more intense and complete form of reconstructed recall and one that brings into therapeutic focus more of the patient's responding apparatus, including affective, perceptual, motoric, and experiential. Psychoanalytic transference is also a kind of regression, but through hypnotic regression we aim at and achieve a similar result. Both require much subsequent "working through," but hypnosis may permit us to arrive at that point much more quickly. Numerous experimental and clinical studies have been conducted on hypermnesia and regression over a period of several decades (As, 1962; A. Barabasz & Christensen, 2006, 2007; Baker, 1983a, 1983b, personal communication to A.F.B., 2004; Barber, 1965; A. Barabasz, M. Barabasz, Lin-Roark, Roark, Sanchez, & Christensen, 2003; Christensen & Barabasz, 2007; Cooper & London, 1973; Dhanens & Lundy, 1975; Fligstein, A. Barabasz, M. Barabasz, Trevisan, & Warner, 1998; Hose, 1930; Kleinhauz, Whorowitz, & Tobin, 1977; Nash, 1987; Nash, Johnson, & Tipton, 1979; Nash, Lynn, Stanley, Frauman, & Rhue, 1985; Orne, 1951, 1979; Udolf, 1983). Our attention here is on hypnoanalytic treatment techniques, so we will not try to review the literature in detail, but rather simply present the consensus of the research findings to date.

1. Suggestions given in the state of hypnosis for improved recall produce a significant increase in reported memories. Hypnosis alone does not bring about any such improvement.
2. The amount and accuracy of recall is related to the nature of the reconstructed memory material. Meaningful memory material, such as reports of entire incidents, are better remembered than isolated words or numbers, e.g., license plate numbers. There is little evidence for hypermnesia in the case of nonsense syllables but there is some data to the contrary (Fligstein, A. Barabasz, M. Barabasz, Trevisan, & Warner, 1998); further research is necessary.
3. Hypnosis facilitates recall of material that is anxiety-provoking. Revivification of recollections through age regression is generally superior to simple verbalizations, as in hypermnesia alone. The process of age regression is not exact. Reconstructed memory material

apparently secured from a regression to age 8 may include events that happened both earlier and later, or may represent the child's adult view of what he or she was like as an 8-year-old. Age regression can produce developmental responses unique to the age regressed, perhaps due to the facilitation of primary process. For example, an adult regressed to age 5 will identify abstract figure pairs orientation in space just as 5-year-olds do to a statistically significant, although not perfect, degree.

4. Age regression need not be complete to be genuine. The ego regulates its own capacity to regression (degree of regression).

5. Tailored hypnotic inductions show significantly greater success at achieving more "genuine" age regression experiences than "canned" inductions. It appears that such individualized induction procedures may facilitate the ego's ability to regulate its own degree of participation. The better matched personality style between therapist and participant takes advantage of the naturally occurring ego-syntonic capacities of the participant, thereby facilitating greater hypnotic responsiveness.

6. There can be a great deal of difference in the material elicited in so-called age regressions activated in the experimental laboratory and those that have been observed during psychotherapeutic sessions. Simply telling a person to go to the age of 5 is not the same as actually focusing on events and situations that are commonly known to 5-year-olds (such as being in kindergarten). Many, but not all, laboratory studies can be criticized on this basis. Regression in an intensive hypnotherapeutic interaction with a trusted therapist is not the same as performing in a laboratory with an objective and usually impersonal investigator. This might account for many of the misleading conclusions of some researchers that regression is simply "role-playing." It may indeed be merely role-playing in their laboratory situation (see J. G. Watkins, 1989).

7. Both hypermnesia and age regression are susceptible to inaccuracies and confabulations, as are renditions of conscious memories.

The data casts considerable doubt about the use of hypermnesia and regression to enhance the testimony of eyewitnesses in court (see Chapter 11 in J. G. Watkins, 1992a). However, research studies provide considerable evidence and justification for the use of age regression procedures in therapy. Hypermnesia functions best in the recall of therapeutically meaningful material, and that is precisely the kind of material we wish to secure in hypnoanalysis. The emphasis is on the meaningful, not necessarily the veridical.

Reconstructed memory material related to anxiety is likely the very best recovered. Anxiety-laden material is often that which is most fruitfully activated and is what we frequently are seeking during hypnoanalysis.

The finding that recall is better using age regression is consistent with the conclusion that genuine insight must involve motor, behavioral, affective, and perceptual participation, not merely intellectual verbalizing. The fact that we may often be securing distorted memories does not contraindicate the value of obtaining them in therapy. It is common that conflicts have their origins in distorted perceptions, and it is in the eliciting of corrective experiences that the therapist achieves the best results.

We need not subscribe to an earlier view of learning as the inscribing of experiences on a kind of digital recorder involved in the brain, hypermnesia being then simply the reactivation of such a hypothetical recording. There is indeed no such recorder capability in the human brain. Some memory traces are simply lost. However, everything that emerges is of value in the conducting of hypnoanalytic therapy, even though part is likely to be confabulated, part may be fantasized, and only part is objective and veridical. These points cannot be emphasized enough when we use hypermnesia and regression. Now the question arises about the source of the incompleteness or distortion.

To experience something, we must first perceive it. Because perception is selective, such material may never have been perceived in the first place; hence, it was never recorded in any way and cannot be reconstructed, much less recovered. Furthermore, because of personal dynamic needs, our selective perceptions may "choose" to see or hear only certain aspects of an experience. This fact alone limits the memory material and the nature of that material that can be recalled. We can't get out what was never there in the first place. Items that are cognitively dissonant with the patient's established sets of thinking, misguided as they may be, simply don't register.

When stimuli of dissonant items are so powerful that the individual cannot protect him- or herself by ignoring them, then distortion and other defense mechanisms will come into play in an attempt to eliminate or at least minimize inner conflict. These same defensive needs may operate to resist recovery by hypermnesia via regression. The recalled or re-enacted material emerges but with the distortions and confabulations produced by the initial defense reactions; just as in fully conscious memories, pathological defenses come into play when confronted with the reality of the situation. The person simply exclaims, "That isn't what I said; I can't believe you ever took me so literally." Hindsight and guilt serve to distort even the most consciously represented memories about significant events.

Hypnosis is not a truth serum, and we should not expect it to achieve anything more than the person's recollections distorted by defense mechanisms. It is precisely such distortions and confabulations that we seek to undo in analytic therapy to facilitate the person's growth into a more fully functioning person, an intrinsically, as well as extrinsically, happy, giving, individual. Accordingly, we welcome the emergence of such distortions and confabulations as have first to be available to us as therapists to make change possible. Despite a patient's constitutional givens and idiosyncratic libidinal needs, horizontal and vertical explorations are hypnoanalytic techniques that enable us to get access to such memory material with both their accuracies as well as their distortions. Obviously, these issues raise serious problems in the use of hypnotic hypermnesia in forensic situations.

Horizontal and Vertical Exploration

Let us refer to figure 4.3 to help us conceptualize the horizontal and vertical exploration strategy when employing hypermnesia and regression to recon-struct memory material that has been repressed. The schematic should be considered only as a useful conceptualization intended for the convenience of the practicing therapist and not construed as our statement of personality theory. Let the experiential life space of an individual be represented by a solid whose upper surface ABCD constitutes the intermediate present, including all current behaviors, experiences, and so on. Let EA be a time dimension running from the moment of conception to the present. Current stimuli impact the ABCD surface and constitute the immediate perceptual experi-ential and behavioral world for the person. The impacts modify the surface and constitute the person's here-and-now. These modifications are encoded and become part of the person's future memory system. As new stimuli from subsequent moments strike, new surfaces evolve, superceding and covering over older ones. The time-line dimension, AE, lengthens. Data inscribed at earlier periods tends to shrink below the level of awareness. Probably recall suffers first, then recognition as the new experiences retroactively inhibit the

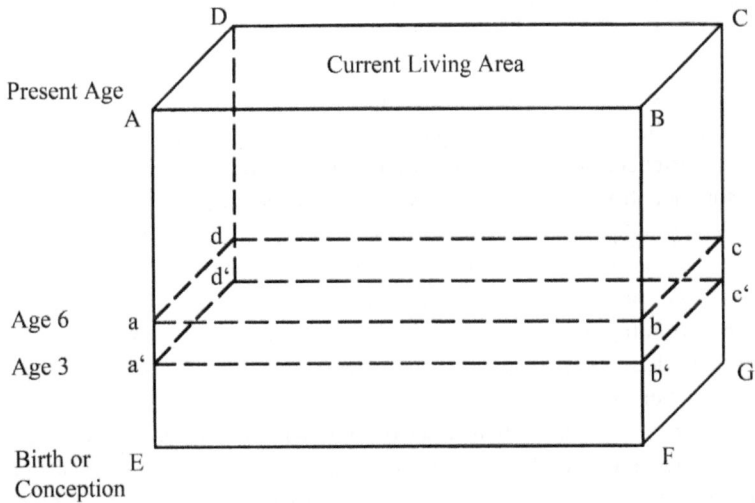

Figure 4.3 A schematic conception of "life space."

activation of earlier ones. According to older "recording machine" theories of learning and memory, all impacting stimuli would make specific traces, and these would be retained unchanged. Accordingly, to recover them all, we would have to regress an individual to the appropriate age level, and we could secure an objective and veridical account of exactly what happened at the time. By regressing him or her to, say, the 6-year-old level (ABCD), we could then get a true picture of his or her life and conflicts at that time. Such a view would simplify greatly the job of the analyst, psychoanalyst, or hypnoanalyst.

As we have learned from the previously cited research findings, the situation is indeed much more complex. We can still use our conceptual formalization shown in Figure 4.3, but we must consider more carefully just what goes into determining the makeup of the life space solid.

Some of the stimuli involved in the current experience of the here-and-now (plane ABCD) were sufficiently strong as to make specific impacts of which the individual was quite aware. Other stimuli, either because of their lesser magnitude, or because they were in conflict with previous experiences and motivations, made contact, but their impacts were not sufficient to evoke that experience we call consciousness. They were encoded in memory, but being below the perceptual threshold, they became part of the person's "covert" or "unconscious" behavioral repertoire. This was studied experimentally by E. R. Hilgard (1986, 1992). We cannot emphasize enough that some of the stimuli may never have been encoded at any level, covert or overt. The person simply cannot remember them, because he or she never learned them in the first place.

The situation is still more complicated by findings that the impacting stimuli may reach below the surface (ABCD) and modify underlying layers. What happens today may change the person's memories of what happened yesterday. Furthermore, the process of modifying memory traces not only is influenced by the impacts of immediate stimuli, but also continues (after experiences have once been inscribed) through the influence of "internal stimuli." These may represent needs, motivations, traumatic or other previous experiences, attempts to eliminate anxiety and achieve more cognitive consonance, transference experiences with earlier significant figures, and so on. Perceptual psychology (A. Barabasz & Dodd, 1978; Kubovy & Pomerantz, 1981; Hochberg, 1978) explains that we tend to organize experiences into patterns or Gestalts. Accordingly, newly received impacts may, by associations, be incorporated into earlier encapsulated patterns. The patient regressed to eighth grade sometimes reports memories or shows some responses appropriate to earlier or later age levels. Experimental studies have often noted that the regressed participant may describe experiences of his or her earlier period in language more appropriate to an older person. As discussed earlier, we do not have to accept the naïve assumption that for regression to be genuine, it must be complete. However, these same findings support the position that communications from individuals regressed to periods before they had learned language may not be merely verbalizing fantasies when they speak in terminology appropriate to a 5-year-old of an event that happened before they could have learned such words.

It is common for the debunkers of hypnosis to dismiss as pure fantasy reports by clinicians of the recovery of very early experiences, such as those occurring during the first year of life (Cheek & LeCron, 1968). These experiences were presumed to have occurred prior to the acquisition of language. The child at the age of 1 may not have learned the word "burn," but he or she can experience the pain and, at a later age, after having learned the meaning of the word "burn," can attach it to his or her earlier experience and more easily communicate it to the therapist. The fact, therefore, that recalled and re-enacted data doesn't derive from the exact age to which the patient had been regressed in no way negates our use of it in hypnoanalysis. Quite the contrary, it only calls on us to use greater care and caution in interpreting age levels as we build up a therapeutic picture of the patient's life experiences. The horizontal and vertical exploration techniques are just two ways of investigating the person's "life space."

Horizontal exploration involves regressing a person to some specific age level and then conducting a case history interview at that regressed age. The technique for regression is to ablate the present and then move the patient in his or her experience back to the desired age. For example, one way to proceed might be as follows:

> You are forgetting all about how old you are, what year it is, and where you are. You are going back through time, and becoming younger and younger, younger and younger. You are 18 years old, 17 years old, younger and smaller, 16, 15, 14, 13, 12, younger and smaller still, 11, 10, 9, 8, 7, 6. You are now 6 years old, and you are in school in the first grade. You are sitting at your desk. You can see all your classmates around you and pictures on the wall. Your teacher is standing in front of you. What is your teacher's name?

The steps include the following:

1. Ablating the present.
2. Moving the patient back step-wise to the earlier age.
3. Rebuilding his or her experiential world in the regressed age with much vivid description.
4. Testing the adequacy of regression by asking for a specific item (the teacher's name).

Once regression has apparently been secured, we then treat the patient as if he or she were a 6-year-old and we talk accordingly. We explore "horizontally" the surface (ABCD) as it was presumed to have been at that time. Our purpose is to try to secure reports on the patient's relationships with parents and siblings, his or her reactions to school, friends, play and hobbies, worries, conflicts, and so on. In other words, we are trying to get a picture of the patient's life as it was perceived by the patient at the age of 6. We hope that as much of it as possible will represent actual objective reality, but all we really know is that it does represent some kind of subjective reality to our patient. In general, what is important to the patient is what is represented. If the patient claims he or she was mistreated by an older brother and then constantly feared him, we accept that information (at least at first!) on its face value. At some level of the patient's being, the patient feels fear of the older brother, and therapeutically that must eventually be dealt with. This is the key item to place in our chart notes for future use.

We have already noted that the patient apparently has a good relationship with this brother at the patient's current age of 21. We wonder what has happened throughout the years. What changes have occurred in this brother relationship and why? We may choose now to move to "vertical" exploration. Keeping to the brother relationship as a common thread, we regress the patient up and down the time line (AE) to find out what happened and when: "You are no longer 6 years old. You are becoming younger and younger. Five years old, four years old, three years old, yes three years old. You are now 3 years old. Do you have a brother? What does he look like? Tell me about him. How do you feel about him?" Notice we do not ask, Do you like him, but rather, How do you feel about him? We move to (A', B', C', and D'), the 3-year level.

We now note that this brother was especially jealous of the patient during the patient's early years, because the patient was perceived as the favorite of the parents. Later, the brother came to the patient's rescue in a traumatic situation, and the patient perceived the brother in an entirely new light. The patient lost the fear, and they became good friends. Through "vertical" exploration, we have traced the development of this brother relationship (as in hypnosis the patient recalls experiencing it) and can be better prepared to deal with any "unconscious" blocks that disturb the patient's present interaction with the brother stemming from the transference feeling the patient held at age 6.

The patient's experiential life space is, in a sense, examined with a kind of "mining" process along both horizontal and vertical shafts. Using such procedures, we can systematically explore the three-dimensional living space of our patients, throughout their growth and development. Psychoanalysis is more than "strip mining," where we merely scrape off the top layer as in so many nondepth therapies. With the psychoanalytic approach, we scrape off the top layer, then the next, then the next, and so on. No matter whether we use the classic psychoanalytic technique of free association or the hypnoanalytic techniques of horizontal and vertical exploration, we may still only get a role-playing, a partial regression, or hopefully a more complete regression. All regressions are incomplete to some extent (see A. Barabasz & Christensen, 2006, 2007; Christensen & Barabasz, 2007; Kluft, 1987; Kris, 1956). Because a more complete regression is what we prefer, the question is, "How can we maximize the chances for as complete a regression as possible? What procedures can we follow to expedite this reaction?"

It is naïve to simply tell a hypnotized person to go back to some desired age level, although this may occasionally achieve that result with certain patients. One suspects that a number of the research studies that have reported negative results may have used such a simple suggestion and got nothing more than simple role-playing. To protect the guilty, we shall refrain from listing those studies admitting to just that practice. A far better process is to remove, as much as possible, the interferences of the present by ablating current orientation, allowing time for the participant to return to an earlier experiential age, and then describing most vividly some event that took place at that time. As described by A. Barabasz and Christensen (in press), the change that can take place is most likely topographic, in the sense that we are eliciting primary process responses rather than temporal ones, as an actual regression in time might produce.

It is also important that we use the present tense: "You are there. What is happening?" not "What happened when you were 6?" In light of the findings regarding hypermnesia for entire incidents as being far better than sentences and words, the skill of the hypnotherapist in attaining significant regression probably hinges on his or her first securing a reasonably deep state of hypnosis, and then on his or her fluency in picturing a true event at the regressed age. A school scene is one typical way of going about this, because we can assume that the patient was in school at that time. Regressed reliving is enhanced when the therapist can visualize him- or herself in the same experiential time frame and coexist with the patient. The patient's here-and-now becomes, for the moment, the hypnotherapist's here-and-now. Visualize and experience the classroom situation as the patient might have as a child, but without suggesting details. It is essential that you avoid suggesting details, because you do not want to create the patient's responses by suggestion, you want to learn about what the patient encoded, which was important at that period in his or her life. Don't put words in the patient's mouth! For example, "You are back in the first grade. Look around and tell me what you see. Where is the teacher? What is your teacher's name? What does your teacher look like? Yes, it is Mrs. Thorp [the patient has told you this], she is standing in front of the class. Mrs. Thorp is standing in front of the class. Now what is she saying?" and so on. Build with the specifics and the details based only on the ones that the patient furnishes to you, not ones that you imagine might have occurred. It is important to make the setting as vivid as possible, without suggesting items that may or may not be accurate. One cannot guarantee in any way that the patient's reconstructed memories will be objectively correct without some confabulations or fantasizing in response to the therapist's "demand" to remember, but the more the patient is nondirectively induced to involve him- or herself in the regressed situation, the more likely it will be that the hypnotically regressed experience is truer to what really happened, but more importantly truer to what the patient encoded as a possible basis of current conflicts at the present time.

Ideomotor Finger Signaling

Over 40 years ago, Cheek (1962) suggested permitting a participant to answer questions while in hypnosis by nonverbal means, rather than having to answer questions orally. This form of communication may be considered partly "dissociative" and partly "projective," but it is certainly "hypno-diagnostic." This extension of interviewing in trance asks the patient to answer questions by finger signaling, rather than verbally. Cheek conceptualized the procedure with Leslie LeCron while observing demonstrations of Chevreul's pendulum (see Barabasz & Watkins, 2005, pp. 91–94). Cheek adapted it to the diagnostic understanding and treatment of a wide variety of conditions with refinements continuing for a quarter of a century thereafter (Rossi & Cheek, 1988).

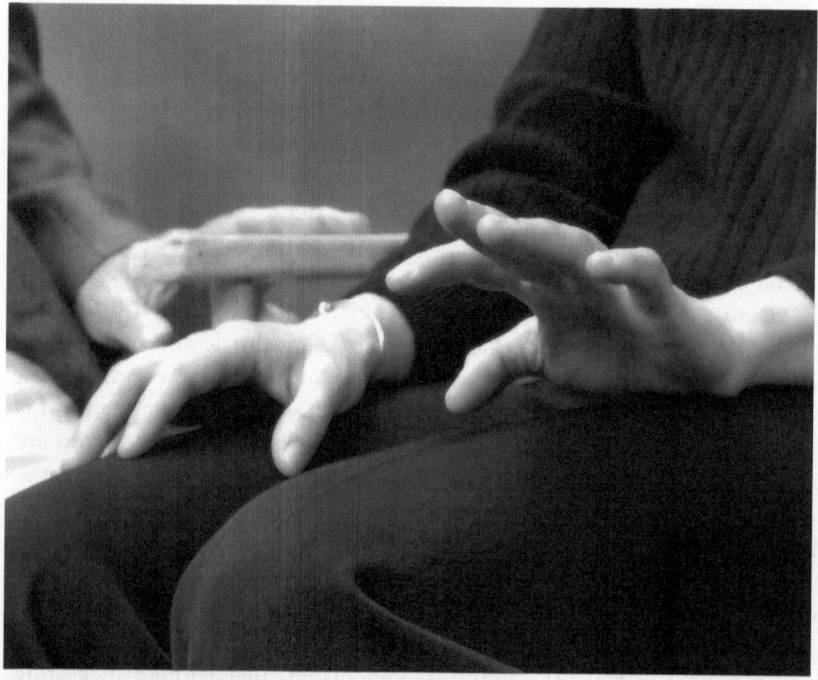

Figure 4.4 Ideomotor signal for "yes."

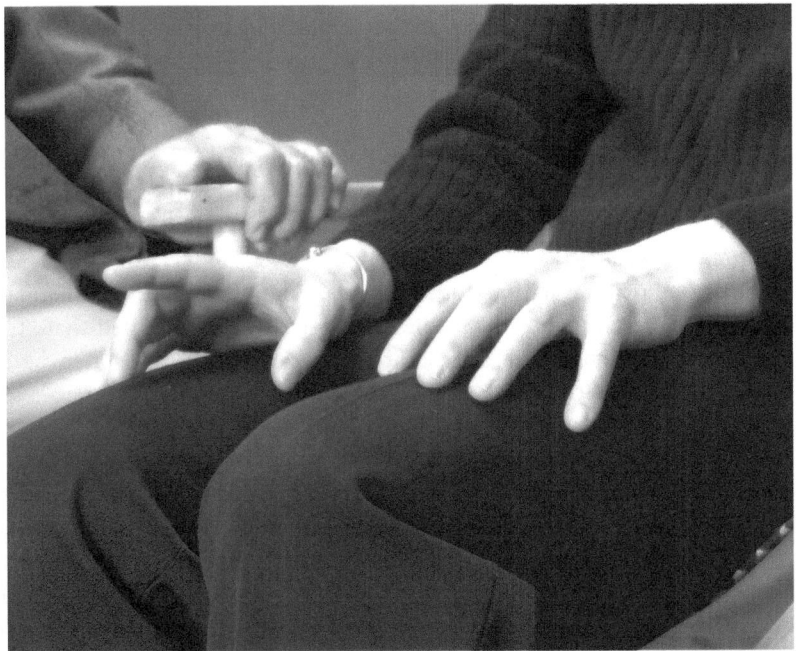

Figure 4.5 Ideomotor signal for "no."

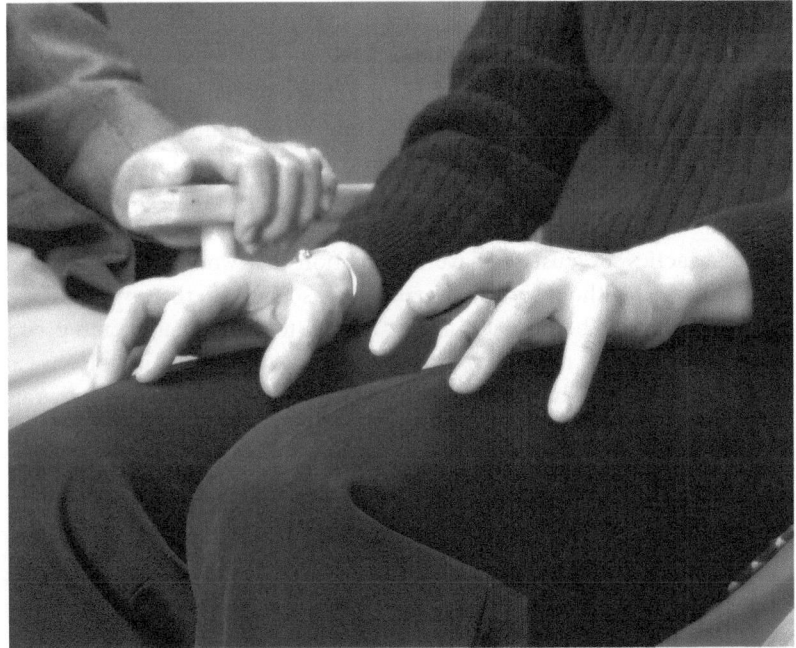

Figure 4.6 Ideomotor signal for "I don't know," or "I don't want to tell."

Ideomotor signaling involves the principle of informing the patient that his or her "subconscious mind" can answer questions without conscious participation by lifting the first finger if the answer is "yes," the second finger if the answer is "no," and the third finger if the answer is "I don't know" or "I don't want to tell." Rossi and Cheek (1988) tell the patient to "let his fingers talk for him," asking the patient to think "yes-yes-yes" and see "which finger will lift" to signal "yes." The same choice is then offered for the "no" response and for an "I am not ready to know consciously yet" answer. This refinement of the procedure is an attempt to reduce the directivity of the hypnotherapist. Despite the lack of empirical studies, Rossi and Cheek reported that "true unconscious, ideodynamic signals are always repetitive and often barely visible." They have extended the motor communication to arm signals and have reported a number of research studies relating to ideomotor signaling. Despite the lack of empirical support for the notion of true, unconscious, ideodynamic sources, the procedure is certainly a valuable one in getting information past conscious censorship, because the participant does not have to formulate a verbal response. Our view is that the process of formulating a verbal response can often lighten the state of hypnosis and, thereby, facilitate the mustering of the very defense mechanisms that we are wishing to circumvent.

Summary

Understanding and diagnosing a patient is a continuous process, not completed in the initial interviews. Hypnosis can aid in inquiry by accessing areas of personality not normally available to conscious questioning. Specialized hypno-diagnositic techniques, such as interviewing in the hypnotic state, "in–out" technique, hypermnesia, regression, and ideomotor signaling, offer the hypnotherapist ways of bypassing normal criticality, repressions, and other defenses. This can help us substantially in our planning therapeutic strategies and tactics, because we have information that would not be otherwise easily obtained without spending many more sessions in therapy. The data so gathered is limited because it is always subject to confabulation and pseudo-memories. However, regardless of its veridicality, it processes a subjective and experiential reality, which is the basic material with which the hypnotherapist and participant need to meet the goals of analytic treatment.

5

Advanced Abreactive Techniques

Meissner's (1991, p. 41) *What Is Effective in Psychoanalytic Therapy* noted that the therapeutic results of abreaction are undeniable; it is from abreaction that analysis was born, and some psychotherapists rely on it almost exclusively. Abreactions are an integral part of many different approaches to therapy including psychoanalysis (S. Freud & Breuer, 1953; Ferenczi & Rank, 1924; Reik, 1933; Reich, 1949; M. V. Kline, 1958), hypnoanalysis (D. P. Brown & Erika Fromm, 1986; Meissner, 1991; J. G. Watkins, 1949, 1955, 1961, 1992a, 1995), primal scream therapy (Janov, 1970), and behavior therapy (A. Barabasz, 1977; Stampfl, 1967; Wolpe & Lazarus, 1966). As noted in Gunnison's book on hypnocounseling (2004), modern adaptations of person-centered therapy also make provisions for abreaction.

Abreactive techniques bring about emotional catharsis as a special form of release therapy. It is by this form of treatment, performed with the use of hypnosis, that Freud discovered unconscious processes and proceeded to the development of psychoanalysis. The principle involves the revivification of an emotionally disturbing experience that happened to an individual much earlier and the release of the affect that has presumably been bound up in that experience. When successful, the result is a great feeling of relief to the patient and often the dramatic disappearance of the patient's psychopathology related to that experience. Unfortunately for the state of therapy today, Freud abandoned the procedure and developed the free-association technique of psychoanalysis, because at the time he felt the results of hypnotic abreactions were only temporary. A close reading of Freud's work informs the reader that he, in fact, felt uncomfortable at having to deal with powerful unbound emotions, and his abandonment of the procedure is much more likely to have been based more on his own personal problems with it (S. Freud & Breuer, 1953; M. V. Kline, 1958). In a discussion of the effectiveness of abreaction, Reik (1933) supported the view that maintaining the "elements of surprise is the most important part of analytic technique." Such surprises were, of course, less than ideally compatible with Freud's personal approach to therapy.

Despite Freud's issues, Nunberg (1932) concluded that abreaction is one of the component factors in analysis. First, there is the improvement brought about by abreaction in the usual sense of the word, which he attributed to the relief of endopsychic tension due to a discharge of accumulated affect.

Secondly, he reported a similar relief of tension on perhaps a smaller scale arising from the actual process of becoming conscious of something hitherto unconscious. This thinking is entirely consistent with Freud's statement (1920) that the very act of becoming conscious (bringing underlying issues to conscious awareness) involves a discharge of energy.

The abreactive procedure derived from Freud's "principle of constancy," in which he argued "that an individual seeks to keep stimulation as close to zero as possible. His principle is difficult to comprehend as it conflicts with the common observation that people often seek out states of excitement and consider them pleasurable" (Greenberg & Mitchell, 1983, p. 26). After periods of sleep, organisms rouse themselves to experience increased stimulation. This reasoning is cited as a rationale by traditional analysts supporting their skepticism of abreactive techniques. Indeed, traditional analysts such as Meissner (1991), who in the same volume recognized the "undesirable" positive outcomes, still regard abreaction as "an occasional adjunct to analysis, no doubt a useful one, and possibly even as an inevitable accompaniment of mutative interpretations."

It is our position that the "principle of constancy" must be modified here to suggest that what is actually sought is not an absence of stimulation, but rather an optimal degree of stimulation, one that alternates over time. Thus, when we have worked too much for too long, we enter sleep, where stimulation is greatly lowered. After a period of sleep and understimulation, we awaken with renewed energy and eagerness for new experience.

Let us explain further by an analogy. Say you wish to boil some water in the microwave oven. If you set the heat too low or the time too short, the water will not boil, you will see no bubbles or steam, it is "understimulated." The water needs to reach 100 °C (212 °F) or greater. If it is to boil, additional heat (simulation) must be applied. However, if too much heat is applied to the water in a glass container with a very tight lid, then this cannot be translated into escaping steam. Stress and tension will develop in the vessel. Likewise, when a person has received excessive stimulation (such as in trauma), and it has been inadequately released (or completely repressed), then the person suffers from tension (anxiety and likely a number of maladaptive symptoms). Abreaction is like a safety valve on our vessel of water (Watkins & Watkins, 1978). It operates to release excessive stimulation stemming from the pressure of increased tension. The individual emotes, and the amount of tension or stimulation is lowered to a more comfortable level. In other words, there is a better balance between excessive stimulation and understimulation. The symptoms disappear, at least for the moment. As we will discuss later, this is why a single abreaction is almost always insufficient to bring about a permanent resolution of symptoms, an observation that Freud made. This is why Freud felt that therapeutic progress made with abreaction was only temporary. There was no evidence that he pursued multiple abreactions to test his conclusion. It is this balance of equilibrium between overstimulation and understimulation that we seek in helping our patient to a more adaptive, more comfortable, and more meaningful existence.

Such release procedures are both spontaneously and naturally engaged in during sexual orgasm. Thus, abreaction is one of an individual's own self-adjustments for the acquiring and maintaining of a desirable equilibrium. Abreactions occur spontaneously to relieve uncomfortable tensions and reduce excessive stimulation as part of normal human self-maintenance. It is only when the "safety valves" have been unable to open overtly and spontaneously, and release the bound affect, that a psychotherapist must initiate the procedure to help the patient surmount the blocks that prevent his or her natural defenses from operating. Therefore, abreaction is a therapeutic technique for dealing with tension caused by excessive stimulation, which is bound and which has not been released through normal channels of behavior and experience.

Despite Freud's failure to continue exploring hypnotic abreactions, Pierre Janet (1907) did explore them further and became convinced of the value of emotional discharge. He employed the procedure extensively to test the effects in a variety of ways, often inducing crying spells in patients, which he felt needed considerable repetition if the relief from the symptoms was to be permanent. Wilhelm Reich (1949), one of Freud's closest associates, contributed his work on character analysis and "character armor," which increasingly emphasized the release of affect bound in the patient's "muscular armor." Others followed Reich's contributions relating to the release of affect (Lowen, 1975; Rolf, 1978).

Earlier still was the work of Simmel in Germany, which was based on his treatment of "combat fatigue" soldiers in World War I (J. G. Watkins, 1949). He used hypnosis to help these men release rage by attacking and destroying dummies dressed in enemy uniforms. Another active user of hypnotic abreaction therapy during the same period was William Brown (1920). Brown treated several thousand cases of war neuroses and maintained complete and rigorous chart notes to track progress, successes, and failures. He concluded that the cathartic liberation of pent-up feelings brought dissociated segments of the personality back into contact with the ego, thus resulting in a reintegration of the patient. Only after such therapy did the patients begin to move toward full functioning again. Brown deserves credit for recognizing that emotional release must be intensive, continued to exhaustion, and repeated. He also recognized that such releases must be followed by reassurance and interpretation if symptomatic release was to be permanent. These are remarkable and incredibly accurate conclusions based on the treatment of thousands of cases of war neuroses.

It then took the Second World War, and the work of Grinker and H. Spiegel (1945a, 1945b), to provide further data on the effects of abreactive technique. Grinker and H. Spiegel conducted many abreactions with Air Force personnel who had developed anxiety reactions following bombing raids over Germany.

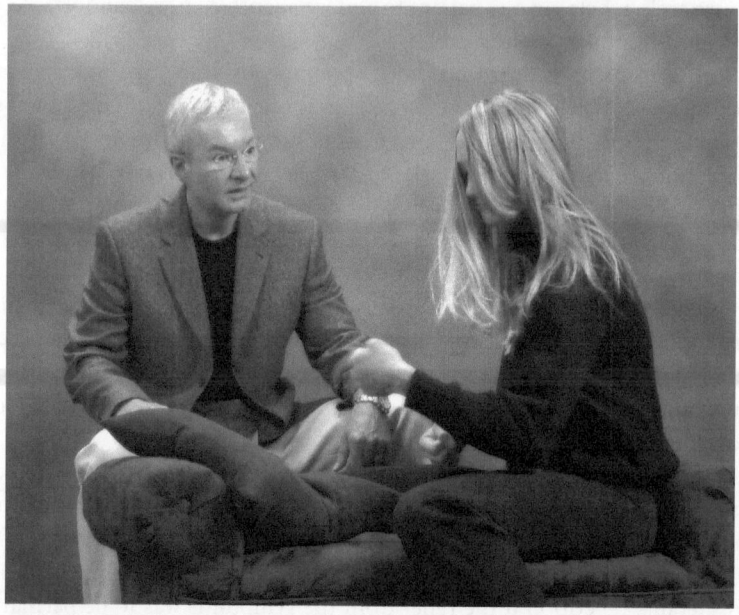

Figure 5.1 Arreed Barabasz and Ciara Christensen demonstrate hypnotically induced abreactive release of bound affect.

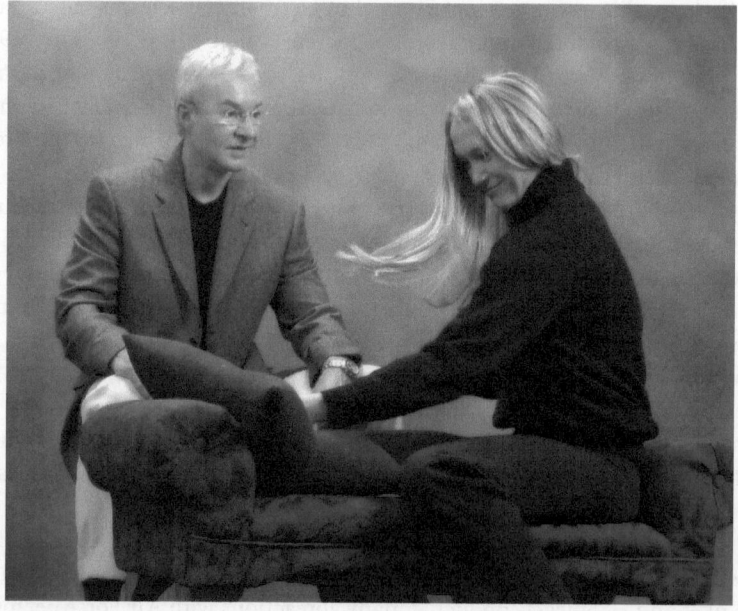

Figure 5.2 Combining the therapist's ego strength with hers allows Christensen to overcome a threatening person from her past.

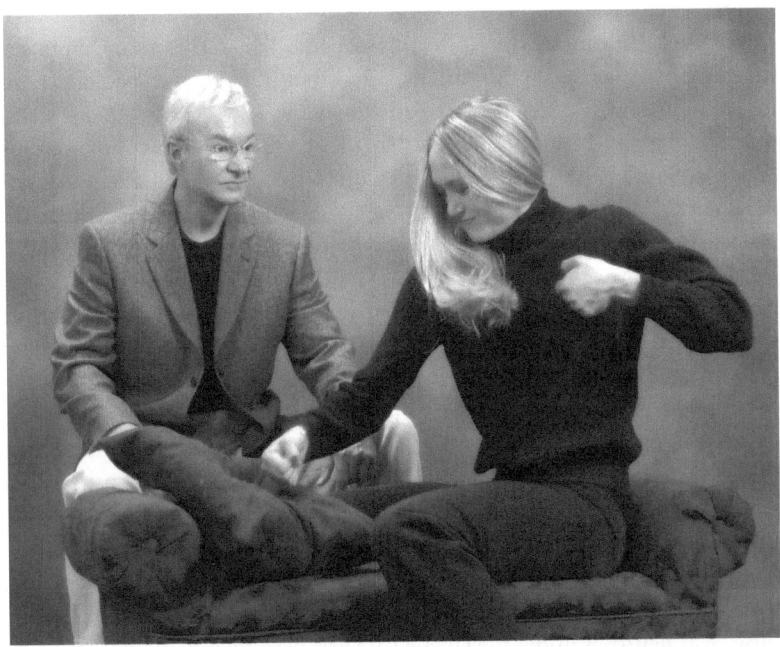

Figure 5.3 The therapist must confidently be able to handle the "heat" of the expression of anger. Failure to do so prevents an adequate release of the bound affect.

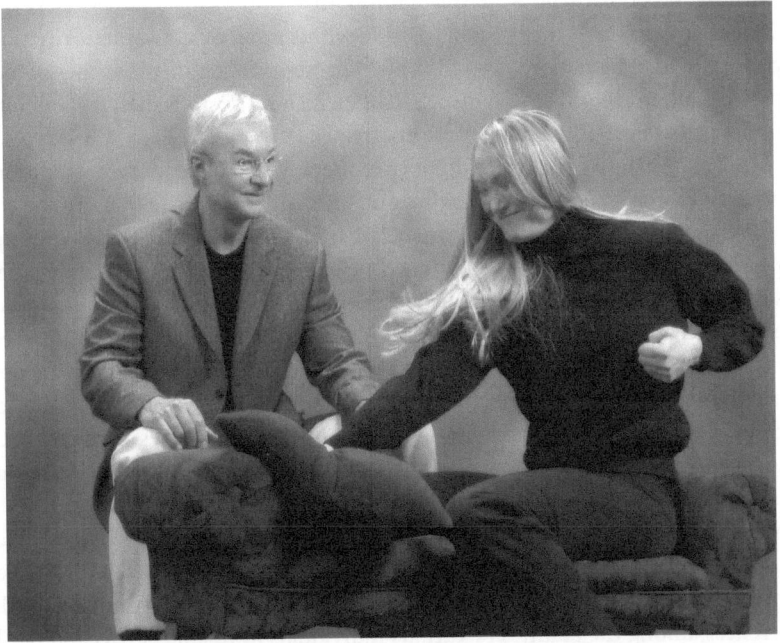

Figure 5.4 Anger and fear released allow the emotion of joy to take their place.

Unfortunately, their emphasis was on the use of the "truth serums" available at the time, sodium amatol and sodium pentothal, rather than hypnosis. It was during this same World War II period that J.G.W. developed and refined the technique with a number of patients at the U.S. Army's Welch Convalescent Hospital in Daytona Beach, Florida. Hypnotic abreactions were used almost exclusively in treating patients who were hospitalized after "emotional breakdowns" during combat on both the Italian and French battlefronts. These classic cases are described in *Hypnotherapy of War Neuroses* (J. G. Watkins, 1949, 1951, 2000). During the war, J.G.W. (1942a,b. 1943, 1951) was active in using psychology for "psychological warfare" to promote emotional dysfunction in enemy populations (J. G. Watkins, 1942, 1943a, b). After he entered military service, this changed into the goals of promoting psychology to enhance and improve emotional adjustment in soldiers suffering from war neuroses.

The trauma neuroses of war that J.G.W. encountered during and following World War II are now included within a broader category, called post-traumatic stress disorder (PTSD), as noted in the *Diagnostic and Statistical Manual IV-TR (DSM IV-TR)* of the American Psychiatric Association. PTSD encompasses all the symptoms that are caused primarily by exposure to very stressful situations, such as fire, explosion, accident, loss of loved ones, rape, hijacking, torture, and child abuse. War neuroses under the label PTSD first became well known throughout the United States after the Vietnam War. Today, Jews who were incarcerated in Nazi concentration camps still report suffering from this disorder.

The symptoms found in civilian cases are, in fact, not unlike those exhibited by those in combat who were treated in both World War I and World War II. They include anxiety, depression, schizoid withdrawal, psychosomatic reactions, phobias, and dissociations, as well as overt psychotic reactions. The egos of these patients have received severe insults, from which recovery is difficult and often prolonged, especially when they are not treated in the acute stage. A wide variety of techniques have been tried: supportive therapy, directive therapy, traditional analytic therapy, humanistic therapy, and ultimately, ego-state therapy.

Personalities suffering from dissociative identity disorder (DID) (multiple personalities) and amnesias (discussed in our Chapter 9) almost always have severe stress experiences in their backgrounds. The earlier the traumas were experienced, the more severe the ego damage, and the more difficult the treatment. Some of the most difficult cases are ones unlucky enough to have a genetic background with some probability of psychosis. Nonetheless, even with these cases, J.G.W. had remarkable and well-documented successes in treating the war neuroses. Many of those patients revealed histories reflecting nontraumatic childhoods. Their first contact with severe stress, and sometimes feelings of abandonment, was when they entered battle. Until that time, they had relatively intact egos. Still, one encountered patients who broke down under the mild stress of merely being inducted into military service. Overall, there are enormous differences among the abilities of various individuals to tolerate stress and not be damaged; hence, their "ego strength" shows them to have enormous resilience.

Daniel Brown and the late Erika Fromm (1987) produced what is perhaps one of the most elegant and detailed descriptions of PTSD conditions, their etiology, and psychodynamics. The authors also considered in-depth treatment strategies from both cognitive-behavioral as well as psychoanalytic viewpoints, which included object-relations theory. Conservative treatment approaches were emphasized. They seemed rather pessimistic about outcomes and did not recommend abreactions as part of the therapeutic tactics. Erika Fromm (personal communications, AFB, 2001) was very complimentary about affects that could be wrought by abreactions. However, she indicated she just couldn't bring herself to turn up the heat and act in as direct a manner as is required over prolonged periods to use the technique effectively.

Our experience seems to be at variance with the emphasis on conservative treatment advocated by D. Brown and Erika Fromm. Although J.G.W. has treated many war neuroses, and particularly the acute ones that were seen in a hospital over a period of many years, he has also treated a substantial number of civilian neuroses related to severe traumas that occurred both during early childhood and later when the patients were adults. The results with such cases have been regarded as fairly good. The majority of them have long records of maintaining recovery over time. We believe that abreactive procedures, when properly conducted, are almost a sine qua non for PTSD patients, and we have no persuasive evidence to the contrary. The appropriate and successful treatment of PTSD patients requires more than the prerequisite skills one must have in hypnosis. It also must involve techniques that go beyond merely releasing affect. Such techniques are essential if abreactions are to be long-lasting in their positive effects.

More than half a century ago, Wolpe and Lazarus (1966) were two key figures in ushering in the revival of interest in release therapies. They used procedures similar to abreactions by presenting some of the first systematically collected data supporting the behavioral techniques of "flooding" or "implosive therapy" (Stampfl, 1967). The humanists were not long to follow with Janov's "primal scream" (Janov, 1970), an abreactive-like approach that involved regressing patients to the earliest years of their lives and reliving the early pain of parental rejection. The importance of emotional release as a key to the attainment of cognitive insight was also emphasized by Perls (1969) as well as Rose (1976).

Sometimes confusing to counseling and clinical psychology graduate students is the tendency of Wolpe workers to utilize their own unique terminology rather than calling these releases abreactions. However, most good therapists recognize that emotional release is essential to good therapy in the context of some form of reliving. Some hypnotize their patients, others do so without knowing that they have induced the state, whereas others have avoided hypnosis altogether. Let us again recognize that when therapists use techniques that emphasize the focusing of attention, concentration, and imaginative reexperiencing, they are in all likelihood inducing trance states indirectly without realizing it. In fact, hypnotizability is recognized as being essentially a universal feature of PTSD sufferers. We have yet to see a PTSD patient who did not score above average on the standardized clinical scales of hypnotizability such as the Hypnotic Induction Profile (H. Spiegel & D. Spiegel, 2004) or the Stanford Hypnotic Clinical Scale (Morgan & J. R. Hilgard, 1975).

Freud's self-reported inability to secure a more permanent relief of symptoms through abreaction appears to have been the result of his comparative inexperience with unconscious processes at the time of his early acquaintance with hypnosis, and his failure to follow through the emotional release with reassurance, interpretation, and reintegration. Traditional psychoanalytic therapists might well profit from taking a second look at abreactive procedures that include these key features.

Another criticism of cathartic therapy comes from studies that appear to show that the acting out of experimentally induced anger in a participant not only fails to provide true release, but may even increase angry behavior (Keet, 1948; Berkowitz, 1973). However, when Nichols and Zax (1977) continued with a controlled study involving actual patients, they concluded quite the opposite and found "definite support for the effectiveness of emotive techniques in stimulating catharsis and at least partial support for the effectiveness of catharsis to produce improvement in psychotherapy."

One of the problems with attempts to study the effects of release of "repressed rage" in the laboratory is that such studies, rather than relating in any way to repressed rage, are all set up to meet the demands of a laboratory situation rather than a clinical one, in which immediate frustrations are experimentally induced. This is not at all typical of symptom-causing in patients and cannot in any realistic way be compared with neurotic, long-term, repressed affect stemming from childhood abuse or other trauma. In none of these laboratory studies did they continue the anger release to the point of physical and emotional exhaustion! Furthermore, there was no interpretation or egotization of symbolic meanings to achieve reintegration afterwards. It is difficult to see how any such findings could be generalized to therapeutically designed abreactions (Olsen, 1976).

The techniques that we describe here for conducting abreactions are unlike those in the artificial laboratory situation. On the basis of a substantial number of clinical reports, clinical trials, and the few research studies extant, we tentatively conclude that in general the following holds:

Cathartic therapy, involving the thorough release of affect, is an effective therapeutic procedure for a wide variety of cases.
To obtain the best results, the trauma situation must be circumscribed.
Acute rather than chronic conditions are likely to produce the best and longest-lasting result.
The technique is most effective when treating symptoms that have been precipitated by specific traumatic situations.

Abreactions may not be effective in treating neuroses that have developed gradually over the years and are firmly entrenched through the practice of maladaptive behaviors that have had much reinforcement, particularly when a pathological significant other has been involved in the person's life over a long period of time (J. G. Watkins, 1992, p. 54)

Indicators for Abreaction

Before beginning an abreaction, it is essential to determine whether or not the conditions are favorable for a cathartic procedure. The best indicators are as follows:

1. Acute rather than chronic conditions.
2. Specific symptoms that seem to be related to specific conflicts.
3. "Sufficient ego strength" in the patient to undergo severe emotional buffeting.
4. A therapist who is both willing and able to coexperience the traumatic event with the patient. (This is absolutely essential to producing the most likely positive lasting outcome.)

We think of symptoms as acute if they are recent in nature. However, that is not always important. The fact that they appeared rather suddenly, particularly after a period of adequate functioning, may be of far greater significance even though the traumatic incident occurred many years before. If the patient told us that certain symptoms such as headaches, anxiety, prolonged irritability, phobia, or depression first appeared after a very emotionally upsetting experience, or one we would have expected to be upsetting to most people, we would have a reasonable basis for inferring some causal relationship. However, proximity alone does not determine cause. It suggests a relationship, and this is usually worth investigating.

Let us assume that the patient has said, "When I was 7 years old and my mother died, I didn't cry. Everybody told me what a brave little girl I was." An "Operation Iraqi Freedom" soldier might have reported: "I got separated from my buddy. When I found him, he was dead. Then, Doc, I began to have these headaches."

The two situations above both suggest acuteness and specificity and, therefore, are more likely to respond to abreactive treatment. They might be regarded as emotionally unfinished business. A situation that would normally precipitate strong emotions has occurred, yet the affect did not appear, at least overtly to the patient or others. In some way, the situation should have caused an emotional response at the time it was presented, but the normally expected response was blocked (frustrated). But where did these emotional responses go? It has been argued by Reich (1949) that the emotion was still present, but that it was now frozen or bound in the person's character armor, thus creating enormous tension, anxiety, and ultimately neurotic symptoms. Your job as the hypnotherapist then is to unbind the frozen affect, release it, and achieve closure of the previously unresolved conflict. A normal reaction was not completed at the time of the event, so employ a hypnotically induced abreaction to reexperience it, and add your ego strength to that of the patient. Allow the patient to, at last, complete it.

Obviously, these patients had blocked off or dissociated the emotion in the first place, because neither the little girl nor the trained combat soldier could express them at the time, could not afford even for the sake of self-preservation to experience it, nor did they feel the emotion at that time. Our job as therapists is to confront them with it. But we need to know that they have sufficient ego strength to cope with it, experience it, and master it. In the majority of therapies, we usually have a number of "positives" going for us. Because we have a therapeutic relationship with the patient, there is the benefit of adding the therapist's ego strength to that of the patient's. We (together) can endure now what the patient could not face alone. We present the patient with a trusted therapeutic guide in a kind of "with-ness." The patient is then much better able to confront the previous trauma and come out the winner. At the time it occurs, neither the little girl nor the combat soldier could deal with it by themselves, and accordingly, they had emerged neurotic losers. It is also likely that if the trauma had occurred when the soldier was a child, as an adult, he himself would be likely to possess greater ego strength.

Nonetheless, there are times that we may be faced with a patient with a poorly developed ego, who is barely able to cope with normal frustrations. Overt irritability amid a thin veil of politeness and coping is just one constellation that we may see in a patient. Recognize that the patient in such cases is very fragile and might break into an acute psychotic reaction if forced to confront more than he or she can handle. It may be wise to first study the patient further, perhaps with the aid of psycho-diagnostic instruments like the Minnesota Multiphasic Personality Inventory (MMPI) II, Rorschach, or House-Tree-Person. Recognize that this situation does not occur often, but when it does, abreaction is at least temporarily contraindicated in favor of a period of psychological testing and re-evaluation. Rogersian therapy conducted with the frequent use of incomplete thought and reflection of content that seems relevant to the disorder can provide a diagnostically useful period of relief from the pressure of more directive therapy.

Recognize that an important factor here can be the insecurity of the therapist. If we as therapists can't take the heat of the full abreaction, how could we possibly expect the patient to do so? Sometimes the problem is one that you, the therapist, must first solve within yourself.

Abreaction Induction

There is no half way. You either start an abreaction or you do not. Once the decision is made, go into it with all the feeling you can muster. Unlike fractionation (Kluft, 1992, 1999), don't get partway into the release of affect and then decide it's too violent. This usually means that you can't take it as the therapist. To be of value to your patient, once you open up the patient's bound affect, it is essential that you continue until it has been fully released. Would a good surgeon open up his or her patient and then decide, "Oops, I can't go through with this, I am not prepared to cope?" Would only part of a tumor be removed because he or she feared cutting too deep when the only cure was to remove all of it?

Assume that through previous sources of information obtained from our horizontal and vertical explorations, you already know much about the probable trauma, where it occurred, and the age of the patient at the time. Generally, the best tactic is to induce as deep a trance as possible, while maintaining full interactive contact, and then use regression procedures to take him or her to that time and place. Your background on the situation should provide the information to make the determination as to whether or not it may be desirable to regress the patient to a point in time prior to the traumatic event and then gradually work up to it. Such a procedure can be valuable in that it provides an evaluation of the patient's pretrauma functioning and perhaps whether there might have been another event that had occurred, which might have reduced the patient's general level of functioning before the primary traumatic event. Sometimes there has been an erosion of the patient's functioning due to a variety of factors prior to the trauma. The patient is then essentially ripe for the trauma with less resilience than is typically available.

Revivify the regressed scene using distinctive mental images, but drawn only from the information provided to you by the patient previously. Use the present tense. You might say, "It is June 5. You are 7 years old. Your mother has just died and you are at the funeral. You feel very alone, very very alone, and sad, very sad. That feeling is getting stronger and stronger, stronger, and stronger. You want so badly to cry. Your father has told you, 'Try to be brave!' You are trying to be brave, trying to be so brave, but you just can't hold back the tears any longer. Let them come, they've needed to come for such a long, long time. Just let them come."

Combat veterans from the Afghanistan liberation and Operation Iraqi Freedom may present histories with many common background themes. Revivification of the traumatic situation can be enhanced by the use of soundtracks of combat noises, such as a helicopter, rifle, machine gun, mortar fire, and rifle-propelled grenades (RPGs). These can serve as strong instigators to assist in the elicitation of regression and reliving. Kolb (1988) reported success in using such methods to elicit reliving regressive experiences in his Vietnam veterans with PTSD. It is legitimate to use essentially every modality possible to help build up an experiential return to the traumatic episode, so long as you don't go beyond what you know the scene to be about. Don't fabricate information.

The crucial factor in ensuring success of the technique is to revivify it until there is a breakthrough and the feelings begin to flow with nothing to inhibit them. Persevere! Let the pounding, shouts, and screams occur. The more and more intense the response, the more effective the abreaction will be. The only constraints, of course, are that we must protect the patient from hurting him- or herself or, for that matter, the therapist. Other than that, there should be essentially no restriction on the patient's movements or outcries. It is necessary that we avoid trying to calm the patient or asking the patient to "take it easy," or "don't get so upset." These latter techniques are indicative of an insecure or, at least, less than ideally confident therapist. These are precisely the points we wish to avoid conveying to our patient. The key factor is that we want the patient to be as fully upset as possible during the abreaction process.

A client A.F.B. saw who came from Europe explained that her previous psychologist "had been doing abreactions with me but I couldn't get the demon out, I felt he wouldn't accept me and didn't want to upset him."

Continue the experience until the patient is completely exhausted, not only psychologically but physically as well. Once the tears, anger, or fear has subsided, then and only then comes the time for interpretation and calm reassurance. Timing is of key importance. As you have been coliving and coexperiencing the emotional experience, you too will have taken an emotional buffeting. It is time for both of you to reach a state of calmness and peace. And it is time for the patient to secure an understanding of what this is all about. The therapist must bring meaning through interpretation. But the bound energy that had previously kept this understanding from egotization has been spent. The resistance is now, at last, down. At this time, the interpretations can be accepted and integrated by the patient. With defenses at their lowest, this is a key point of opportunity for interpretations to take hold. The interpretations should then, obviously, immediately follow the emotional release. This is no time for a break. In a short period of time, perhaps a few days or even a few hours, the defenses will be re-established, and the opportunity for a more permanent resolution of the patient's conflicts will be lost, or at least substantially reduced. Genuine insight can more easily follow after the emotional resistance to it has been exhausted.

It is usually desirable to repeat the abreaction several times during the same session. Repeat it the next day, a week later, perhaps a month later. The affect will eventually be exhausted, and a time will come when the attempt to stimulate it again arouses no more feeling in the patient whatsoever. It has become a neutral experience, remembered of course, but no longer capable of causing anxiety or other symptoms. Occasionally, a single abreaction can be sufficient, but this is the exception and not the rule, so be prepared to do repetitions if there is insufficient symptom change after the first or second abreaction. B. F. Skinner, the famous learning theorist, observed that rats who had learned to press a bar to receive food but then were extinguished from the response when the food was no longer provided (they learned to stop pressing the bar) would "spontaneously recover" from the extinguished response weeks later, pressing the bar again when put in the old cage. Humans who have years of practice behaving in the service of their repressed emotions may have the same ingrained habits, thus requiring a few repeated exhaustions just as Skinner's hungry rats did.

When J.G.W. (J. G. Watkins, 1992a) was working at the Army hospital in Daytona Beach, Florida, back in World War II, a battalion surgeon who had a tremor in his right hand was referred to him. The physician had diagnosed himself as having Parkinson's. However, as one of his medical colleagues said, "He didn't know his neurology too well." It wasn't Parkinson's but rather a hysterical tremor.

J.G.W. noticed whenever he had to salute a commanding officer, the surgeon's hand would shake violently. The surgeon told him that he hated the colonel, who was the commanding officer of his hospital detachment. The surgeon then said, "If I could ever get that son of a bitch on my operating table, what I wouldn't do to him." This patient was over 6 feet and 6 inches in height and weighed over 240 pounds. However, with perhaps some trepidation, J.G.W. decided to do an abreaction. So he closed the door and put a table in front of the patient; the patient was hypnotized, and the table simulated his operating table. A pillow was placed on it, and the visualization given to him in the abreaction was that of his commanding officer lying there. "Here he is. What are you going to do with him?" And for the next few minutes, he and J.G.W. committed murder. He was stabbing and cussing "that son of a bitch," ripping with his imaginary scalpel, and J.G.W. was standing by him shouting, "Give it to the son of a bitch. It's what he deserves."

J.G.W. and his patient committed psychological murder over and over again. Finally, "we" were exhausted. The patient's cussing and screaming ceased, and his body relaxed. Reassurance was given, followed by interpretation about the resemblance of the commanding officer to his own father. He was then brought out of hypnosis. Holding his hand up, he was smiling. At last it was steady, there was no trace of a tremor, and the cure was lasting.

Silent Abreaction

Hypnocounseling, such as may be the norm in both community mental health counseling centers and university counseling centers, needed a form of abreaction that could fit the physical limitations of the therapist's office. Professional buildings are seldom soundproofed to an adequate level; they are built for quiet consultations. Shouting, cursing, and screaming patients simply would not be understood by the university administration or, for that matter, many colleague therapists. Few are prepared for such violent displays of feeling.

While at the University of Montana counseling center, Helen Watkins (1980) recognized the need for an alternative to the full-blown, loud expressiveness of the typical abreactive procedure. Yet, at the same time, it was clinically advantageous to develop a procedure that offered many of the therapeutic advantages of a full abreaction, but somehow without involving loud noise and violent behavior. She called it the "silent abreaction." An added benefit for the hypnocounselor who may be less experienced is that it can be more easily initiated than a true behavioral abreaction. It does not submit the patient to as severe an experience and is considerably easier to carry out, yet it can in many cases still be highly effective. It is subject to a number of limitations that do not apply to regular abreactions, but it remains especially useful in dealing with repressed anger when the physical surroundings do not permit openly expressing feeling with such violence for fear of discovery or embarrassment. Under these conditions, a silent abreaction is the preferred alternative.

Another advantage of the silent abreaction is that it can be a first step leading to a full-blown abreactive therapeutic intervention. It becomes a safe, early releasing of emotion that does not require such complete bodily involvement. The partial release of affect through a silent abreaction makes it easier for a patient to feel less afraid. He or she is more able to involve his or her voice and body overtly in reliving the traumatic event later. Because a partial release of the expressed feeling has already taken place within the silent abreaction model, its violence in the full-blown abreaction is typically reduced. This is because there has been a partial pre-exhaustion of the emotion in the silent abreactive phase.

Given that the silent abreaction is primarily effective in the discharge of anger, rather than other emotions, let us focus on anger that needs to be released because the patient was unable to express it during some early experience in life. The patient has buried, encapsulated, and repressed that feeling, using enormous energy that needs to be freed for more constructive purposes and appropriate non-self-defeating adaptations to real life. Given that the patient was unable to release the anger during the original experience, he or she must have been taught something like "it's not nice to be angry" or had fears of retribution if the anger was expressed. Some who perceive a threat that is not related to present-day reality obviously inhibit the expression of rage, especially when it deals with events of the past. What the silent abreaction offers is an opportunity to unlearn such suppressive messages, which were acquired early in life and have been reinforced over a period of several years by pathological partners (see J. G. Watkins & H. H. Watkins, 1997). But after abreactive therapy, the new dictum for the patient then becomes, "It's all right to feel angry; it's important to rid myself of the angers of the past, so they won't bother me in the present."

The silent abreaction is conducted in three distinct phases: Following the initial hypnotic induction and deepening, the hypnotherapist describes a scene in which the patient and the therapist are walking together, along a path in the woods. They come to a large boulder, which blocks the path. The patient is told that a large branch is nearby on the ground and is asked to pick it up and give the boulder a powerful whack. Hypnotic depth is reassessed, and a suggestion is made that the boulder symbolizes everything that has frustrated the patient, and that it can represent a specific person, a traumatic experience, or whatever else seems appropriate. The idea is to convey that the boulder indeed symbolizes all the frustrations ever experienced by the patient and that they are all wrapped up in this single mass of stone. The therapist may say something like this:

> In a moment I want you to start beating on that boulder, hitting it harder and harder until you are completely exhausted, and when you're worn out and too tired to go on, signal me by lifting one of your fingers. You won't be heard in this office; you can yell, scream, and do or say whatever you wish in this place of ours beside the boulder. I will make sure no one will intrude in our scene in the woods.

The patient starts to beat the boulder in fantasy while the therapist urges him or her to exhaustion. Check the clock. This can take 3 to 5 minutes or, in many cases, even longer, during which time the therapist urges the patient to "come on, hit it again, harder; keep on going; more and more; come on, let's go; don't give up on it; keep hitting it." The ideomotor finger signal tells the therapist when the patient is just too tired to continue.

The second phase of the technique involves a picturing of the therapist and patient walking up a small rise to a meadow filled with wildflowers. This is accompanied by a vivid description of the sun shining, the breeze gently blowing, and a clump of trees under which the grass is so very plush, so very green, so soft and inviting. The patient can then be told, "Before we can go to the third and final phase of what we are doing today, I need to hear you say something positive about yourself." The issue here is that many if not most people have been taught not to express anger, and to feel guilty, very guilty if they do so. Accordingly, this hypnotic suggestion is focused on teaching the patient that "it's all right to get angry." Basically, whatever the patient says is accepted, even if it is a very mild self-compliment like "sometimes I am nice to people."

After the positive statement is made, the stage is set to begin the third phase. In this phase, the patient is asked to

> Pay close attention to your toes. You'll soon note a warm, glowing, tingling sensation there, and when you notice that feeling, let me know by lifting a finger.

This sensation is then spread throughout the entire body: up the legs thoroughly; into the trunk; through the body, the shoulders, the arms, the neck, and so on. An excellent alternative to this is the simple progressive relaxation model, particularly for both resistant patients and those with the greatest level of pent-up anger. A.F.B. developed the microcosmic orbit meditation hypnotic induction using university student volunteers as well as a clinical patient population (the rationale and details of the procedure, along with exact protocol for induction, appear in Barabasz & Watkins, 2005, Chapter 14, pp. 323–334).

Following either procedure, the therapist then tells the patient that he or she is now aware of an increasing, warm, glowing sensation of well-being. The patient is asked to recognize that this sensation comes from the patient's own positive feelings about him- or herself (this is particularly facilitated with the meditation-based microcosmic orbit induction), from his or her inner resources, and from confidence that he or she can solve his or her problems. The patient is asked to signal the therapist by lifting a finger when he or she is increasingly aware of these sensations of warmth and glowing. Then the hypnotic suggestion is given that the tingly warm sensations will become stronger, and again the therapist asks for the finger signal acknowledgment. When the ideomotor signal appears, the therapist says:

> This additional warm glowing feeling comes from another wellspring. It comes from me, as a measure of my belief and faith in you that you will be able to solve your problems.

Coming after the release of anger bound up in the body for so many years, it is a reward for letting go of that anger. The patient is then brought out of hypnosis slowly and carefully with the suggestions that the tingling feelings are slowly lessening and will be gone, but the glow will continue. The silent abreaction can be repeated by the patient on his or her own through self-hypnosis again and again until any remains of the anger have dissipated.

Remarkably, despite the availability of this technique since it was first published by Helen Watkins (1980) and taught throughout the world in literally hundreds of workshops on hypnotherapeutic techniques, there is still no empirical data extant comparing the silent abreaction, which is partial, with the full-blown one involving overt and motor behavior. It would seem, on the basis of face validity, that a full abreaction, which enlists the patient's total expressive behaviors, would be better than one that involves only an inner experience. Nonetheless, we have heard from hundreds of therapists who continue to report many good successes with silent abreactions. Our position remains that we recommend the more complete catharsis when such is not contraindicated by the limitations of the therapy setting.

The Affect Bridge

As we listen to our patients in therapy, the sensitive analyst or analytically oriented counselor learns to listen to fluctuations in the train of associations and to infer from these areas of repressed conflict. Chains of related ideas are sometimes drawn toward the centers of conflict or memories repressed from consciousness, yet at other times they move sharply away from such centers as the forces of defense and resistance seek to protect the patient from the anxiety that would result from contact with such material. Quite frequently, the patient shows that his or her symptoms are related to repressed affect, but, alas, we do not know from what time and place in their life they start. We are not informed of any specific traumatic experience that seems relevant. What can be done if we do not know just where to regress the patient? Of course, through horizontal and vertical exploration, we may in time locate the precipitating incident, but if we knew just where to go now, the treatment might be expedited greatly.

In 1958, J.G.W. tried a novel procedure on a patient for the first time, which produced surprisingly effective results. *The affect bridge* was first published in Spanish (J. G. Watkins, 1961) and later with enriched explanation in English (1971). In both psychoanalysis as well as analytically oriented counseling, the stream of consciousness moves from the present to recollections of the past along chains of associated ideas. The patient says, "I remember when I was 10 years old, and that reminds me of another time when I ... ." Memory A leads to memory C, because both of them overlap with memory B. Memory B is a "cognitive bridge," which can move us from A to C. Memory A can lead to memory C, not only because they are both embedded in the common cognition B, but also if they are both related to a common feeling or affect. When we are grief stricken, we are more likely to remember other situations in which we experienced a similar grief feeling.

When such analytic therapy has not succeeded, failure has often been caused by the intellectualization of the therapy. It has dealt only with ideas and has not elicited feelings, emotions, or affects. Thus, the forgotten or pathogenic experiences that may lie at the very basis of some conflict are not revealed in their true, living, experiential colors. In a sense, they are seen as an old monochrome (black-and-white) film with the volume turned down instead of in vivid color with full sound effects. If this is to be understood, integrated, and controlled, a forgotten experience must be lifted from repression in all or at least most of its original vividness, its original "feelingness," or, as the existentialists hold, its "beingness." Insight, to be genuinely therapeutic, must be total and must involve full visceral and muscular, as well as cerebral, responses. In other words, we must feel it as a known entity if we are to have insightful understanding that is likely to result in positive therapeutic change.

The problem with traditional psychoanalytic therapy and analytically oriented counseling is that it relies far too often on these chains of ideas, and because the "bridges" that connect these ideas are almost invariably intellectual thoughts, there is a tendency for treatment to become emotionally flat and sterile and be confused with depth. Analytic hours go on interminably day after day, week after week, month after month, with the patient repeating in words over and over his or her "memories" but not undergoing what has been termed by Alexander and French (1946) the "emotionally corrective experience." The analyst's instruction, "What does this make you think of?" or "What does this remind you of?" constantly directs the patient's attention to his or her intellectual processes rather than the crucial emotional processes that were encoded at the time the memory was taken on. It is the associated emotion that is the key, not merely the intellectual recording of a happening. Associations move in ideational circles, leaving untouched the zone of feelings where the really significant origins of the patient's pathology may be found.

A way of breaking through the interminable stalemate of intellectualized therapy is the affect bridge. It employs hypnosis to cross time lines from present to past more rapidly, and it emphasizes the use of common elements, that is to say, "bridges," between present and past experiences, which are affective or emotional rather than intellectual in nature. The patient is encouraged to make his or her associations along chains of "affect" instead of chains of "ideas." Therefore, when repressed experiences do emerge into consciousness, they are usually accompanied by much more vivid feeling and reliving. This provides a basis for a truly emotional corrective experience.

The affect bridge (Watkins & Watkins, 1997, pp. 120–121) differs from traditional hypnotic abreactions in the way the reliving experience is initiated. Once the earlier situation has been revivified, the rules that govern the successful working through of emotional abreaction are then applied. As with traditional abreactions, the technique bears resemblance to flooding (Wolpe & Lazarus, 1966) or implosive therapies (Stampfl & Levis, 1967). This allows us to break out of a sterile intellectuality into the feeling and experiential realm of emotional change and growth.

A 35-year-old woman was referred to J.G.W. for weight reduction following the birth of her child because she had been unable to attain her prepregnancy weight. She reported several months had elapsed since the delivery, but that her weight had receded very little from what it had been immediately prior to the birth of the child. She would regress into lapses of greedy, if not actual binge eating, behaviors. Direct hypnotherapeutic interventions had little immediate effect despite her ability to enter a fairly deep state of hypnosis. Posthypnotic suggestions controlled her eating for only a few days, during which these periods would be followed by sudden outbursts of eating and gaining back the very few pounds previously lost. Her craving would "overcome" her, and she would rush into the kitchen to satisfy herself with anything she could find.

Her eighth session is particularly interesting, first, as an illustration of the affect bridge technique, and second, as a basis for comparing it with the more traditional analytic approach as to the number of sessions usually required to elicit repressed material. Starting the session nondirectively, the patient opened the hour by describing an incident that had happened the previous Tuesday afternoon. She was in the nursery taking care of her baby, when she felt an overwhelming urge to eat. She "rushed" into the kitchen and began gobbling cakes, cookies, and sweets. When she was filled almost to the point of sickness, a great sense of guilt overcame her. At the time she went into the kitchen, she was so overcome by craving for food that she could not control her urge. The eating and gorging was not described as dissociated such as is common among bulimic patients (M. Barabasz, 1996).

Hypnosis was induced and, with little effort, achieved at least a medium level of depth. She was asked to return to the previous Tuesday afternoon when she was in the nursery. In this brief regression, the situation was vivified with much description. She soon began to experience intense craving. The feeling was accompanied by swallowing movements. She was then given the following hypnotic suggestions:

> Your craving to eat is becoming more intense. It is so strong that you can think of nothing else. You feel confused. The room is fading. Everything is a great blur. The only thing you can experience is craving, craving, craving, CRAVING! The world is full of craving.

The craving was intended to represent the affective element that might be the common bridge between the present incident and some earlier significant and likely pathogenic experience, where she might also have experienced such craving. The hypnotic suggestions were aimed at intensifying this feeling and ablating other elements in the Tuesday afternoon situation. She was induced to pay attention only to this affect and experience it most strongly. The affect of craving was treated as the common bridge between the present and the past, and the patient was moved over this bridge into some as-yet-undetermined situation in the past, which it was believed might, through transference, be unconsciously determining her present behavior. She was instructed as follows:

> Now you are becoming younger. You're going back, back, back into the past, down a road consisting of craving, craving. Everything is changing as you go down the road except the craving. The craving is the same, always the same. And you are becoming younger and younger. You are going back to some time in your life when you first felt this same craving. WHERE ARE YOU? WHAT IS HAPPENING?

Unlike traditional abreactive procedures, the patient is selecting the time and place in the past to which she will move, rather than the therapist. What you are doing hypnotically is simply conveying your belief that the patient will move to some such time and place.

At this point, the patient replied, "I am lying in bed. There are slats up and down. I want to suck my thumb, but mamma's tied a cloth on it with bitter black medicine."

Through their common affect of craving, situation A, the incident that Tuesday afternoon in the nursery, and situation B, the frustration of an infantile need to suck, are seen to be related. Something about the care of her own baby must have reminded her unconsciously of the earlier experience and, through transference, stimulated the affect of craving, just as she felt it in her childhood.

The patient was now allowed to gratify this need:

Mary, you can take off the bad cloth now and suck your thumb if you wish. [Notice this is kept permissive. She is told she can suck her thumb if she wishes rather than she must suck her thumb.] Go ahead, suck your thumb. Go ahead and suck it if you want to.

The patient made motions of "removing the cloth" and placed her thumb in her mouth. Then she lay on the couch and assumed a partially fetal position while vigorously sucking and slobbering. For 15 minutes, she continued this sucking as she was encouraged to enjoy this regressed experience to the utmost. Finally, she removed her thumb:

I don't want to suck anymore, I feel so yummy.

The craving had been traced hypnotically through an affect bridge to this childhood experience of frustration. But is this connection sufficient to account for the patient's overeating? Or must we know much more to effect a cure? Let's see now: She no longer feels the affect of "craving," but she does feel the affect of "yumminess." This is a key upon which we will need to build another affect bridge to discover some even earlier significant experience. The additional affect bridge was created as follows within the same hypnotic session:

Mary, Mary, you are now forgetting all about being in the crib with the slats. You are becoming even younger. Going back, back, back. But the world is filled with yumminess. You feel so yummy as you become younger. You are going back to sometime when you first felt yummy. [It is essential to avoid suggesting a specific scene because you have no basis, as of yet, to suggest with any specificity where she is going. To do so would create an entirely artificial situation for the patient, which would likely be therapeutically ineffective.]

At this point, the patient said nothing, but, putting her hands near her mouth, she clutched at some object in front of her. She began opening and closing her mouth and sucking through protruding lips. The therapist only said, "Do you know where you are?" There was enough retention of the adult ego remaining that the patient could understand and nod. Nothing more needed to be said. Both of us were aware that she felt she was nursing at the maternal breast and that this was what felt "yummy."

Needless to say, there can be substantial argument that the brain is not sufficiently matured at that point of life to develop memory traces as we think of them now. We are not attempting to make statements about the veridicality of this reconstructed memory, but the point is that this is what the patient encoded as "feeling yummy." We need not know whether or not the patient's mother had, for example, allowed her to suck her nipples at a later age, say at 3 or even later, when such memory could be encoded. The important issue is that the patient had successfully crossed the affect bridge to something symbolizing maternal breast-feeding.

The patient was next asked, "Do you think you would like to remember all of this, and bring it back when you are awakened out of hypnosis? Are you ready to understand it?" This is a question, not a command. It was used to test the integrating ability of the conscious ego, and to allow the patient to maintain complete control to choose whether or not she was ready for this insight. She indicated agreement again by nodding.

> All right, you can slowly return to the present time and alert yourself as I count to 15. You will bring back with you all the memories, the feelings, the experiencing, and the understanding of this, which you have indicated you are now capable of handling. [The count out of hypnosis was then initiated.]

The patient opened her eyes and burst into laughter: "Now I know why I crave to eat cookies and cakes. I don't want to have a baby, I want to be a baby."

In the following 8 weeks, the patient lost 30 pounds and returned to her pre-pregnancy weight of 132 lb. Let us recognize that this rate of weight loss exceeds the ideal substantially, versus the normal healthy weight program loss of no more than 1 to 1½ lb per week (see Barabasz & Watkins, 2005, Weight Reduction with Hypnosis, pp. 371–377). She maintained the weight loss for several years of follow-up after treatment and reported little difficulty with craving to eat.

Recognize that it is important we specify that the patient is to return to a point where he or she felt that same affect (craving, fear, anger, etc.). All angers may not be psychologically the same, even though they have similar physiological bases. Some cravings may well be qualitatively different from other cravings. The task at hand is to activate that specific affect, in this case craving in the here-and-now that is apparently related (transferred) to a critical earlier incident in which it was originally experienced. If J.G.W. had not specified the same affect, the patient might have returned to some other similar experience, but not the one that was sought.

The craving affect she was experiencing in the nursery was the same as the affect of craving when frustrated by being unable as a child to suck her thumb. Hence, it served as the affect bridge between the two and took us from the present experience in the nursery with her own child to the past one, wherein the patient herself was a child in the crib.

She was then told to "remove the cloth" and given permission and encouragement to suck her thumb, which she actually did for some 15 minutes. The affect must be satisfied in its original regressed-experiential setting. In this case, the craving was satisfied essentially to the point of exhaustion; she no longer wished to suck her thumb, but felt "yummy."

Now, the new affect has replaced the craving. It is the feeling of "yumminess." Another affect bridge had to be run. All experiential content except the affect of "yumminess" was ablated and she was told to go back to the first time she felt "yummy," whereupon she said nothing, but cupping her hands in front of her mouth, began with protruding lips to "nurse."

Then she was asked, "Do you know where you are?" On receiving an affirmative nod, she was then asked if she would be willing to return to the present and bring with her the understanding of what her craving represented, the memories of the crib and the cloth, plus what the experience of "yumminess" stood for. She agreed, again with a nod, and upon emerging from hypnosis in a fully alert state, she broke out into laughter.

The affect bridge is not in any way an entire system of therapy. It is merely a single hypnoanalytic method that can often facilitate the process of association, helping the patient to move from present transferred experiences to earlier origins. It can often shorten the treatment process very substantially, and it assists in revitalizing insights by stimulating the affect components of "relived" experiences. In these ways, it will likely be a valuable addition to the armamentarium of the analyst as well as the analytically oriented counselor.

The Somatic Bridge

The somatic bridge is a modification of the affect bridge developed by Helen Watkins (1997, p. 121, 2000). The somatic bridge asks the patient if he or she feels tension in any part of their body. If the reply is, for example, "a tightness in the chest," "butterflies in the stomach," or something similar, the patient is asked to concentrate on that part of the body, and after induction of hypnosis "go back" to an earlier time when that same sensation was first experienced. Quite often the patient will actually enter hypnosis at the first suggestion without a further formal induction (Nash, 2005) and will regress to an earlier experience, which is then dealt with as in the affect bridge.

Experimental Evidence for the Affect Bridge

Literally hundreds of clinicians report to us every year their successes with a number of techniques that we have recommended and taught in workshops over the years. The affect bridge has almost always been prominent in reports of successful treatments, yet, as is usually the case, virtually none of these clinicians have presented their work or published their findings even as case studies. Nonetheless, there is experimental evidence related to the phenomenon, consistent with experimental studies regarding mood retrieval of memories (Bower, 1981; P. C. Watkins, Matthews, Williamson, & Fuller, 1982). Memories of the happenings during a party may return to the time when the mood feelings of parties are again being experienced. From an ego-state theory perspective (discussed in Chapter 10), this would be explained as the reinstatement of a former ego state. As such, the experience is directly consistent with studies of the affect bridge (J. G. Watkins, 1971). The normal changing of ego states is also illustrated in bilingual people who have learned one language in childhood, but who now as adults reside in a different country and speak, often fluently, the new language of their present residence. Helen Huth Watkins is just one very personal example of that experience.

Born in Bavaria, Germany, Helen spoke no English before age 10, at which time she and her mother moved to the United States to live with an uncle and aunt in Pittsburgh (after her father had died). The public school to which she was sent had no facilities for foreign-speaking students. She was left to learn English entirely on her own, as do small children first learning to speak. This did not involve the usual methods of a foreign-language class, when a word in German is equated with the same word in English; for example, "baum" equals "tree." She simply created a new ego state, an English-language one in which she learned the words as if for the first time. She became quite fluent in English without a trace of an accent. Consistent with the affect bridge when, she traveled to Germany with J.G.W., she spoke German to store clerks, who took her for a native. This required a switch of ego states, which J.G.W. tested by asking her to say what month it was when she and her mother came over on the ship; she responded instantly with "Juli" (pronounced "Yuli" in German). Her thinking had moved to a German-language ego state!

In a significant contribution to learning theory a quarter of a century ago, Bower (1981) and Bower, Monteiro, and Gilligan (1978) hypnotically induced moods (happy or sad) to create an experimental analog of affect-state dependent learning. For example, subjects were taught two lists of words, one while happy and the other while sad. The tests for recall were given later, when the subjects were in the same or the opposite mood. State dependency appeared as better recall of the same-mood list and worse recall of the opposite-mood list. This finding held when mood was either happy-happy or sad-sad (retention better) and the opposite was happy-sad or sad-happy (retention worse).

In a separate investigation (summarized by Bower, 1981), they induced a happy or sad mood in their participants and asked them to describe a series of unrelated incidents of any kind from their pre-high-school days. They reported that "happy subjects retrieved many more pleasant than unpleasant memories, a 92% bias, whereas sad participants retrieved slightly more unpleasant than pleasant memories, 55%, a bias in the reverse direction." When subjects were asked to describe their childhoods, they reported that memories "were enormously dependent on their mood at the time." These findings support the notion that J.G.W. should not have been surprised when, in his first affect bridge patient, the state of craving returned to an earlier incident (a crib) in which she experienced the same craving. In yet another study, Bower and his colleagues (summarized in Bower, 1981) found that when given stories to read, happy readers tended to identify with happy characters and to remember more details about them, whereas sad subjects tended to identify with sad characters and to remember more about them. Teasdale and Fogarty (1979) found that happy participants recovered happy memories faster than sad ones, whereas sad participants recovered sad memories faster than happy ones.

Bower (1981) hypothesized an "associative network theory of memory and emotion" to account for these findings. He suggested that an event is represented in memory by a cluster of "descriptive propositions," which are the basic units of thought. These are connected to each other within a somatic network. The somatic network presumes that each distinct emotion has a specific node or unit in memory, which collects together many other aspects of the emotion that are associatively connected to it. The emotional feelings, behaviors related to them, and verbal labels assigned to them are connected with the various events in which they occurred throughout different times in one's life.

The common affect provides an associative bridge that permits us to move from one emotional event to another that possesses a similar affect. The theory can be extended to account for such phenomena as mood-contiguity effects, mood state-dependent retention, and even dissociation (which will be discussed at greater length in Chapters 9, 10, and 11). Bower concluded that he had "described two basic phenomena: first, the mood-contiguity effect, which means that people attend to and learn more about events that match their emotional state, and second, mood state-dependent retention, which means that people recall an event better if they somehow reinstate during recall the original emotion they experienced during learning."

In their chapter on practice guidelines for the treatment of traumatic stress, Cardeña, Maldonado, van der Hart, and D. Spiegel (2000) discussed the most efficacious treatments for PTSD. They noted that hypnotic responsiveness varies somewhat throughout the life cycle, and individuals are more highly hypnotizable during their late childhood years. Hypnosis was recognized as most important in treating PTSD patients because they are easily hypnotizable and it can be integrated into various approaches to help patients recollect traumatic events. They reviewed data that showed that age regression, including specific reference to affect bridges, was an important part of an eight-process model to treat PTSD.

Vaillant (1997) discussed the source of psychopathology as the impairment of human emotional experience and illustrated as well as recommended the use of how affect bridges can be used with great effectiveness to bridge the gap between intrapsychic and interpersonal issues.

McKenzie (1994) reported on the case of a 40-year-old woman with vomiting phobia and secondary infertility. Investigation revealed that she was afraid of holding a baby in case it might vomit on her. The use of the affect bridge as an exploratory technique rapidly revealed relevant traumatic child-hood memories, which facilitated her treatment and resolved the phobia with lasting results.

Bills (1993) outlined the use of the affect bridge in hypnosis for the manage-ment of a major dental phobia, which allowed the patient to undergo required dental procedures without undue anxiety. Jiranek (1993) used hypnotic age regression emphasizing the affect bridge, followed with self-hypnosis to treat a 39-year-old woman who was experiencing guilt. The affect bridge made it possible to reveal substantial levels of repressed guilt that strongly affected the patient's present coping abilities. Hypnosis allowed the client to access repressed material via regression concerning sexual advances by an uncle, of which she was apparently not fully consciously aware. The case was reported as successfully resolved. Malmo (1990) explained how hypnosis is compatible with the feminist approach to therapy when control of both the hypnosis and the hypnotherapy is turned over to the patient. She described step-by-step use of the affect bridge technique for tracking feelings or bodily sensations. She provided numerous examples as to how it had successfully uncovered repressed memory material of traumatic events in childhood, leading to suc-cessful therapeutic outcomes. Milne (1985) described a case of a 26-year-old woman with unreasonable jealousy who achieved the critical therapeutic breakthrough with self-hypnosis after an apparently unsuccessful therapy session using the affect bridge method of hypnosis.

In a remarkable attempt to deal with pedophilia, Stava (1984) used hypnotic uncovering techniques emphasizing induced dreams and the affect bridge to reduce inappropriate sexual arousal in a male pedophile. Pedophiles in treat-ment are normally highly resistant to any form of lasting cure. In the present case, treatment effects were examined on objective criteria including test bat-teries using the MMPI, the Personality Research Form, and the Rorschach, as well as direct physiological measures of penile tumescence, which resulted in a significant reduction of sexual excitation to slides of prepubescent children as well a reduction in defensiveness and sexual anxiety with regard to adult women.

Degun-Mather (2003) focused on the use of ego-state therapy including the affect bridge in the treatment of binge eating disorders with a patient who had a complex history of starvation through adolescence and adulthood, alternat-ing with binging. The patient had been resistant to several other therapies, was confused about herself, and had no clear sense of her identity. She recognized that there were parts of herself that seemed to separate from each other. Ego-state therapy with hypnosis provided her with an understanding of the cause of her compulsive state binging. The affect bridge was the key that enabled her to access another child part of herself concerned with a fear of starvation and abandonment as well as wanting to remain "solid" but not fat. Treatment produced great improvement in her eating behaviors, which she had never experienced before. Accessing the ego states using the affect bridge was the key to starting an inner communication, which made cognitive and emotional changes possible. These therapeutic gains were reinforced later with cognitive therapy, from which the patient had never previously gained benefit.

Emmerson (2000b) emphasized that finding the origin of the client's presenting problem is imperative for the discharge of unwanted symptoms. Discovering and processing the unresolved trauma that is associated with a current pathology is the key. He recommended combining his own resistance deepening technique and the affect bridge to reduce the client's resistance to hypnosis as a focus to achieve a medium to deep hypnotic state.

The Corrective Emotional Experience

In an attempt to speed up psychoanalytic treatment, Alexander and French (1946) stressed the importance of achieving what they termed the "corrective emotional experience." By that, they meant reactivating an early emotional situation within the analytic transference that had been marked by the patient's inability to cope effectively or to master the situation. By reexperiencing it through transference onto the analyst, it was thought that the patient had a new opportunity to understand it, to perceive its relevance to present-day situations, and then to master it. This enables the patient to respond realistically to other people in their environment and more adaptively to similar situations.

The concept stressed the necessity that the situation be reexperienced and given a more favorable outcome. Psychoanalysts focus on doing this by way of the transference reaction, whereas our focus is to attain the same objective via abreactions. When it comes to reactivation, the goals are identical between the two variations of analytic approaches. As first pointed out by J.G.W (1954), hypnotic trance is in itself a form of transference phenomena. At the very least, it provides an altered state of consciousness in which such phenomena can be more easily initiated.

Within trance and the hypnotic relationship, we strive to achieve the identical result advocated by Alexander and French (1946), a corrective emotional experience, but our focus is on providing a more favorable outcome of the reexperienced situation via abreaction rather than depending to any significant degree on the effects of transference. No doubt, transference occurs. However, we do not see that this phenomenon is essential to account for the variance in personality reconstruction and eventual adaptive responding we achieve when using abreactive techniques with resonance.

We usually obtain a corrective emotional experience in the patient when all the steps for conducting a successful abreaction are carried through to completion. However, J.G.W.'s late wife and colleague, Helen Huth Watkins, insisted that something is lacking, both in the model of Alexander and French, and in the procedures described in this volume for conducting an abreaction. Indeed, both models advocate correction through reliving, relief of bound affect, and new understanding through interpretation, one within the analytic transference and the other within the state of hypnosis. However, Helen Watkins held that for true reintegration to take place, interpretation is not enough. She maintained that there must be a redoing, a corrective action, either in fantasy or in reality, which must be more than a cognitive understanding. The patient in the regressed state of hypnosis must make a specific behavioral move to change the situation and leave it not as a failure but as a favorable memory.

Let us take the patient who has abreactively reexperienced a childhood molestation and released her fear or anger. She must now, within the memory, experience herself as pushing back the molester and this time successfully protecting herself (H. H. Watkins, 1978). The therapist has a key role here, by adding to the patient's ego strength. The presence of the strong therapist with the patient in the situation enables the sufferer to now master the experience more surely. Let us say that the individual has been traumatized by a very fearful experience. The hypnotherapist (after the releasing abreaction has been secured to exhaustion) must, in fantasy, take the "little girl," hand in hand, back into the feared situation to show her that now she has nothing to fear. The actual physical holding of the patient's hand helps to secure this critical "with-ness."

Whether or not the patient remembers the corrected version or both versions when she is realerted out of hypnosis apparently is not important for lasting therapeutic effect to take place (A.F.B.'s preference is for the patient to recall both, but there is no data to suggest this is better). The key is that the corrected version be the one that remains in her "unconscious." It was the original version of what happened, whether or not this was actually true or fantasized, or whether it took place in reality. It must now be corrected. That corrected version of the event takes the place of the failure that she experienced as a child. In the corrected version, she overpowers her molester. The successful coping is established and remains in her inner personality structure, so that it, rather than the earlier failure experience, will be the determining agent of her day-to-day behaviors and adjustments.

Some time ago, one of J.G.W.'s psychoanalytic friends remarked to him, "My God, when you hypnotists start twisting the memories of patients, we psychoanalysts will never get them straightened out." Our point here is that when memories are altered through later positive therapeutic influence, the original version may well be permanently lost. The experimental research of one of the most staunch opponents of reliving-type experiences with hypnosis, Elizabeth Loftus (1979), clearly found in the data she presented that once suggested memories had been "frozen" in a participant's mind, they may permanently modify the original veridical trauma recollection(s). This is our therapeutic goal. The implementing of memories will probably remain controversial for some time, but many others have presented similar findings, the first of which after Loftus being Udolf (1983).

What is really important here is that in psychotherapy, our concern is with the improved mental health of patients, which involves psychological reality and not objective reality. If a veridical memory causes symptoms and maladaptive behaviors, it would seem obvious to even the most casual observer that its replacement by a more benign recollection is in the interests of our patient's welfare. As the ancient philosopher Epictetus (1952) pointed out more than 2,000 years ago, it is the view that we take of things, not what happened, that determines our reactions. Similarly, the father of modern cognitive therapy, Albert Ellis, adopted this view more than half a century ago (1962), and it remains today as the key basis for cognitive behavioral therapy. Indeed, Aaron Beck's cognitive therapy approach to the treatment of depression (1976) is apparently effective because his therapy has taught people to reframe situations. It is what we think we have perceived and experienced that determines the way in which we adapt to the world around us. It is indeed the view we took of what happened to us at an early age, even into our 20s, and it is that view that must be corrected if we are to achieve health and adjustment.

It is preferable to permanently destroy a pathological memory and replace it with a health-giving one. We may not always be able to do this. However, the psychological reconstruction of a traumatic emotional experience is a legitimate therapeutic goal. More important is that patients take some specific restorative act to correct the continuous impact that their harmful memory has on their self-image and maladaptive defense interactions.

In an audio recording published by J.G.W. and H. H. Watkins (1978), in which Helen Watkins included an excerpt from an abreactive session, a patient, regressed to the age of 3, relived a situation in which his mother had locked him in a dark closet ("filled with monsters"), because she said he had stolen some cookies. The poor little boy's terror was so great that he passed out and, in fact, had awakened later in bed, regressed in his behavior to a much earlier level. In remembering and reliving the situation, he emerged from hypnosis with a severe headache. He could not cope with the powerful and punitive mother.

Helen Watkins said to the hypnotically regressed patient, "I think it is a horrible thing to do to a child. Feel. Feel that feeling of resentment and anger. Let it come through, and your headache will stop. Get in touch with that anger. It's all right to be angry. Go for it." But the patient couldn't do it.

He replied, "I can't, dammit! There is something blocking it. There is something that says, 'Absolutely not.'"

Something happened at age 2 that kept the patient from being able to express anger.

He explained, "I just stopped getting mad, that was the last time I got mad at anybody, really."

He was then rehypnotized and regressed to "that experience that happened to you just before you turned off your anger." He responded with some anger, but not very strongly.

"That's not fair." [Hitting the couch.] "Mommy! You fooled me."

With too much fear to continue his anger, he started crying and whimpered, "I'm not suppose to be mad."

The session continued as follows:

"She hit me with a big belt."

"She hit you with a big belt?"

"She told me when I got mad at her; she was going to beat me with the belt."

The therapist now tried to strengthen the child state so it could cope with Mommy by suggesting the child's increase in size.

"You're going to grow up a little bit now. You're gonna get bigger. Can you see? Mommy is there with the belt? Now she's gonna hit you with that belt. But you're bigger and bigger and you can get mad, you can get mad."

This technique did not work either. The child still felt too weak to confront Mommy.

"No, I'm just a little tiny kid."

The therapist tried another tactic. This time she strengthened his ego by allying with it.

"Now I want you to pay close attention. I'm not going to let her hit you anymore. I'm going to hold her back and you can get mad at her; you can get mad at her. Can you see me holding on to her? She has a belt in hand, and I'm not gonna let her hit you. And you can get mad."

The patient with a therapist-strengthened ego now can take the necessary action to redress the wrongful Mommy.

"Can I take the belt and hit her with it?"

"Yes. Don't be afraid to. I am not gonna let her hit you."

The patient began to laugh and flailed his arms, beating the couch hysterically time and time again, at the end of which he spontaneously emerged from hypnosis. Even when it appears that a patient has spontaneously emerged from hypnosis, use all the normal cautions to assure full realerting.

The therapist now interpreted: "It's all right; you can be mad now, you don't have to lock yourself into the closet or lock in your feelings. All those feelings can come out now."

"God damn. You're right, my headache's gone."

The therapist responded with, "I knew if we got the anger out, your headache would go away."

The patient can now fully verbalize his rage.

"God, what a bitch. God, what a bitch."

He continued on with a plethora of memories about the mother's mistreatment. The therapist finally said, "You will remember more and more of these negative experiences. The energy you have used to repress all of this now is available to you for more constructive purposes." The patient looked up with a grin: "How come I feel so tired?"

Laughing resonantly with the patient, the therapist replied, "Well, that was a lot of work. You beat the hell out of my couch."

Poison Pen Therapy

Abreactions focused on hate can also be conducted through written catharsis, either with or without hypnosis. J.G.W. first termed this "poison-pen therapy" (1949).

A very depressed and, in fact, suicidal woman awoke one night and spontaneously typed such a letter to her parents. She brought a copy to me in therapy. Excerpts from the letter follow:

> Momma and daddy, I hope this letter sears your souls and sends you to everlasting hell which you so well deserve and which you gave to all your children. You two beasts were so busy fighting all your lives that you did not give your children the slightest love and understanding. How could you expect to raise children in that hell that you did and get anything but children filled with hate, hate, hate, and confusion? I was a perfect child, never spanked, wasn't that wonderful? Like hell it was. You held your affection up as the bone I must jump for, and I was always good because I wanted to be loved, not because I wasn't spanked. I never vomited my food as a small child because I feared the lack of affection it would bring. When I got older I could only retaliate by vomiting. Truly you are hating people and you will die hated!

The letter was much longer and, unfortunately, was actually mailed. Even though its writing brought great relief from both depression and the imminent danger of suicide to the patient, we suggest that this technique only be used when the patient can be trusted to honor the request to bring the letter to treatment, not mail it. One can visualize the reaction of her parents. The reaction might well have created worse reality problems. The value of such a cathartic, abreactive release comes from expressing the anger at the parents that exist within the patient, not the old people who exist in reality, who now would not remember such actions and simply would not, at this date in life, comprehend this message.

Criticisms of Classical Abreactive Techniques

Meissner (1991) reviewed criticisms of abreaction, citing Rado (1925). He noted that abreaction may be opposed in its function to analysis. He also asserted that the therapeutic effect of catharsis may be attributed to the fact that it offers the patient an artificial neurosis in exchange for his or her original one, and that the phenomena observable when abreaction occurs is akin to those of a hysterical attack. These criticisms are essentially twofold in that abreaction, as thought of in this manner, may well cover two alternative processes, the discharge of affect and libidinal gratification. The first grants abreaction nothing more than an occasional adjunct to analysis, although clearly a useful one. The second is seriously critical of the procedure; it regards it with great suspicion in that it promotes the belief that the event is likely to impede analysis. In cases in which the predominant etiological factor is an external event, the effects of abreaction might not be permanent. We are basing the procedure described in this book on the encoding or embedding on memory of some external event. Nunberg (1932) saw abreaction as a component factor in analysis, whereas Freud himself (1920) recognized that the act of becoming conscious involves a discharge of energy.

If abreaction is merely viewed as a flooding of affect, and nothing more, then obviously it may simply be a repetitive acting out. However, David Spiegel (1981) demonstrated convincingly that hypnotically induced abreactions were very effective when followed by "working through." We are in full agreement with this, except that we define "working through" as the detailed and rather complex process of reassurance and reintegration.

D. P. Brown and Erika Fromm (1986) reviewed both hypnotherapeutic and hypnoanalytic techniques in great detail; this is a must for all serious analytically oriented hypnotherapists, as well as for those using hypnocounseling techniques. However, we disagree strongly with their views regarding abreaction in that they stated it may be of limited use only in certain cases of acute stress symptoms. Contrary to our findings and the procedures described herein, they go on to advocate a very cautious and conservative approach intended to avoid "acting out" and other "emotional expression."

Our experiences, as well as those of Helen Watkins and many therapists whom we have taught over the years, have reported quite the contrary experience. Beginning as early as J.G.W.'s work with World War II soldiers (1949), followed by over 15 years treating veterans in hospitals and clinics, plus a lifetime thereafter of private practice with many dissociated cases (A. Barabasz, 2003b; J. G. Watkins and H. H. Watkins, 1984, 1997), we have seen very few of the hazards of which D. P. Brown and Erika Fromm (1986) warn. Although we, like all other therapists, have had our share of failures, many of our most outstanding successes were the result of profound hypnotic abreactions. The results have been lasting, with many years of follow-ups of cases that we treated with resonance, reassurance, and reintegration/egotization.

Why, then, the disparity between our experience and the recommendations of D. P. Brown and Erika Fromm (1986) and similar concerns expressed by Frederick (2005)? We regard dissociated affect, such as is found in trauma and child abuse cases, as representing a quantum of pathology that requires ventilation, expression, and release, coupled closely with a resonant therapeutic relationship as well as interpretation and working through. Our experience is that one can release this quantum violently within a short period, or slowly and over an extended period of time. But this quantity must be released in full and worked through, one way or another.

Obviously, a hazard that exists is the amount of affect released. Will it be too painful to the patient? Will the patient be overwhelmed? It is essential that the therapist is ready to carry it through to the end without being overwhelmed him- or herself. Some therapists are emotionally ill-equipped to do this and, therefore, should avoid abreactive therapy. In this respect, an abreaction is like a "battle" between the "good guys" and the "bad guys." An old principle of military battles is that victory goes to those who reach the conflict area "the firstest with the mostest." In the abreaction, it is important that the contact between the dissociated "bad" affect and the ego be strengthened and reinforced with greater power on the side of the patient's ego.

The strength or weakness is not a constant, inhering in that structure. It is measured by the strength of the therapeutic "we-ness," that is, the combined strength of the patient and the therapist, "me and my big analytic father (mother, brother)." This is, in a sense, an ego loan and is related to the amount of resonance offered the patient by the therapist. The weaker the patient's ego, the more intense must be the therapist-patient resonance. The strength stems directly from the clinician's therapeutic self. It is the therapist's commitment and willingness to "walk in the shoes" of the patient that counts. If the hypnotherapist is not willing to submit him- or herself to the buffeting of violent coexperience with the patient in the released affect, then the regressed patient remains like a small child. The patient recognizes that his or her ally, his or her "therapeutic parent," is not willing to accompany him or her into the dark closet, "into the jaws of hell." The patient's ego is then not sufficiently strong to prevail. Unaccompanied contact with the released affect simply should not be undertaken. A key to successful abreaction is combining the ego strengths of both the therapist and the patient, so that the patient can prevail in reliving the event. (Watkins & Watkins, 2000).

In our experience, even when the most powerful acting out has taken place, the patient seldom emerges from it worse. There has been an emotional release, resistances are down, and the time for reassurance, interpretation, and reintegration is at hand. The dire warnings of negative consequences by traditional psychoanalytic practitioners and therapists seldom take place. The personality reorganizes, newer more appropriate ego defenses take place, and the patient moves forward more adaptively. We have yet to see a permanent psychosis so initiated. Yes, there have been transitory psychotic reactions that appear, but in every case we have found these to have a healing effect, so long as the therapist does not panic. As Marin Orne once quipped (in a personal communication to A.F.B., 1990), "If something like that were to happen it is routine. It must always be routine for the therapist." Although we are not sure that the word "routine" may be the best label, we can rest assured that these effects are not only infrequent, but transitory at best and have the potential for healing.

Cursing and screaming, a young woman proceeded to throw every book in J.G.W.'s professional library (several hundred), smashed an ashtray, and then stormed out, shouting, "I never want to see you again as long as I live." A traditional therapist would never tolerate such acting out and might have even insisted on hospitalization. This young women had a longtime chronic character disorder involving depression, hostility, constant smoldering anger, and a schizoid manner that lent itself to the precipitation of such overwhelming rage.

J.G.W. simply let her go, and wrote her a note saying, "Dear Trude: I shall expect you at our next regular hour. With kind regards, Jack Watkins." She came to her next therapeutic session, profuse with apologies but beaming all over. Her emotional avalanche had swept away years of depression, repressed anger, and narcissistic character traits. She had accomplished more in that 1 hour than in years of conservative, supportive, and psychoanalytic treatment. With the release of all this bound affect, her resistance was greatly lowered. He could now interpret the transferences from her father and her brother and she could now accept such interpretations.

For this patient, it was the start of an entirely new stage of personality growth. Contrary to what might be traditionally predicted, this remarkable progress was not subsequently lost during the many months in which J.G.W. had contact with her. She resolved a life-long hatred of men, married, and built a new life for herself. Had I panicked, stopped her, rejected her, or returned to a "tiptoeing on eggshells" approach, she would never have taken this step forward. We had won a decisive battle in her therapeutic struggle.

This is another example of a self-initiated abreaction. It demonstrates the healing value of emotional release, the communication of desperation, the revolutions of self in which lifelong neurotic patterns of character and behavior can be swept away as the entire governmental structure of the ego is reorganized. The therapeutic opportunity to snatch victory from the jaws of chaos and defeat, and of therapist self control with courage are important, but the intensive relationship and total commitment to one's patient are most important.

Such is an example of one of numerous similar cases in which greater character change followed destruction of lifelong maladaptive behavioral patterns. The neurotic patient who is close to a psychotic break may also be close to a "cure"!

Abreactive therapy can be somewhat dangerous, but it is a very powerful therapeutic technique. Surgery is dangerous as well; merely the use of the general anesthetic puts the patient at risk of death, even before the cutting begins. But if surgery is required to keep the patient alive and is the only alternative, dangerous or not, the treatment choice is obvious. Emotional release, and even acting out, can be turned into a great therapeutic opportunity in treatment rather than a liability, if the hypnotherapist is willing to take advantage of it. You have to have the guts to carry it through. The patient must also be protected, either by the restraint of hospitalization if absolutely necessary, or the restraining hand of the hypnotherapist's "therapeutic self." As in any other investment, one must evaluate risk versus possible gain. Yes, you may have been taught, as we were in our first graduate classes dealing with therapeutic interventions and ethics, that hospitalization is safer, but just for the moment. The restraining hand of your therapeutic self brings with it greater risk, yet it is more healing if you have the skills and can trust yourself and your relationship with the patient.

A minimal level of ego strength in the patient is necessary, but it appears that the reported "failures" of abreactions are due more to the limitations of the analyst, rather than to the technique. If you cannot commit yourself in an intensive coexperiencing of the violent affect, then don't. If you can't take the heat, stay out of the kitchen! If you can't handle the required level of intense involvement with your patient, abreactions are not for you, and you and your patients would be better off to follow a safer release procedure such as the "slow burn," which will not be so threatening but will take longer. This brilliant, less threatening approach was conceptualized by Richard Kluft (1986), which he termed the "slow leak." The patient is instructed to release the anger gradually over a period of time. It is indeed an elegant alternative. However, it involves so much activity on the part of the therapist in controlling it, rather than permitting the patient to regulate its speed.

The Slow-Release—Slow-Burn Procedure

Even with the closest resonance of which we are capable, and the utmost of therapeutic commitment to our patient, there are times when the abreaction has become so violent or the pain so strong that the patient's ego cannot apparently tolerate its full intensity. Infrequently as this may occur, it can and does occur, and in those cases the patient regresses. Long term, the possible gains may outweigh the risks, but nonetheless, we hesitate to precipitate such reactions on purpose and prefer to play it more safely, because we are not certain we can bring the patient back to a more normal and adaptive functioning. There are times when the patient will even inform us that he or she would prefer to suffer at a lesser intensity over a longer time than become deeply involved and get it over with immediately. Such patients are often good judges of their ability to tolerate anxiety. We recognize that some are simply "therapeutically lazy." They lack courage, or want only comfort and further support of their maladaptive defensive reactions to life. Ask the patient in hypnosis about his or her ability to endure these emotional releases, and make it clear to the patient that it requires courage on his or her part, as well as on yours. In any event, repressed affect must be released and integrated. This can be accomplished either in chunks, with noticeable and sometimes remarkable advances during each session, or in small conservative bits.

Our therapeutic alliance with the patient (Konzag, Baandemer-Greulich, Bahrke, & Fikentscher, 2004; Lorentzen, Sexton, & Hoglend, 2004; Miller, 2004; Frederick, 2005) is the most effective element in toning down the intensity of the release when using the slow-burn approach. In one example, a hypnotically activated "cotherapist ego state" contracted to desensitize a fear ego state and do the job over a period of 3 days. H. H. Watkins (1978) did just that and eliminated a constant source of tension. Again the results were lasting.

A.F.B. and J.G.W inform their patients that therapy is indeed hard work if it is to be effective in a reasonable length of time and that it involves "blood, sweat, and tears." To get well, the patient must commit him- or herself to it, but as the therapist, you also agree to make the identical commitment by clearly indicating that "I will not abandon you." Helen Watkins referred to this as a "love" for your patient, while A.F.B. refers to it as "unconditional love." In this sense, I try to convey the point that, although a patient's behaviors at times may be completely unacceptable, I will always accept the patient as a person, and this is part of my commitment to his or her wellness. In a few cases, it has meant hundreds of hours and many months of free therapy as recalled by A.F.B., J.G.W., and H.H.W. We remind our patients after a painful but productive emotional release, as did Frieda Fromm-Reichman (Greenberg, 1964), "I never promised you a rose garden." The patient usually feels so much better afterwards and commonly thanks us for having carried through therapies "to the other side" and cosuffered it with them. The therapeutic alliance is indeed a renewing of our "we-ness" relationship.

When abreaction is used to relieve the severe suffering that, for example, a dissociative identity disordered patient (multiple personality) experienced as an abused child, we may find that an incomplete resolution of the dissociated rage can precipitate a stage of self-directed anger, with an enormous number of accompanying maladaptive behaviors (easy outs for the moment with great prices to pay in the future). In the extreme, some of these patients go so far as to make suicidal gestures or some form of self-mutilation, such as with cutting or trichotillomania. We must protect our patient from these behaviors, and in extreme cases we may have to resort to hospitalizing our patient. Recognize it is as a last resort and a sign of a failure on our part to convey the unconditional nature of our therapeutic alliance with the patient.

Kluft's Fractionated Abreaction

Both Kluft (1986) and Comstock (1986) emphasized the indispensable necessity for abreactions in the treatment of such cases. They also provided specific ways to mitigate the patient's suffering or to reduce its intensity to a tolerable degree. Obviously, such measures are essential with patients who have lived much of their lives with the disorder and are now at the point of suffering from physical conditions, which may include cardiovascular risk. Let us not precipitate a myocardial infarction with an abreaction where the patient is cured of his or her neurosis at the expense of clinical death.

Kluft developed the approach in the treatment of elderly patients whose dissociation had existed for an extended period of time and who were no longer strong enough to face the full fury of their long-repressed rage. In these cases, the release was so slow that the patients involved scarcely felt any discomfort. The reaction was continued over an extended period of time. In yet another brilliant approach to the goal of reducing the intensity of the abreaction, Kluft (1990) developed the "fractionated abreaction." In this approach, emotionally laden material is brought to awareness in manageable bits through a variety of uncovering techniques. The feelings that would be associated with the memories would actually emerge at other times in "solitary moments." One key to his approach was the use of hypnotic "time distortion," so that the patient could experience the painful emergence of the affect with lower intensity but over a much longer duration of time. Kluft developed these procedures in his treatment of dissociative identity disordered patients (multiple personalities) but they are equally applicable to many other conditions.

The Split-Screen Technique

The split-screen technique developed by Herbert Spiegel and David Spiegel (2004) is projective in nature in that it implies that the patient will "project" sensations, images, and thoughts onto an imaginary screen of the patient's choosing (e.g., computer screen, surface of a calm lake, clear blue sky). It is intended to separate the painful sensations and thus attenuate traumatic abreaction as may be encountered in the reconstruction of traumatic early memories.

Patients learn they can control the intensity of content by adjusting the size of the images or their proximity to the screen. They can also manipulate the images by changing colors such as creating a monochrome (black-and-white) image rather than a more intense full-color image. Patients can also turn the screen off if the image of the memory becomes overwhelming. Given this level of control, the technique provides a new assurance of security and sense of control. The Spiegels also use a variation of the technique that asks the patient to divide the screen in half. Then they can project a left sinister side—the trauma itself—and then a right side, a picture of how they could now protect themselves and stand up to the abuser or adaptively handle the incident.

Therapists who do regressions to discover conflicts in the early life of their patients seldom go back earlier than the age of 2 or 3. The argument is that if they don't have language, they cannot communicate with a therapist. Accordingly, few therapists try to regress a patient to birth or earlier, and our experimental colleagues maintain that it is impossible; the brain does not yet have enough maturation. We (J.G.W. and H.H.W.) have argued that a child at birth has the experience of pain if scalded on its arm. Then, 2 years later, when it has acquired words, it can communicate that experience to a therapist (see Watkins & Watkins, 1997).

H.H.W., who refused to be governed by establishment thinking, had been initiating "birth abreactions" (and even earlier) to many of her patients, with exceptional results in many cases (Watkins & Watkins, 1997). In some instances, she regressed her patient to pre-birth times (pp. 217–222). This technique is controversial, but she used this technique in a number of cases where her patient was in conflict as to whether to have an abortion. She took neither the position of advocating nor of discouraging the patient's decision, but often helped her to resolve the conflict.

Summary

The neglect of abreactive procedures until recently can be attributed to the widely disseminated misconception that the results obtained are limited or temporary and somehow, therefore, are incomplete or inconclusive. When this has occurred, it is now recognized that practitioners who have released affect have done so but failed to fully exhaust it without giving the necessary reassurance, interpretation, and integration. Failures with the technique can also be traced to lack of full commitment and confidence on the part of the therapist and an unwillingness to commit one's self to the unconditionality and "we-ness" of the therapeutic alliance, which is the most crucial element in the psychotherapeutic relationship (Barber, et al., 2000).

Failures have also been due to the fact that the need for repeated reliving has been neglected, and the therapist has lost confidence in the procedure because the "miraculous" results did not occur after a single rendition. Finally, they have often failed to make the necessary commitment to the patient and invest themselves in an intensive, resonate relationship, in which they, too, coexperience and co-suffer with the patient (J. G. Watkins 2000; Watkins & Watkins, 2000). These therapists have misjudged the patient's ego strength and have not presented him or her with a strong ego ally.

Abreactions provide critical as well as valuable therapeutic leverage when they are applied to specific traumatic events that the patient has consciously known to occur and which have resulted in repressed affect, inadequate mastery of the precipitating situation, and resultant ego damage. When the abreaction is carried through to completion, the results are undeniably positive in most cases. Abreactions are especially indicated in the treatment of post-traumatic stress disorders. However, they are not without hazard. They require considerable sensitivity, skill, patience, and courage on the part of the hypnotherapist as well as the patient.

Not only must the therapist and the patient have enough strength to coexperience them; not only must the affect be encouraged and prodded to complete exhaustion; and not only must this be followed by reassurance, interpretation, and reintegration, but the entire experience from beginning to end must often be repeated several times if complete release and extinction of the bound affect is to take place. Healthy ego and object representations will be established clearly, and the ego will be better able to cope with stress in general. Interpretation by itself is frequently inadequate to secure a genuine emotionally reconstructed experience. The patient as well as the therapist must take positive action together to correct the memory of a negative or a failure experience and restructure it into a successful one. It is a matter of ego strengthening and trauma resolution, rather than the creation of a bland artificial façade of a cure.

The loud shouting and violent emotional behavior that characterize abreactions can easily scare off the timid therapist. A number of therapeutic settings in office buildings and university counseling centers make it unfeasible to carry out such procedures. In these cases, silent abreactions may be useful. In these settings, the patient experiences a perceptual release of anger without the motor and verbal accompaniments that preclude the use of the full abreactions. There is considerable clinical experience reported by a number of practitioners suggesting that these are effective, but as yet the data are relatively sparse comparing their effectiveness with full-blown abreactions.

We are often unable to determine exactly where and when the critical incident occurred, even when we are quite certain that the patient is experiencing transference feelings (Seruda, 1997), inappropriate to the present. When an abreaction is therapeutically indicated, we need to know just where in the patient's past to initiate it. The affect bridge is a procedure that has been developed to deal with this problem. It allows us to return to a previously unknown event in which the patient experienced a feeling state similar to that which he or she is feeling in the present. The procedure has been demonstrated to be a very effective therapeutic technique and has had considerable validation and support from both clinical and experimental studies on the relation between mood and memory, as well as direct clinical studies on its effectiveness.

A written abreaction technique termed "poison-pen-therapy" (J. G. Watkins, 1964) encourages expression of affect in letters that are not mailed. Kluft's fractionated abreactions and the slow-leak or slow-burn release are approaches that spread the reaction at a lowered intensity level over a period of time. The Spiegels' split-screen technique provides another very effective alternative. These procedures are indicated if the patient's ego is considered to be too fragile to handle the full abreaction and/or if the therapist's personality does not lend itself to full involvement as a coexperiencing, cosuffering agent with the patient in a full-blown abreaction.

Abreactions have been criticized on the basis of claims that they are ineffective, that they encourage the patient to "act out," and that they are possible hazards to the patient or the therapist. When both the therapist and the patient have a close therapeutic alliance, when there is a constructive relationship, and when the therapist is resonating with the patient, these criticisms are no longer compelling. When carried out skillfully, abreactions can frequently advance therapeutic progress with great rapidity. They are extremely potent treatment procedures in the hands of the skilled and dedicated hypnoanalytic practitioner.

6

Sensory Hypnoplasty and Hypnography

As a young graduate student, J.G.W. once took a course in the history of modern music during an intensive summer-school session. The instructor was the composer Edwin Stringham, a distinguished visiting professor from Columbia University. He proved to be a most innovative teacher. His goal was to give us an understanding of impressionism. Rather than merely lecturing on its objectives, its history, and the lives of its composers, he also played impressionistic music (Debussy, Ravel, and Stravinsky). Still not content, he brought in samples of impressionistic poetry, showed us prints of impressionistic paintings (Degas and Monet), and photos of impressionistic sculpture. He showered us with what many years later became known as "holistic teaching." Unlike other instructors, he stimulated our imagery as well as our cognition, and we derived a true insight into the meaning of "impressionism" because he presented it through many modalities: verbal, auditory, visual, and kinesthetic (J. G. Watkins, 1992a).

The Use of Art in Hypnoanalytic Technique

This chapter plus Chapters 7, 8, and 9 bring to you a group of procedures that, although different, have much in common. Each is related to the other, and when brought together, each enhances the other. Any one of these chapters could have come first. Each chapter includes descriptions of techniques that involve fantasy, imaging, projection, subject-object dissociation, and motor communications (nonverbal communications) both real and hallucinated. The order we have chosen here involves a rationale of beginning with the more tangible and concrete approaches, proceeding to the techniques that emphasize projective fantasy, then describing those that center on dissociation and ego splitting. This leads us more naturally into the complex techniques of hypnoanalytic ego-state therapy. Each of the chapters prepares us for rewarding work with patients conceptualized within ego-state theory and therapy, as well as hypnoanalysis.

Once completed, the ground for an understanding of covert personality entities, as compared to true, overt multiple personalities (dissociative identity disorder), has been laid. The significance of the separation of defenses, as broadly based throughout a continuum extending from normal personality structures at one end to severely dissociated personalities at the other end, becomes more clear. This also teaches "third ear" sensitivity (Reik, 1948).

Consider the example presented by J.G.W. above, where as a young student his insight was derived based on many modalities, both verbal and nonverbal. This type of teaching was similar to the concept of holistic teaching. Sonnier (1982) proposed a model, which was based on the research of Levy (1974), of the functioning of the left and right hemispheres of the brain. Levy's contribution lay in his demonstration that these hemispheres do more than control opposite sides of the human body. According to Levy, each hemisphere has its own unique mode of thinking and its own mode of consciousness. The left brain was thought to reason logically, expressing our understandings in verbal terms as well as analytical. The right brain was thought to preside exclusively over such functions as spatial relations, imagery, metaphors, and dreaming. Presumably, in the engineer and the scientist, left-brain activity is prominent. In the artist and musician, it is the right brain that primarily processes the data. In any given experience, one or the other may be dominant, or the two may collaborate. This is especially so when the more intuitive and feeling aspects of our perceptions are brought to consciousness in the form of verbalized "insight." Of course, the latest research data on brain function shows that the left-brain/right-brain concept is greatly oversimplified. There is a complex interplay between the hemispheres via neuronal integration and a number of other processes. Nonetheless, for our purposes here, let us continue to use the left-brain/right-brain concept metaphorically.

But how do the two halves then collaborate? The corpus callosum, most easily thought of as a cable of fibers, connects the two halves and provides the exchange of impressions necessary for an individual to integrate these two models of consciousness. There are gender differences. Females are thought to have greater interconnectivity between the two hemispheres than the majority of males (there are some dramatic exceptions to this generalization, in that a small percentage of males who have histories of early life accomplishments possess considerable cross-talk between hemispheres). But generally, it is males rather than females who are operating from primarily one side or the other. This may be why some males avoid, at nearly all costs, emotional reactions leading to the level of crying. When they do so, they are totally engaged in single-hemisphere involvement.

By contrast, it is not usual to find a female able to balance her checkbook while tears stream from her eyes over the death of a dear friend. Such behavior is almost an impossibility among males. When connecting links are severed surgically (Sperry, 1973), the individual is in considerable conflict, as right-brain information may be verbally mislabeled by the left brain. Something of this same nature appears to occur when there is a repressed unconscious process (which may be more right-brain mediated). A patient's efforts to acquire conscious, logical left-brain (i.e., primarily verbal) understanding requires effort on the part of the psychotherapist.

Dissertation research conducted by Wilson (1986), one of A.F.B.'s PhD students, measured EEG power spectra in each hemisphere concurrently during "holistic" and "nonholistic" learning tasks. The asymmetry hypothesized by Sonnier (1982) was not demonstrated. We concluded that there must be much more to the holistic concept than simple left-brain versus right-brain differences. The matter became even more complex when we looked at the power response patterns that increased for nonholistic versus holistic teaching styles. In post hoc analysis, a laterality effect was indicated when left-brain/right-brain EEG power ratios were compared separately for participants grouped by right or left versus integrated orientations, but only on a learning style self-report preference inventory. The interaction with differences in hypnotizability remains to be studied, because the brains of these 30 college students were obviously not acting according to Levy's theory.

The last 20 years brought with it exponential increases in technology, which made it possible to determine (for all but a handful of role-play model theorist holdouts) that hypnosis can produce physiologically demonstratable brain function/reaction changes that cannot be produced by suggestion without hypnosis or by role-playing. These national and international award-winning studies of EEG event-related potentials (ERPs), magnetic resonance imaging (MRI), and positron emission tomography (PET), were reviewed in Barabasz and Watkins (2005), chapter 3, Theorizing about Hypnosis (Rainville, Duncan, Price, Carrier, & Bushnell, 1997; Rainville, Hofbauer, Paus, Duncan, Bushnell, & Price, 1999; Rainville & Price, 2003; Ray & De Pascalis, 2003; D. Spiegel, 2003; Szechtman, Woody, Bowers, & Nahmias, 1998; A. Barabasz & Lonsdale, 1983; A. Barabasz, M. Barabasz, Jensen, Calvin, Trevisan, & Warner, 1999; A. Barabasz, 2000; D. Spiegel, Cutcomb, Ren, & Pribram, 1985; D. Spiegel & A. Barabasz, 1988; Kosslyn, Thompson, Constantine-Ferrando, Alpert, & D. Spiegel, 2000). Certain of these studies also provide information reflecting on the role of the anterior cingulate as involved in a type of executive functioning that allows one to focus on or pay attention to a set of cues (Aston-Jones, Rajkowski, & Cohen, 1999). An example would be a person fully absorbed in listening to a lecture, watching a movie, or reading a book who may be dissociated from distracter cues that might otherwise trigger arousal (J. R. Hilgard, 1974, 1979). But how does this reflect on differences in presentation of material, and how is it that those with hypnotic capacity have a greater degree of receptiveness?

Horton, Crawford, Harrington, and Hunter-Downs (2004) reported the first experimentally controlled magnetic resonance imaging research demonstrating differences in brain structure size between low and high hypnotizable persons. Participants were stringently screened for hypnotizability with two standardized scales and then were exposed to hypnotic analgesia and painful stimuli. Consistent with the state theory conceptualizations of hypnosis, only the high hypnotizable participants in the hypnotic condition had significantly inhibited attentional and other responses to the stimuli and had larger (31.8%) rostrum corpus callosum area involvement between the prefrontal cortices as compared to the low hypnotizables. As foreshadowed by A.F.B., Crawford, and M. Barabasz (1993), these results provide support for a neuropsychophysiological model that high hypnotizable subjects have more effective frontal attentional systems, implementing control, and monitoring performance, as well as greater ability to inhibit unwanted stimuli from conscious awareness, than do lows.

These findings converge on the nature of what we have long observed to occur between repressed unconscious processes (which are attentionally mediated by the brain, and patients' conscious efforts to bring them to consciousness with logical, verbal understanding). The effectiveness of a skillful and sensitive hypnoanalyst may derive from his or her ability to "tune in" on the patient's brain communications (associations, metaphors, postures, gestures, images, and dreams) and communicate with them in logical, verbal interpretations, where they become both conscious and under the patient's control. In a sense, such a hypnoanalyst becomes a bit like J.G.W.'s music history instructor, who integrated artistic understanding with scientific understanding and brought both into the subject's awareness.

Communication between therapist and patient is the heart of psychotherapy. Like psychotherapy, the essence of hypnotherapy is the communication between patient and hypnoanalyst through the exchange of meanings, usually in the form of words, but also in communications that take place without words. Our posture, our gestures, our inflections, as well as facial expressions and openness or closeness, in fact, all our nonverbal communications, are just as important as our verbal ones. Thus, we transmit our meanings to others concealed from our own normal awareness. Such indirect communications often reveal meanings that are from the unconscious.

Inner meanings communicated by artists are brought to us through sculptures, drawings, and paintings. The later paintings of van Gogh—through vivid oranges and blacks, and agitated landscapes—portrayed, so well, the storm of depression that was sweeping over the artist at the time, and which finally led to his suicide. The medieval painters, in their productions of angels, Madonnas, and devils, displayed the religious conflicts that pervaded that age and in their own selves. Such art productions have been used in psychological projective tests, such as the draw-a-person test (Machover, 1948) and the House-Tree-Person test (Buck, 1948). These devices provide the psychologist with ways in which patients can express their fantasies by drawing images that may portray something related to their personality structure, as well as their inner motivations. Carl Jung (1916) and Otto Rank (1932) analyzed the work of many artists in an attempt to understand their psychological processes. Naumburg (1947, 1950, 1953) as well as Stern (1952) reported the use of drawings and paintings in implementing psychoanalytic therapy with both neurotics and psychotics. Grof (1975, 1980, 1985), a quarter of a century later, administered graduated doses of lysergic acid (LSD) to volunteers, and their productions were extensively analyzed in comparison with their normal states.

Because of the lack of apparent positive therapeutic outcome results, art therapy enjoyed only a brief time as a popular mode of treatment, although there are many reports of its use (see, for example, Kramer, 1971; Levick, 1981; Wadeson, 1980, 1982). Unfortunately, the lack of its success (patients just doing artwork without therapeutic interpretations) in providing positive treatment outcomes also led to ignoring its use in the diagnostic sphere. Thus, it has not received the attention it warrants in helping us to evaluate our patients' personality structures and/or pervasive mood states. Given that hypnosis offers a wide avenue for providing direct access to unconscious phenomena, most hypnotherapists, hypnoanalysts, and hypnocounselors have preferred to rely on communication through words rather than through art productions. The literature in this area is, therefore, rather meager. Nonetheless, a range of greats in the field have touched on this modality. Sensory hypnoanalysis, as it was termed by M. V. Kline (1968), was one avenue that extended the early approaches developed by Ansile Meares (1957), called hypnography, and later hypnoplasty (Meares, 1960).

Hypnography

Meares used clever and creative interventions that are difficult to replicate. He found hypnotized subjects were more amenable to projective painting than those in their normal state of alertness. At first, Meares had his patients draw with a simple pencil, but later found that black paint proved more effective than either a pencil or his attempt to use a full range of colors (Meares, 1957).

Following these early explorations, he developed a fairly standardized procedure to facilitate replication. He spoke of a "critical depth of hypnosis" as a prerequisite that usually required several sessions of practice with hypnotic inductions. Then, he would have patients hold the brush very loosely as hypnotic suggestions were administered, such as: "Here is a paintbrush. Here is a paint book. I dip the brush in the paint. Your hand takes the brush. It paints it. Your hand will now paint whatever is in your mind." Note the importance he attaches to deep hypnosis, and the initiation of specific highly directive suggestions, which conclude with the open-ended one: "Your hand will paint whatever is in your mind."

Meares persevered as patients had difficulty getting started, a situation that also often occurs when using automatic or dissociated handwriting. (This will be discussed in our Chapter 9 on dissociative hypnoanalysis.) He continually urged the patient with repeated hypnotic suggestions until the painting movements began. When the brush got dry, Meares would simply say, "The brush is running dry. I take the brush and dip it in the paint." This activity on the part of the therapist was often necessary with very passive patients. Furthermore, when patients were asked to dip the brush themselves, they frequently knocked over the paint jar or spilled the paint! This reflects the inhibition of motor control for many individuals while experiencing hypnosis. Once the paintings were completed, associations to them were elicited before the patient was brought out of hypnosis and back into a state of normal alertness. For some undisclosed reason, Meares' standardized procedure included a recommendation of a half-hour sleep for the patient after the session before dismissing him or her. Presumably, after that rest period, Meares ensured normal conscious alertness before allowing the patient to leave his office.

Paintings produced while in hypnosis appeared most often to resemble children's productions and, at best, initially represented the outline of some object. Once again, there is evidence of a regressive process in hypnosis that is essentially topographic, rather than temporal, in nature, where the patient moves to primary process responses. This is supported by the fact that the patient's prior skill in drawing or painting was apparently not utilized in the hypnotic productions. Meares spent up to several sessions developing a critical depth of hypnosis, so it seems reasonable for us to assume that these sessions were all conducted at the deeper levels of hypnotic responding. Obsessive-compulsive patients in a normal state of awareness displayed much neatness, yet became very sloppy in their hypnotic productions. This tended to validate the presumed psychodynamic defenses of excessive neatness as opposed to its unconscious opposite or, as Freud hypothesized, a regression to anal smearing. This finding suggests that hypnographic paintings do tap unconscious motivations at some level.

Consistent with concrete thinking as shown by children and psychotics, the paintings of an object tended to refer to very specific meanings. Thus, the painting of a house did not represent any house but rather a very specific house that was significant in the patient's life. At other times, the object represented a symbol. The house might constitute a symbol of a woman, a very specific woman, such as the patient's mother, as is commonly found in a psychoanalytic dream. Meares found only rare exceptions to this rule. The paintings almost always represented something that was very important emotionally to the patient. The paintings provided an entirely new dimension with the potential of greatly shortcutting therapy time and enhancing treatment outcome.

The paintings provide an exception to the rule that free associations to the paintings are just as important as the productions themselves and can often be helpful, if not essential, to the interpretations of their meaning. Accordingly, it is best that the association immediately follow each rendering. The best way to facilitate this process in the shortest possible time is to provide a posthypnotic suggestion at the end of the painting, such as, "You won't wake up completely while I talk to you," or "You can talk as if in a dream. What is it that the hand has painted?" Notice that the painting is credited to the "hand" and not to the person. The essential concept is to dissociate the hand from the response involved.

The defensive process enables us to express a covert or unacceptable meaning and suppress that meaning from consciousness at the same time. Hypnography affords a modality whereby a patient can reveal to the hypnoanalytic therapist what he or she has felt a need to conceal from him- or herself.

Thus, the associations that we elicit are more completely "free." "What do you think about concerning this painting?" Another way of doing this is to use what J.G.W. refers to as a "radial approach" by mentioning specific items in the picture, such as, "Tell me everything which comes to mind related to the small tree there." The associations are especially essential when the painting refers to traumatic incidents in the patient's life. Such a painting, in fact, may be just the stimulus required to induce a regression to the emotion-laden experience and precipitate the abreaction. The manner in which the product was made may also be the patient's way of expressing his or her underlying meanings rather than the apparent content of the picture itself. Watch them as they work; look for aggressive motions, sexual motions, and so on. Give these same considerations to that of gesture, posture, and facial expressions, and take these into account as you would in any therapeutic interaction whether hypnotic or nonhypnotic.

A patient referred to A.F.B. with a "working diagnosis of borderline personality disorder" had a history of fleeing from career opportunities "just when they looked the brightest" and leaving other jobs for a wide variety of defensive excuses. At the age of 32, she had had a series of 2- to 5-year relationships with immature, jealous, and controlling men who had similar rationales for moving from one job to another. She presented with an awareness of her poor relationship choices and her rejection of "objectively" more rational ones, with the defense that she "loved him" (the current childlike male was a year older than she). Despite obtaining considerable historical information ripe with superficial reasons for job and schooling changes, I could make little progress even with the addition of hypnosis. The bases for insights seemed to be there, but unexposed and not circumscribed. I was pessimistic about the potential use of abreaction and the potential outcome of my treatment attempts.

Given that she had had formal training as an artist, A.F.B. asked to see her artwork. A repeated theme, "I just can't express right," was her light pencil drawings of a ship on dark gray paper or on canvas with a shaded "blue wash" background. Other than the fact that in each case, the ship had clear lines on it dividing its compartments, they were all very faint renderings. At an apparently deeply repressed level, she was aware of the divisions, her different selves, and at the same time recognized the ship was lost at sea in the fog. In light hypnosis, she noted, "It's just out there in the big ocean going nowhere, the engines are running, and it seems to be going somewhere but it might as well be drifting." (Unfortunately, these remarkable renderings were all too faint to be reproduced in a figure here.)

In another very different rendering, a drawing of a woman's face, she said, "This is me torn to pieces. My dark side did this" (not saying it was the tearing up or the drawing itself). "This is all that is left." She gave me the torn bits of beige paper as if still trying to hold on to something; the repressed material was, I thought, momentarily near consciousness. I said, using a tone of voice I frequently use for hypnotic inductions, "It's O.K., it's O.K." I lowered my head slightly while still looking at the bridge of her nose and assumed a slowly closing bodily posture, my nonverbal signal for going inward. Her eyes closed and I assumed, without testing, she had attained at least a light trance state.

My hypnotic suggestion was simple, direct, and concrete: "It's still all there; all its pieces are there; you can put the face back together. Your 'dark side' has goodness, too, and can help you do whatever you need to do." After alerting, I carefully put each piece of torn paper into an envelope for her. The next day, rather than bringing in a reassembly of the torn pieces, she brought a rather large oil painting on canvas rendered in dark to light brown tones. The work, no doubt, must have taken her all night and showed abstractly a "torn vagina." She said, pointing to an apparent clitoris, "Even it's torn—can't work right," thus alluding to her loss of what was earlier described as "great sex" responsiveness. She seemed at last to reach a level of some communication among her distinct personality entities similar to a borderline dissociative identity disorder (DID) rather than a borderline personality disorder or full-blown DID patient. She also recognized at some level that her immature defensive reactions (allowing her to have "great sex") were also failing.

Encouraged, I asked her to go into hypnosis. She appeared to enter a rather deep state within a brief period of time. The hypnotic suggestion I used was to tell her, "Even broken things can work, sometimes better than new lucky unbroken ones, because they have to be more creative to get the job done without all the parts working just right." Before I could figuratively pat myself on the back, she alerted herself spontaneously and told me to take my hypnohocus pocus and do with it what would require me to assume an anatomically impossible position. The colorful, four-letter profanities I had never heard her utter before came out more and more loudly as she stood up to leave. She then grabbed a heavy roll of polygraph paper and tossed it at me in what seemed to be a deliberate miss, which instead broke a lamp she knew I didn't like much. It was remarkable to see such ambivalence expressed even in the midst of this dramatic spontaneous abreaction. Accepting her behavior, as few therapists would likely do, I said as calmly as ever, "See you tomorrow, check the time with Linda [the receptionist]." She then slammed my door.

Was there an attainment of adaptive insight in her emotion-filled abreaction and projection of hatred onto me? Before the day was over, she came back to the office and left a package for me. In it was the same torn line drawing of her face but the torn pieces were pasted together on a black background to make a beautiful profile of a black woman's face.

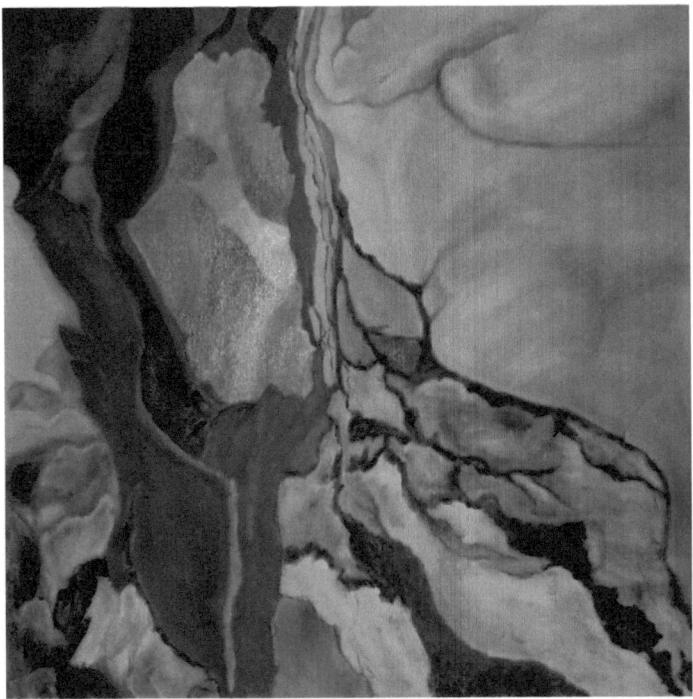

Figure 6.1 Abstract rendering of a "torn vagina" (see text p.102).

Her family tree had an offspring with an African American father, some-thing she had been taught to hate by her parents—whom she now recognized as "screwed up and immature"—even before they split up when she was about the age of 10. Within the next year, she managed to extricate herself from her relationship with the controlling immature fellow and gained entrance to a graduate school of fine arts, where she completed her degree without inter-ruptions. Twenty years later, she was still married to a mature widower whom she had met in graduate school. She had two apparently well-adjusted children who were doing well at school and she had sold many of her paintings and drawings at a growing number of galleries and art shows. She was known for her diverse repertoire and the ability to express artistic styles "as if done by different artists." Her insights had enabled her to achieve an adaptive, reward-ing lifestyle, while at the same time maintaining the creative aspects of her personality. Her husband reported cherishing her spontaneity and energy.

The greater one's experience is in dream interpretation, the better use one can make of the hypnographic technique (J. G. Watkins, 1992a). Meares' exten-sive and in-depth work in this area revealed that both universal symbols and individual symbols were represented. The greatest difficulty in interpretation often lay in the therapist's confusing the two. A.F.B.'s overeagerness to find

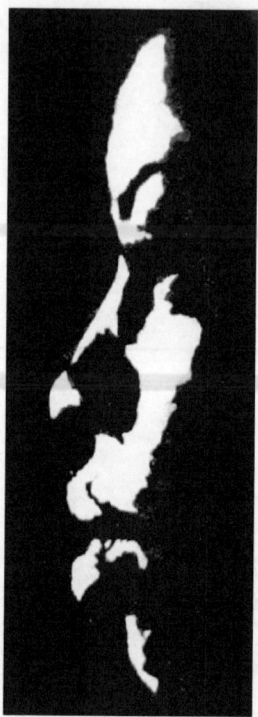

Figure 6.2 Paper tear rendering (see p. 102).

a more rapid solution to the patient's conflicts often led to doing just that. The key to ensure the highest probability of success is to be patient with your patient and yourself until the greatest number of associations has been reached over a period of time.

Given such potential pitfalls and the requirement of considerable experience, the question must be asked, Why should hypnography then be used? The most logical reason would be to employ the technique when a patient is very taciturn and not given to much verbal expression. This situation then is not far removed from the hypnocounseling technique of working with children who are limited in their range of verbal expression, as well as their interests in talking with the therapist. Be just as cautious about revealing to the patient's consciousness heretofore hidden meanings of his or her art productions as you would in working with a child.

The insights are, of course, critical but the patient must be ready to accept such insights. That which is revealed in hypnosis will often come spontaneously to mind in the adult patient's own thinking 2 to 3 weeks later if the therapist can only restrain his or her eagerness to impart this new insight. A.F.B. eventually learned to impart it to chart notes for that moment instead. Typical defenses against verbal revelations may not be operative during art communications, and the patient may often need a period of protection against immediate confrontation.

The majority of clinicians will not find hypnography suitable to their manner of treatment. It is clearly a slower and more cumbersome method of data acquisition than can be secured verbally. But it has the distinct advantage of accessing critical material that often cannot be elicited through words. Hypnography is a useful addition to the armamentarium of the eclectic hypnoanalyst as well as those in hypnocounseling. A modification of hypnography is referred to as hypnoplasty, which is a psychoanalytic procedure first developed by Meares (1960) and refined by Bernard Raginsky (1961, 1962, 1967). This procedure allows the hypnotized patient to express inner conflicts through fashioning clay or plasticine models and extends into other quasiartistic modalities the same principles found effective for eliciting suppressed or repressed material via painting.

Before elucidating this approach, it will be best to gain an understanding of an intermediate approach also developed by Meares, which he termed "plastotherapy." Plastotherapy involves the use of models by patients in their normal state of alertness rather than in hypnosis as a means of facilitating nonverbal communication. Hypnoplasty then is essentially nothing more than the addition of hypnosis to the plastotherapy intervention.

Plastotherapy

Perhaps to oversimplify, give the patient some clay and say, "I want you to model something with this clay, feel it. It's fascinating stuff. Just feel it, now go ahead and model anything." That is all it takes for some patients. For others, the initiation of a response may not be quite so simple. On more than one occasion, further explanation will be necessary to motivate your patient to begin to interact with the clay. You might say, "There are many ways in which we can express ourselves. Sometimes we use words. At other times we can communicate by gestures, facial expressions." (A.F.B. finds it engaging to often portray various facial expressions at that time such as a grimace, bringing an ego-freeing element of humor to the interaction.) "Another way to express things is just in the way we do things and that can be done by you by simply modeling with this clay." (A.F.B. suggests that some people are helped considerably by being reassured that "artistic ability doesn't count here, just go ahead and model"). "Now just let yourself go and make something. I'll be back in just a little while." The therapist should then leave the room, as the patient is less likely to feel inhibited when left alone, at least to begin the process. What is lost by Meares' recommendation to leave the room is the ability to see how the patient interacts with the clay. Is it with light tentative touches, or is there evidence of showing aggressiveness? One of A.F.B.'s patients picked the clay up and slammed it down repeatedly as he left the room before beginning to model it.

A clay model has the advantage that it can be studied and interpreted rather than losing the information with the patient's continued remodeling and remodeling. For those of you who wish to attempt this modality, ordinary modeling clay, potter's clay, and plaster modeling media are available in art shops and many toy stores.

It may be best to wait till a time when the patient seems verbally blocked because of some close-to-conscious conflict. Then be ready and bring in the clay. A swift change in the therapeutic communication is from the verbal symbols, conceptualized as from the left brain, to the more plastic ones of the right brain. When confronted with such a projective task, there is frequently an increase in the patient's anxiety, because the patient senses that he or she may lose some control of the situation. The therapist's physical absence does not, in itself, permit the patient to evade by further questions and verbal interactions. We are accustomed to using words as defenses, and this request to communicate through modeling can represent an assault on one's personality structure. Our most practiced defensive mode of verbal interaction, such as Eye Movement Desensitization Reprocessing (EMDR), another hypnotherapeutic modality, also interrupts verbal defenses (Shapiro, 2001) has been bypassed.

Be prepared for the fact that the initial productions from the patient either are generally quite innocuous or have a symbol hidden, rather than a directly observable meaning. This is especially so in the nonpsychotic patient. Nonetheless, regard these initial renderings as having psychodynamic meanings and recognize that they are subject to interpretation. There may also be an intensification of affect, which can then be used to precipitate an abreaction. You can expect much defensive elaboration from your patient when asked to comment on or associate to his or her production. Typical responses include: "It's really nothing. Just some object which came to mind. It doesn't have any meaning at all. Don't take everything so seriously; this is nothing really." However, if one considers the symbolic meanings, the modality offers a chance for the therapist to observe more readily many of the patient's unconscious conflicts. Indeed, it may be that modeling, like dreams, is also a "royal road to the unconscious" (S. Freud, 1953c). The advantage is that it shortens the time spent in analysis to break down defenses and get at repressed conflicts.

The clay model is an object. Hence, "my" production but not directly "me." The patient is, therefore, not immediately confronted with his or her revelation, as in words that he or she has just uttered. The fact that, unlike a word, the symbol remains in front of his or her senses requires the patient to deal with it. The patient cannot simply dismiss it as with verbal symbols or use any of the plethora of his or her most practiced defense modalities. As a result, new insights will often occur, and they can frequently occur suddenly.

The therapist takes a classical nondirective counseling role but at the same time can come closer to increasing the relationship impact by sitting beside the patient and cooperating in the molding of clay. Such cooperation may be touching the clay without actually molding it or commenting on the patient's production in a reflective manner. A.F.B. recommends the use of client-centered nondirective counseling leads in such situations such as: "Let's see, it seems that you are trying to ... [incomplete thought]," or "I am not quite sure I see what you are doing here" and as the patient begins to model effectively and becomes more interactive with it, simply use nondirective leads like, "Yes, hmm," or simply reflect back, "It seems that what you are doing here is ... ." In all cases, the therapist should remain flexible and open when adding the hypnotic modality, dissociate what's happening from the you/me of the patient, and simply say something like, "The fingers make something" rather than "Our fingers make something." The fingers and one's own self assume responsibility for revealing the conflicts; this is not unlike the drawings in hypnography. The clay models can reflect a wide range of conflicts.

Associations the patient makes about his or her production are, obviously, important. These can often be quite specific. For example, a man is not just any person, but may represent the patient's father; a house may be one the patient lived in as a child. Symbols become more concrete in their communication. At first, as you might always expect, there will likely be denial followed by closer approximations of its true meaning as the associations are extended. If the therapist is analytically trained, the usual principles employed in free association during traditional psychoanalysis can be applied (Glover, 1955). The primary difference is that they start from a tangible clay model and are not completely "free." You may ask your patient to "tell me everything that comes to mind in relation to the object." Alternatively, one can approach the association radially. "What comes to your mind in connection with that hole in the top of the model?" The symbol may be an abstract concept, a wish, a fear, a significant other in the patient's present or earlier life. Such associations to the object, generally, will lead to some significant preconscious or unconscious conflict.

Meares noted that when a patient's defenses are most threatened, there will be an appearance of what he termed "screen symbols," which are like "screen memories," that cover up or elaborate the original repressed material into some sort of temporary disguise. In such cases, be very cautious about using a too-direct interpretation in confronting the patient.

Although the process speeds up the analysis, it does not completely eliminate the need for working through nor the experiential time required to achieve genuine insights. A.F.B. usually remains relatively passive and nondirective, but repeats the associations through simple reflections both to the unhypnotized patient and when the patient is in hypnosis, which seems to speed the process of insight acquisition. When such blockages occur, simply ask the patient to make another model. The associations will generally become more concrete and specific so long as some level of hypnotic depth is maintained. The process of making a second model often reveals the reason for the blockage. If strong affects break out during the associations, the therapist might develop them into a true abreaction.

Recognize that plastotherapy is indeed a projective technique, which can serve diagnostically in a manner not unlike that of the Rorschach or the Thematic Apperception Test (TAT), but unlike such tests, it can be extended directly into the therapeutic procedure. Meares' book of nearly half a century ago (1960) presented a series of photos of many different models produced by patients suffering from neuroses, psychoses, and other disorders. It will be observed that those modeled by the psychotic patients can be very easily differentiated from those of the neurotic patients.

Plastotherapy is not an integrated system of therapy but rather an adjunctive tactic within the basic approach that you are already using in your practice. It has limitations such as the considerable anxiety it often provokes and the fact that patients will on occasion completely reject this method of communication. Earlier practical objections about the use of messy materials have largely been overcome by the nature of the modeling materials now available. The method does reach through defenses more rapidly, can be quite flexible, and affords yet another modality for the therapist-patient relationship to operate in the psychotherapeutic situation.

Hypnoplasty

As foreshadowed earlier in this chapter, from the use of modeling techniques in the conscious state, Meares proceeded to employ these same procedures when the patient was in hypnosis. As in hypnography, Meares believed that a fairly deep state of hypnosis was essential, yet conceptualized hypnosis as "a highly dynamic and constantly fluctuating state of mind, rather than a level of trance." Not too many years later, E. R. Hilgard and Tart (1966) conducted experiments that showed the state of hypnosis as a constantly fluctuating one. Hypnosis is not a special process with a unidimensional brain signature where, when experiencing a hypnotic state, a light bulb of sorts flashes on the participant's forehead, but as the research now shows, reliable neurophysiological correlates, such as event-related potentials, positron emission tomography, and magnetic resonance imaging, reflect the various subjective states perceived by the participant.

Hypnoplasty requires the active movements of the hands just as in hypnography. Therefore, the use of sleep-related relaxation hypnotic inductions are contraindicated. Meares foreshadowed the development of alert hypnosis in his approximation of that by recommending eye fixation or repetitive movement approaches to facilitate the induction rather than a relaxation-type technique. Suggestions included: "You let yourself go, you let yourself go completely so that your body works automatically. Your hands and fingers can do things." The involvement of the fingers was facilitated by such suggestions as, "Your fingers pick up the clay, you do not do it, your hand does." Perhaps it would have been better for him to suggest dissociation of the hand, saying something like, "The hand does it"; notice how "the hand" is dissociated into an object and not a part of "the me." It can be emphasized that the patient will experience it "as if in a dream" yet with their "eyes wide open."

This early attempt at achieving some measure of alert hypnosis was obviously fraught with problems because the state of alertness was not fully developed. The first major advance in alert hypnosis is likely that of Banyai and E. R. Hilgard (1976) with their work in active alert hypnosis, where the research subjects kept their eyes wide open and would pedal bicycle ergometers at moderately high heart rates while attaining the hypnotic state. Hilgard's lab established that responses similar to relaxation-based hypnosis could be achieved using such methodology and used responses on Stanford Hypnotic Susceptibility Scales as criteria. Miller, A.F.B., and M. Barabasz (1991) went on to demonstrate that alert hypnosis was in fact equivalent to the relaxation hypnotic inductions on the criterion measure of cold pressor pain. Pain was administered in both relaxation and alert hypnotic conditions with hypnotic suggestions for analgesia with hand and arm immersed in circulating ice water. These advances, although important from a theoretical standpoint in that they established the equivalence between alert and relaxation inductions as effective ways of inducing hypnosis, still fell short of providing a method that could be used reliably for hypnoplasty.

In figure 6.3, Ciara Christensen demonstrates an example of hypnoplasty while in alert hypnosis. Although the photo is a simulation, it is very typical of what the therapist can expect using this therapeutic intervention.

Alert Hypnosis Induction Protocol

In modern instant alert hypnosis (A. Barabasz, 1994; A. Barabasz & M. Barabasz, 1994a, 1994b, 1996; Wark, 1998), the Barabasz technique involves an initial brief training phase. Patients are taught to roll their eyes up, as if trying to look at their foreheads. The eyes are also led to this position by instructions to focus on the therapist's thumb. The thumb is then moved slowly from 10 to 15 cm in front of the patient's nose to approximately the center of the forehead. The speed of movement should be carefully coordinated with the patient's ability to follow without swimming of the eyes or obvious loss of focus. In cases when the eyes dart or focus seems to be lost, interpret this as a form of resistance. Simply and calmly reinitiate the procedure. Keep that interpretation to yourself, at least for that moment. Normal adults seldom have a problem but a few defensive patients will bring their own idiosyncrasies to the experience, as will children when asked to get their eyes as rolled up as far as possible and then keep them steadily rolled up, as is required for successful instant alert hypnosis induction

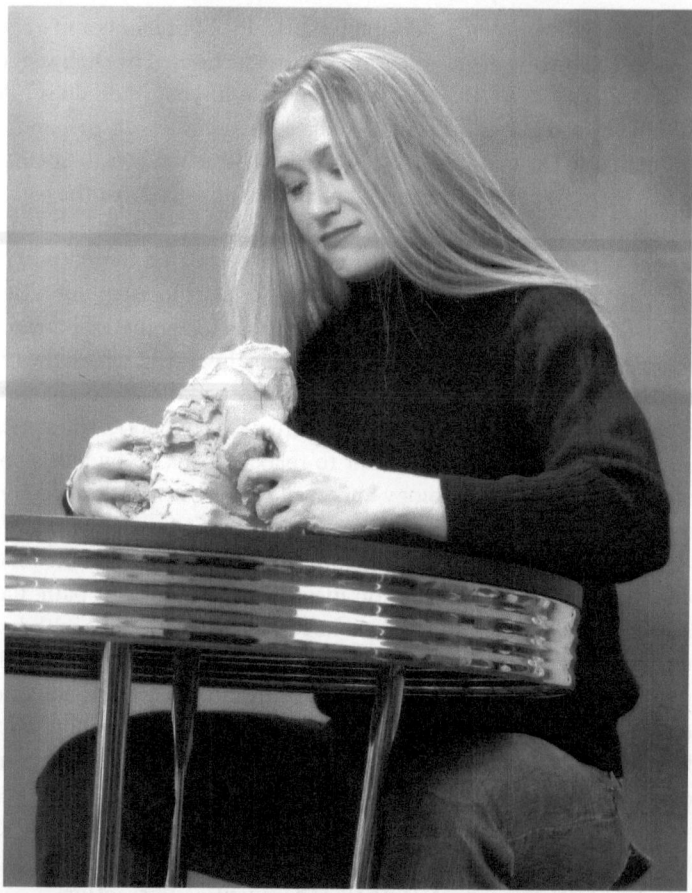

Figure 6.3 Ciara Christensen demonstrates hypnoplasty via alert hypnosis.

effects. Allow ample therapy time for practice trials using verbal reinforcement as the patient approximates the eyes held in the rolled-up position.

Once the eyes are fully and steadily rolled up, it is time to provide instructions to take notice of breathing, to relax, and to feel the calm confidence yet complete eyes-open alertness that will be felt at this point. Once subjective signs of entry into the hypnotic state are observed by the experienced clinician, the patient may simply be asked to raise a finger upon the perception of the suggested responses: "Just lift a finger on this hand [therapist touches one of the patient's two hands] when you feel the comfortable, relaxed, special calm alertness and readiness." Then you may say something like, "In this special state of alertness, you will be able to focus your attention and you can concentrate completely. Now go ahead, pick up the clay. Let the hand do it. It's as if the hands are fashioning the clay as if in a dream. And as you know, dreams can be very, very exciting and you are fully alert."

Features of Hypnoplasty Renderings following Alert Hypnosis

Clay fashioned in the state of alert hypnosis will tend to show much more primitiveness and much more disorganization, and resemble those of psychotic productions than in the simple alert plastotherapy procedure. Meares delineated four different types of symbols: (1) representational, which contains the element of some significant object but a poor likeness; (2) conventional, which might be a person with a head, two arms, two legs, and so on; (3) individual, which is a symbol peculiar to the individual and might include something quite strange or bizarre, the meanings of which will be difficult to determine; and (4) universal, including traditional Freudian sexual symbols as those representing Jungian archetypes.

As in plastotherapy, hypnoplasty is interwoven with traditional psychoanalytic procedures and hypnoanalytic therapy features, including free association and dream interpretation. But in hypnoplasty, they are carried out entirely within the state of hypnosis, and abreactions can be initiated, affects released, and interpretations given. Again, without experimental data, but with much clinical trial experience, Meares believed that analytic therapy proceeds far faster using this modality, yet he cautioned against initiating too much anxiety during the abreactions. It is not known precisely what he meant by this. As we know, abreactions must be brought through to the full if there is to be catharsis and therapeutic progress in most cases.

Figure 6.4, "the devil," was accompanied by this patient statement: "I don't know why I did it. It came when I mixed the clay. While I was doing it, I was thinking of Hermaphrodites." As it turns out, this devil is at this same time the patient's husband. He has the horns and cloven hooves of the devil, and a leering, mask-like face. His male sex organs are shown clearly, but yet he also has the large breasts of a woman, and huge flabby buttocks. The patient had recently been accused of being sexually abnormal. The veridicality, truth or otherwise, of this is not known. The rendering may be merely a matter of the psychological projection of the patient's own unexpressed bisexuality.

Barabasz' Photo-Digital Hypnography

Given that the final products of hypnography, hypnoplasty, and plastotherapy provide symbols that remain in front of the patient's senses and require dealing with it rather than merely dismissing it via verbal defensive symbols, the final production may well be quite abstract in its symbolization of a wish, fear, or significant other in the patient's present or early life. Such associations contain the clues to preconscious and unconscious conflicts but may be disguised by screen symbols. Observations of patients as they work with the clay show greater transparency in the revelation of conflicts that become screened or disguised in the final product. A.F.B. believes that the manner in which a patient handles materials such as the Rorschach gives greater clues to his or her psychopathology than his or her verbal responses, which may be lost if one

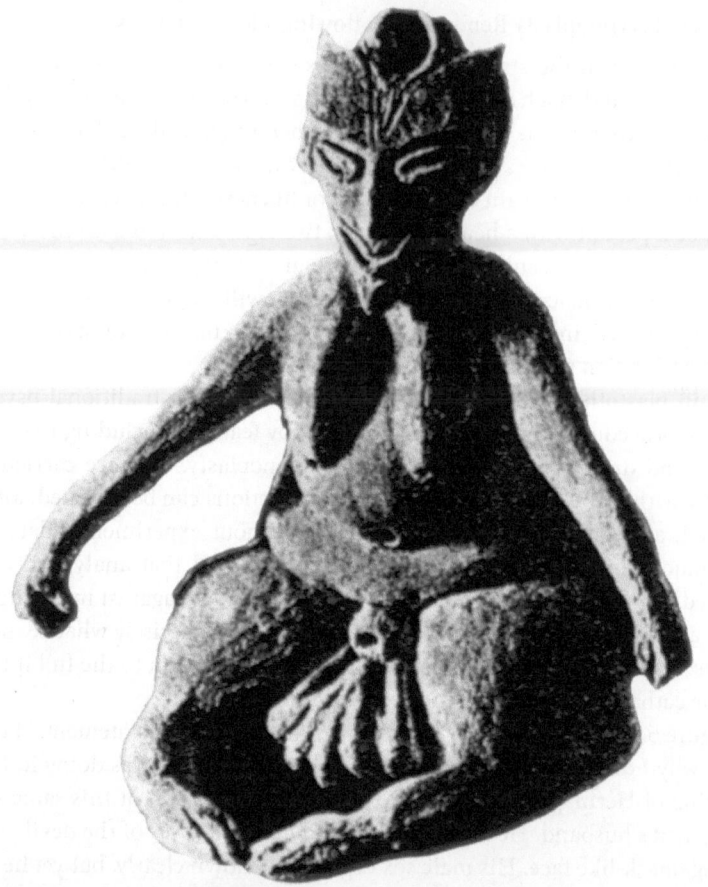

Figure 6.4 Patient's rendering projecting unexpressed bisexuality. (see text p. 111).

looks at only the final hypnoplasty production. Indeed, as Meares noted back when he was working with his plaster of Paris models, the hard object can be studied later at leisure. Nonetheless, it is the final rendering, and a disguised one, more likely than not. Certainly, there was a need for a therapeutically efficient method of producing samples of the patient's process of modeling for the therapist's later study.

Full-motion video recordings were first attempted but as all therapists know, it takes as long if not longer to review a recorded session as it does to conduct the session in the first place. An alternative that A.F.B.'s practice pioneered involves the use of digital camera photographs of the renderings as they are produced. Meares would leave the room after giving hypnography or hypnoplasty instructions. In the digital photographic hypnography or hypno-plasty, we advocate moving to a far corner of the room, well away from the patient.

Figures 6.5 through 6.11 show the progression of a hypnographic painting session. Note the changes as Ciara Christensen demonstrates how the progression of painting the face of a "threatening person from the past" to her demonstration of a typical abreaction that might follow. If only the final product were available, for, as in Meares' method, there would be a comparative paucity of clinical material for the therapist to draw from to make useful interpretations most relevant to the "patient."

Use a moderate telephoto setting (75 to 150 mm) (depending on the size of your consultation office) so that you can obtain close detailed photographs without the invasiveness of close physical presence with your patient while the models are produced. To ensure adequate detail for later study from your digital photographs, it is recommended that you use a camera capable of optical rather than digital zoom so the photo is filled with the model produced by the patient and an image quality (compression ratio) selected with a minimum of 5 MB (this means that a typical 2,592 × 1,944 pixel image size would be comprised of 2,592 pixels horizontally and 1,944 pixels vertically). These are generally considered to be a camera's setting for "fine" or "high quality" rather than "standard image" quality. Photographs produced on your digital printer or via your computer can be attached to your chart/progress notes for later study. Patients who interact rapidly with the clay model at different points can be recorded by most current digital cameras with multiburst-mode shutter settings. Although our data is, at this point, preliminary and waiting further analysis with a greater number of participants, it seems quite apparent that patients reveal many clues to their pathology and underlying conflicts in the process of making the clay production, in fact, more often than the final refined product.

Sensory Hypnoplasty

Extending Meares' procedures, Raginsky (1961, 1962, 1963, 1967) moved the entire approach into another dimension, one that provided more stimuli and at the same time a more specific structure. Raginsky added variations in color, texture, and even odor to the model-making medium, which was in those days referred to as plasticine. He reported that these changes stimulated regression to more circumscribed areas of conflict. Circumscribing (pinpointing), in a sense, the area of conflict is precisely one of the best indicants for a successful abreaction; thus, this methodology is of specific interest to us here.

To stimulate regression to circumscribed areas of conflict, Raginsky used colored clays (plasticine) with the intent of promoting regression to specific areas or levels of development. Thus, he found that the use of red tended to aid regression to oral levels of development or, sometimes in women, conflicts about menstruation. When the red plasticine was quite soft, sexual fantasies were frequently initiated. Soft brown (stool-like) clay brought regression to the anal level and fantasies regarding elimination conflicts. The color white gave

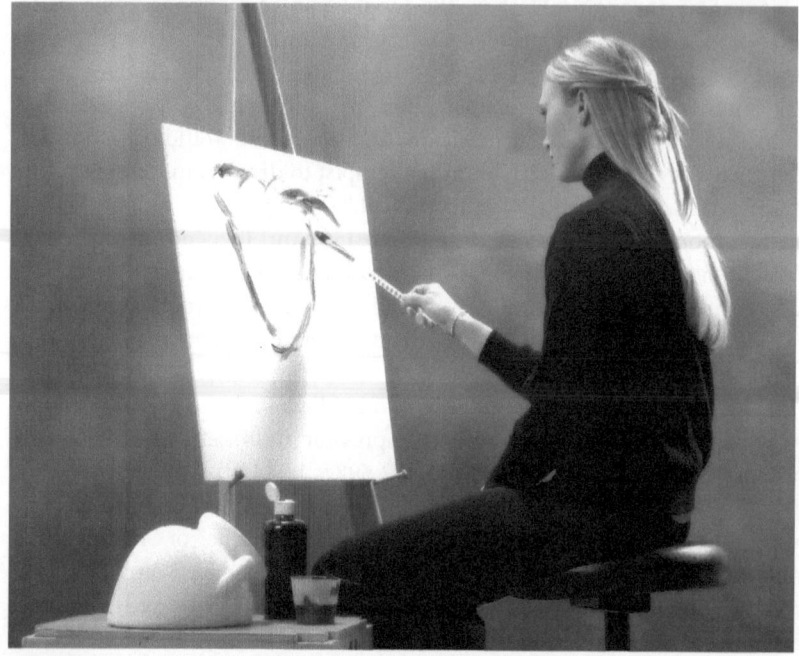

Figure 6.5

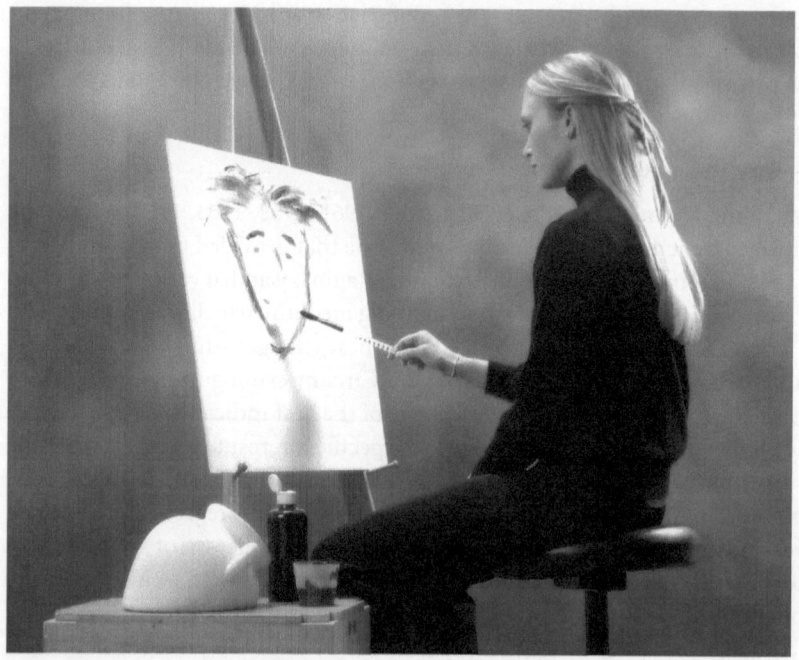

Figure 6.6

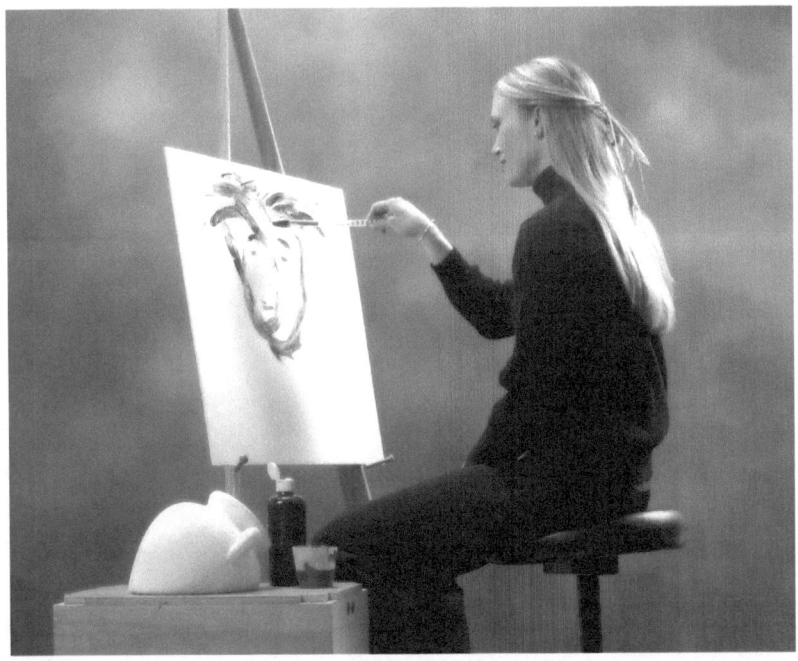

Figure 6.7

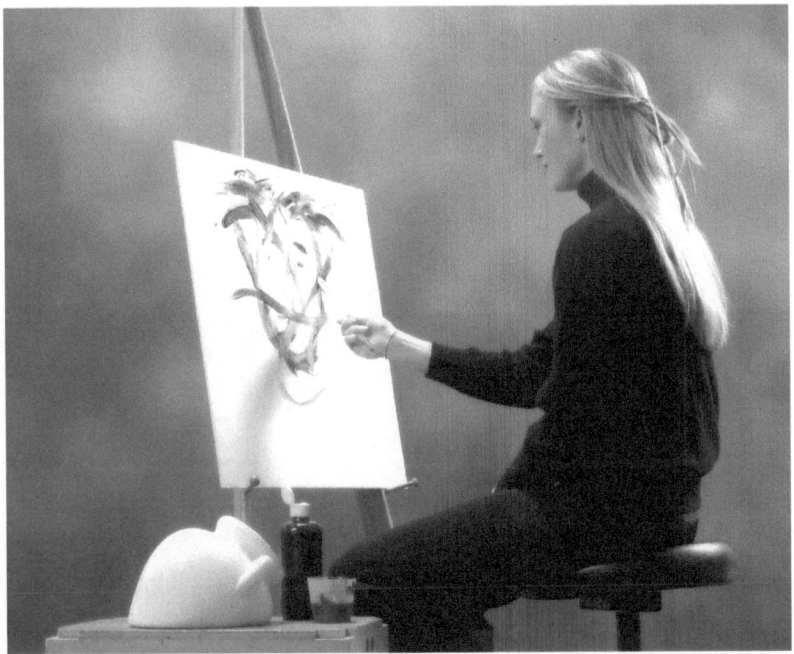

Figure 6.8

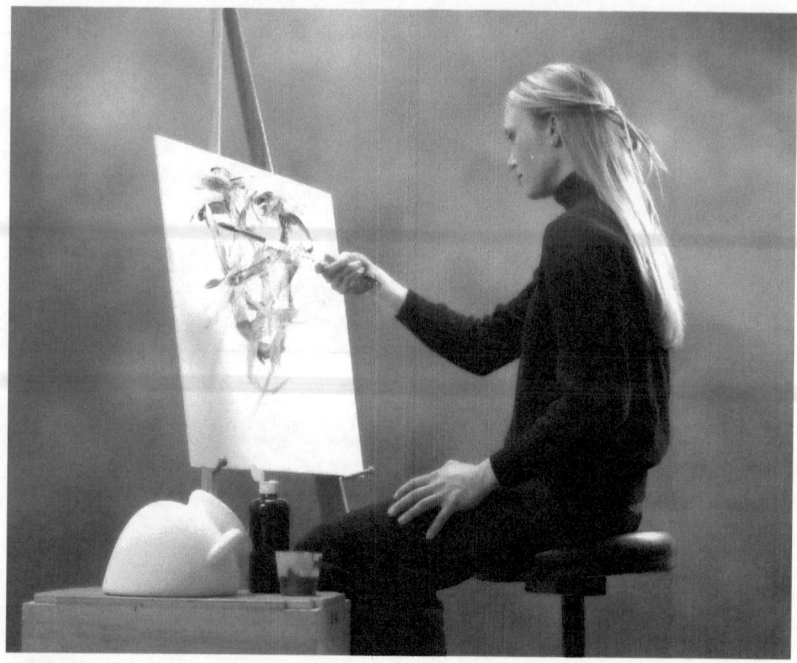

Figure 6.9

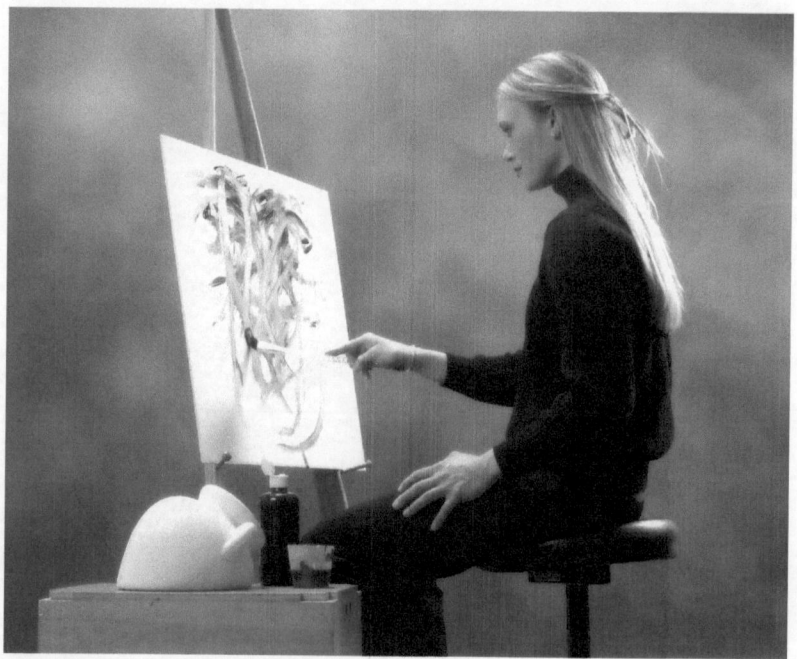

Figure 6.10

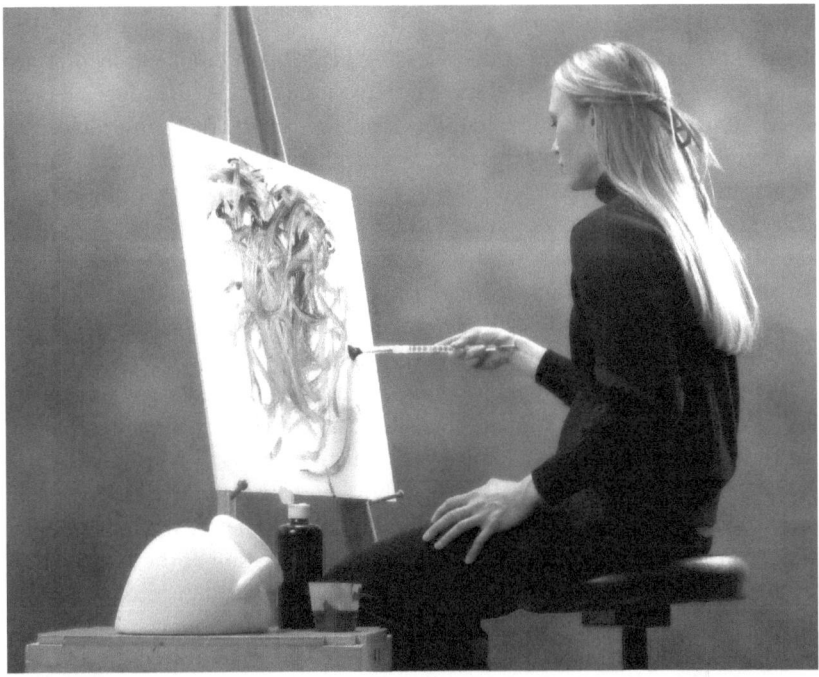

Figure 6.11

patients a "new, clean feeling." To enhance these perceptions even further, Raginsky also added appropriate odors. He found that subjects' associations were most revealing.

Unlike Meares, Raginsky stressed the use of light hypnosis depth. Meares developed the atavistic regression theory of hypnosis, which related the modality to early, primitive levels of function typical of humans as they progressed up the phylogenetic levels from anthropoids to humans (see Barabasz and Watkins, 2005). Therefore, Meares' work emphasized deeper levels of hypnosis. In contrast, Raginsky observed that, because his patients were not so deeply hypnotized, he had less difficulty in getting them to verbalize their associations and, therefore, adopted a technique of maintaining light to moderate levels of hypnosis rather than requiring the deep state used by Meares. Obviously, this makes the methodology available to a greater number of patients, including those who are unable to obtain the deeper levels of hypnotic depth.

Therapists' "interpretations" as well as patients' "insights" require a common understanding of meanings. We know that understandings and meanings can occur within a person that never get verbalized, either to the individual or to others. The personality structure reorganizes around changed meanings on a covert level. Such is the basis of what is thought of by some as "spontaneous recovery." Indeed, the patient "gets well" without either the patient or the therapist being able to explain in verbal terms the psychodynamics of that change. We are not at all referring here to the simple amelioration of surface symptoms because of mere nonhypnotic or hypnotic suggestion or social influence, but rather profound personality reconstruction, which may occur perhaps during such experiences as religious conversions. The majority of therapists who have worked analytically in depth with patients have seen such examples. The patient improves and manifests a profound change of personality during the process of therapy, and there is no reappearance of the symptoms after the therapist's influence and transference relationship with the patient has been terminated. The patient has apparently "gotten well." We can't always explain why, but we accept, with gratitude, the recovery.

Art productions, drawings, paintings, and clay modelings are unverbalized, symbolic communications that create possibilities for therapeutic change like those above. Returning to "third ear" sensitivity described by Reik (1948), we may often be able to translate the symbol's meaning into words. However, sometimes even the most experienced and brilliant analyst will not be able to interpret its verbal equivalent, even though the creation of the symbol and the reactions of the analyst constituted a genuine interchange of meaning between conscious and unconscious levels. Such a change confirmed by her own patient (Renee 1951), Sechehaye (1951, 1956) achieved just those kinds of results in treating a severely regressed schizophrenic patient with a long history using such covert exchanges of meanings through nonverbal symbols. This was later termed by her (1956) as "symbolic realization."

Helen Watkins' Doodle Therapy

Helen Watkins experimented with the use of doodles as a modality of covert communication at the University of Montana counseling center, with clients who had difficulty talking either in or out of hypnosis (J. G. Watkins, 1992a, pp. 89–97). She would inquire as to whether the patient made doodles, and if the response was "yes," she encouraged him or her to bring in such productions. Sometimes the doodling was encouraged with the use of hypnosis, and at other times its meaning was worked out in hypnosis with the patient at a light to moderate level. At other times, the meaning never became verbally conscious to either, but there was significant symptomatic and personality change subsequently. An example of an adult clinical case involving doodle communication was reported by her as follows:

> The woman, now in her 30s, had undergone some 15 years of therapy. Apparently, the traditional psychoanalysts produced substantial gains. However, she reported that "there is still something wrong, something missing, and I don't know what it is." I noticed her writing pad was covered with doodles and I commented on it. She told me that she was an art therapist and that she draws a lot, showing me samples of her work.

I asked about her birth, and she replied that she was adopted. I asked her if her birth mother had tried to abort her, and she replied, "Yes, she told me she was unwed, couldn't keep me, and was embarrassed about her pregnancy." She told me that she was just not ready to have children yet. I then said, "I suppose she tried to do it with a coat hanger?" Startled, she replied, "Why yes, the doctor said I had an injury to my shoulder at birth from just that kind of attempt. But how did you know?" I pointed to her doodles. There were coat hangers covering the page.

I then hypnotized her and suggested that she go back to the beginning, that she would see a small opening, and she would become small enough to easily pass through this opening into a soft, warm, dark room. She lay on the floor of my office, pulled her knees up to her chin, and then scooted herself back into a corner of the room, frightened and huddling. I told her that she was supposed to live and not die, no matter what might be frightening her. She could live without having to run away from situations to protect herself.

Some time later, I described this case to a colleague, who was an obstetrician. He said that when an illegal home abortion is attempted after 6 months of pregnancy, the fetus, with that premature level of development, reflexively will often try to move into the wall of the uterus when a cold, foreign, probing object is introduced.

Regardless of how one tries to conceptualize what happened, theoretically the fact was that the client reported feeling much better and had a sense of completeness that something was now "right." She felt as if her "analysis" was now at last finished. Was this what Alexander and French (1946) recognized and termed "a corrective emotional experience"?

Helen Watkins reported another case in which doodles indicated a destructive relationship and child abuse, which were at the root of a patient's bulimia. (J. G. Watkins, 1992a, pp. 90–91).

This 28-year-old woman was quite depressed at her inability to stop her compulsive binge-purge cycle. Her referring psychologist asked me to use hypnosis to uncover her near-forgotten childhood. She mentioned that she enjoyed doodling and, at my suggestion, brought in a page filled with doodles. In her associations, each of them seemed to be connected to a maternal grandmother. At one point, I asked her to draw a picture of herself and then hypnotized her to achieve a light level of hypnosis and relaxation and report whether one arm felt different from the other. My request came because the right arm had been drawn much larger than the left one in her doodles. She replied that the right hand and arm was larger and much more powerful.

I suggested that it was no longer connected to her, that it was free to move anywhere it wished, and that she could follow it. Whereupon it began to move down the street on which she lived as a child. It proceeded to a house, which she identified as her grandmother's, went in the back door to the kitchen, grasped her grandmother by the throat, and tried to strangle her.

This cued me into a series of abreactions during which she reexperienced many brutal scenes of sexual molestation and cruelty. Her grandmother would alternate between starving her and forcing her to eat until she would vomit. The bulimia was resolved, and she ceased the binge-vomit cycle. It was the doodles that cued me in to the significant experiences, which required abreactions to release wells of deeply repressed anger.

In yet another case of doodle therapy, the patient was unable to talk even with the use of various levels of hypnosis. She would make efforts but then would choke. Her symptom was a lifelong depression. In this case, the doodles were brought in by the patient before each session. Their symbolic meaning could be only inferred. However, using the ideomotor finger signal technique described in chapter 6 (J. G. Watkins, 1992a), Helen Watkins asked questions to find out what age in the patient's life the doodle was supposed to represent. She described the case as follows:

This patient reported to me that she had been depressed since childhood. She hated her critical father and defended her dependent mother. Her parents apparently argued a lot. When I took her down to a "glass-paneled room" by use of hypnosis, she saw them fighting. At the second session, she brought in a doodle made of watercolors.

To me it looked like a womb with a fetus within; however, she had no associations to it but merely said it was just a drawing and had no meaning. I hypnotized her and said, "I'm going to count until you reach the doodle you have made, at which point the index finger will rise." She still could not talk in hypnosis, so I talked to the dissociated hand. When questioned, the index finger would rise to signal "yes." The large finger would lift to indicate "no," and the little finger would respond to communicate, "I don't know." I then talked to the hand as follows:

H.H.W.:	"Hand, is this experience prior to birth?"
Patient:	"Yes." [Index finger lifts.]
H.H.W.:	"Are you able to take her there?"
P.:	"Yes."
H.H.W.:	"Are you willing to do so now?"
P.:	"Yes."
H.H.W.:	"Let me know when she has undone what she needs to do."
P.:	"Yes."
H.H.W.:	"Any place where she needs to go?"
P.:	"Yes."

H.H.W.: "Uterus?"
P.: "No."
H.H.W.: "First year?"
P.: "Yes."
H.H.W.: "You are able to take her there?"
P.: "Yes."
H.H.W.: "Would you be willing to do so right now?"
P.: "Yes."
H.H.W.: "Let me know when she has done what she needs to do."
P.: "Yes."
H.H.W.: "Is it important that she recall at a conscious level what she has just experienced?"
P.: "No."

As the sessions continued, the therapy proceeded via the doodles that she brought in. She continued to respond with finger signals as to what she (the patient) should do and where in her life space she should go. No meanings were ever verbalized. Her conscious experience was that she was in a dark place. Sometimes she felt fear or teared profusely but nothing else. However, at the third session she brought a drawing that resembled a sperm.

When it was asked, the finger signal reported that this represented "conception."

Two weeks later she brought in another doodle; it resembled a fertilized ovum, but no associations could be elicited in either the hypnotic or the conscious alert state.

Following this "fertilized ovum doodle," a profound change appeared to come over the patient. Her depression lifted, her eyes brightened, and her face released and relaxed. Her grades in college improved dramatically, and she complained no more. Her feeling of inferiority seemed to completely disappear, and her sexual relationship with her boyfriend was reported as greatly improved.

More often than not, in similar cases, the resolution of the repressed conflict and the legitimate self-confidence that it thereby releases result also in the recognition by the patient that the relationship with her significant other was one where he contributed to and reinforced her pathology to meet his own selfish needs. It was as if the patient was seeking someone who would punish her and found this (subconsciously sought it) in her relationships rather than seeking mature adaptive ones. Once the issues were resolved, such individuals are able to make far more adaptive choices with a much greater probability of successful interaction over the long term. In the present case, therapy was then discontinued but the patient did return for a single follow-up session 5

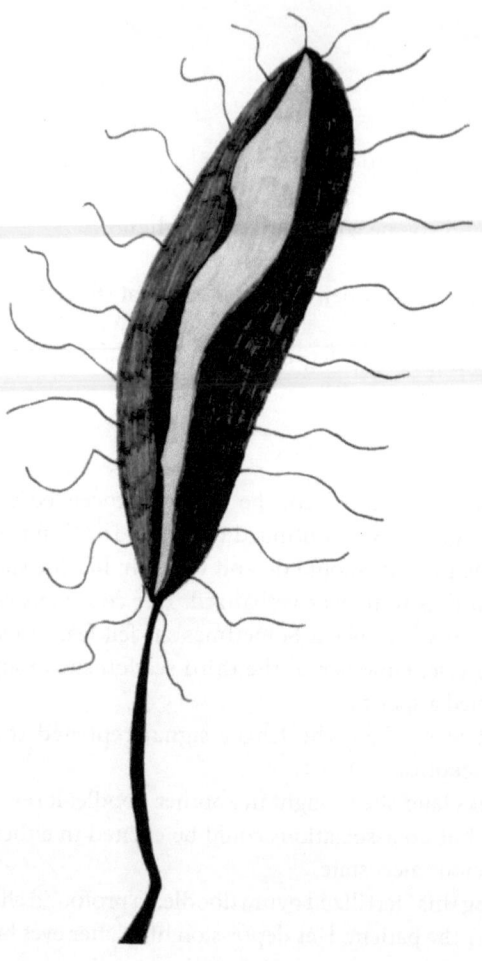

Figure 6.12

months later. All of her gains that were apparently attained in therapy had continued, and further adaptive functioning had been achieved.

But what happened? What communications were exchanged through the doodles and Helen Watkins' relations to them? One can, of course, speculate that the doodles transmitted the symbols of new birth, a new chance, a new sexual relationship, a fantasy of mother and father getting together, and many other hypotheses. But these would only be speculation. What we do know is that the doodles provided a method of covert communication that facilitated constructive therapy, that it was simply not suggestion or social influence on the part of the therapist, and that it endured beyond the time during which a positive transference reaction could normally be expected to hold. At some unconscious level, Helen Watkins' patient had achieved a covert insight through her symbolic communications to Helen and to herself, and she had resolved some inner conflict. Helen chose not to explore the matter any further but to rejoice in the positive changes that took place and were lasting.

Summary

Communication through art productions can provide meaningful therapeutic interaction without the necessity of verbal communication. Drawings, paintings, doodles, and modeling clays are useful media for implementing such procedures. Associations are most essential to get at the underlying meanings of the symbol creations. These may be elicited either in the conscious state or in hypnosis, but hypnosis greatly facilitates the intervention. At times, the use of such symbol productions can help the therapist when the patient is unable or, due to defensive postures, unwilling to communicate by verbal means.

These symbols can also help a patient to resolve inner conflicts by rearranging meanings covertly in such a way that neither the patient nor the therapist knows their true meaning in words. The patient knows them unconsciously and resolves his or her inner conflicts in a situation guided by the therapist. We cannot always explain the recovery that takes place in psychodynamic terms. "Unconscious insight" has made inner sense to the patient, which has resulted in a form of corrective emotional experience.

Meares had his patients sketch images with black paint, with instructions to make whatever they wished and without conscious attention. He called this procedure "hypnography" and reported that it tapped covert processes that could not be expressed consciously.

A.F.B. and his colleagues have experimented with video recordings of hypnoplasty as a promising new development to Meares' original approach. Plastotherapy is a form of treatment in which the patient expresses him- or herself through modeling with clay or similar material. Meares combined this approach with deep hypnosis to develop hypnoplasty.

Raginsky extended the procedure greatly by his use of colored clays and called the new modality of treatment "sensory hypnoplasty." By varying both color and texture of the modeling material as well as sometimes odors, he offered the patient other dimensions in which to express both conscious and unconscious motivations.

Hypnography and hypnoplasty were combined by Milton Kline (1968). He termed his method "sensory hypnoplasty."

Doodle therapy, developed by Helen Watkins, provided another avenue to tap covert processes with patients who are unable to express themselves verbally in a manner that lends itself to a wider range of therapeutic settings. These apparent random scribbles produced by patients and counseling clients without conscious attention are analyzed to determine covert meanings. She provided evidence that they can sometimes lead to areas needing therapeutic abreactions. She also found that it could lead to profound positive changes in the patient even when no associations could be elicited in either the hypnotic or alert conscious state, and that such constructive changes took place that could not be attributed to social influence. These changes endured beyond the time that would normally be expected to hold for a positive transference reaction.

Our point is that a number of nonverbal modalities have the potential to facilitate positive therapeutic change in hypnoanalytic settings.

7
Realities, Dreams, and Fantasies

The French Surrealist poet, St. Paul Roux, would hang a sign on his bedroom door before retiring that read: "Poet at work." A similar belief in nocturnal productivity was expressed by John Steinbeck: "It is a common experience that a problem difficult at night is resolved in the morning after the committee of sleep has worked on it." A shorter version of this has become the cliché "sleep on it." None of these "designate" the dream as spokesperson for the committee of sleep. However, most accounts of solving problems or producing creative products during sleep are of hypnogogic imagery. In the most famous and controversial example, the chemist Kekule reported that his Nobel Prize-winning realization of the structure of the benzene molecule as hexagonal rather than straight came after dreaming of a snake grasping its tail in its mouth. Mendeleev described dreaming the periodic table of the elements in its completed form, and the Nobel Prize-winning experiment demonstrating the chemical transmission of nerve impulses to the heart was conceived by Otto Loewi in a dream. Inventions as varied as Elias Howe's sewing machine needle—with the hole at the pointed end—and Parkinson's computer-controlled antiaircraft gun have reportedly been conceived in dreams. Jack Nicklaus credited a crucial improvement in his golf game to dreaming of a new way to grasp his club. Blagrove asserted that on principle, none of these anecdotes could be accurate. He argued that dreams, by their very nature, can't even intend to solve a problem, much less do so: "The place for problem solving is the waking world" (Barrett, 1993a).

Realities are, in essence, supposed to be responses to the organism's perception of stimuli originating outside of an individual. The scientific method makes much of the need to "test reality" by "objective" observations, yet the kind of reality that psychotherapists and counselors deal with is often internal and subjective. When our patient says she hurts, we cannot directly feel it, experience it, or verify it. We are reduced to accepting the report supplemented by our observation of her overt behavior. Because we, too, have experienced pain, we may "understand" her feelings and perhaps, just perhaps, through resonance (see Barabasz & Watkins (2005); J. G. Watkins, 1978b; J. G. Watkins &H. H. Watkins, 1997), replicate within our own selves a facsimile of that experience. For the moment, then, we may be able to feel and suffer similarly at least to some qualitative extent.

Like our patient's pain experience, dreams and fantasies challenge scientific investigational methods. Some systems of therapy, such as cognitive-behavior modification and those that stress interpersonal relationships, attempt to achieve scientific goals by some form of objective observation. Unfortunately, they do so at the expense of overlooking a vast body of realities that are internal, subjective, yet real to our patient. These subjective realities, no matter how divorced from the veridical world, predict with almost precise accuracy the behaviors, perceptions, and feelings of our patients.

Unlike normal perceptions, such experiences are initiated by that which lies within the patient and are not directly observable or controllable in any way by the therapist. Beahrs (1986) noted that uncertainty, or the principle of interdeterminancy, developed in the study of physics by Heisenberg (1958), must also apply to psychotherapy. We observe, understand, diagnose, and intervene constructively into intangible processes within another individual but with uncertainty and relatively little verified data. To the astute clinician or counselor, the study of dreams and fantasies not only permits insights into the patient's inner processes, but also opens a modality for constructive change. This is because it is the patient's inner and experiential reality, his or her unique perception of events, rather than the external events themselves, which cause his or her symptoms. Perhaps first promulgated by the ancient philosopher Epectitus, and recognized and organized into the first cognitive therapeutic system by Albert Ellis (1962), this observation became the basis for the current preponderance of cognitive-behavior therapies, which were also articulated and systematized by Beck (1976) and Meichenbaum (1977), as well as, of course, by the psychoanalysts (see Wolberg, 1948) many years before the more recent authors reached prominence.

To be effective in therapy, a good counselor or clinician must be adequately experienced as well as trained to "feel his or her way around" in the patient's inner reality. It is like a blind person groping in the dark and relying on other modes of perception to discern the nature of a world in which he or she is trying to bring control over. Freud (1953b) called dreams "the royal road to the unconscious." The present chapter will try to indicate how dreams can be used both diagnostically and therapeutically.

Fantasies, Dreams, Images, and Hallucinations

Although the notion that right-hemisphere brain processes govern images, fantasies, dreams, and hallucinations is overly simplistic (Crawford, 1991; Freeman, A. Barabasz, M. Barabasz, & Warner, 2000), these phenomena have certain attributes in common. They originate primarily from imaginary stimuli (A. Barabasz, 1982), and they are experienced by the individual as if they were visual in nature. They differ in that the images can be produced consciously and represent circumscribed bits of experience. Fantasies are often consciously initiated but may display longer, more story-like productions.

They have more organization than simple images. Both fantasies as well as images are subjective experiences. Unless the person is psychotic, these are sensed as being self-created and clearly a part of one's self.

Josephine Hilgard studied imagining in hypnosis extensively. She found that hypnotizability is highly correlated with the ability for vivid imagination (also see A. Barabasz, 1979, 1982). A.F.B. (1979) found that Antarctic isolation increased hypnotizability, and this was reflected by EEG changes during an individual's wintering-over. A further study revealed that even in the brief summer, Antarctic isolation significantly increased both absorption (Tellegen & Atkinson, 1974) and hypnotizability (M. Barabasz, A. Barabasz, & Mullin, 1983). Antarctic isolation, even for brief periods, was later found to significantly enhance imaginative involvement and hypnotizability (A. Barabasz, 1984). Following these studies, Ramonth (1985a, 1985b) identified absorption as the capacity for total attention in an imaginative activity. Several researchers confirmed the correlation with standardized measures of hypnotizability (Crawford, 1982; Spanos & McPeake, 1975; Tellegen & Atkinson, 1974). When absorption is high, the images become the reality of the subject and outside stimuli are often ignored completely. Such images may be suggested by the hypnotherapist or spontaneously created by the subject (H. Spiegel & D. Spiegel, 2004). They can become a powerful means of communication from unconscious or preconscious processes within a patient as a valuable tool in both hypnoanalysis and hypnocounseling.

Both hallucinations and dreams are subjective phenomena but experienced by the individual as object (the self-object is discussed throughout Barabasz & Watkins, 2005). The person senses them as something that is happening to him or her, not something that he or she is doing. Perhaps the only difference between hallucinations and dreams is that the first occurs during sleep and the second happens while the person is presumably awake and alert. However, at the time they are experienced, the individual "sees" them as he or she would perceive an external object whose image is focused on his or her retina. Such images and fantasies generally occur during normal states of consciousness as well as in presleep hypnogogic reveries, which have many similarities to light states of hypnosis.

Both hallucinations and dreams, on the other hand, appear during some altered states of consciousness such as sleep, deep hypnosis, and, of course, psychosis. They are unconsciously motivated. Both fantasizing and imaging are used by different writers to describe the same class of phenomena. From the hypnoanalytic point of view, images and fantasies represent preconscious experiences. Hallucinations and dreams manifest more "unconscious" and "concrete" mental activity. Hallucinations have often been considered as dreams in the awake state and often have primary process features. The meanings expressed by both hallucinations and dreams are less direct. They employ more symbolism and require often considerably greater effort and expertise to interpret their meaning, manifesting what Freud termed "primary process thinking." Yet, all four represent what we can at least operationally conceptualize as primarily right-hemispheric activity. Thus, different approaches are required to deal with them when we employ hypnoanalytic and hypnocounseling interventions that are conscious verbal communications.

Free association, the verbalizing of consciously controlled thoughts, has been a basic method in psychoanalysis. Fantasy might be considered as a form of free association using images instead of words. The patient withdraws attention from the external world, is passive, and allows a series of visual images to pass through consciousness. He or she usually describes them in words only after the experience and not during it, because the ego activity required for verbalizing (again conceptualized as primarily left-brain activity) is, at least to a certain extent, inhibitory of right-brain imaging (we use the terms "left brain" and "right brain" functioning metaphorically, as the data extant has revealed far more complex brain responses are involved).

Let us think of trance depth lying on a continuum from hypnoidal to light, medium, and deep hypnosis (see Chapter 2, Figure 2.2), where images and fantasies occur during lighter states of consciousness and dreams and hallucinations occur in the deeper states of hypnosis. These conceptualizations are consistent with the experiences of hypnoanalysts and hypnocounselors who are aware that a fairly deep degree of hypnotic depth is required to obtain hallucinatory responses, such as in item 12 of the Stanford Hypnotic Susceptibility Scale Form C (Weitzenhoffer & E. R. Hilgard, 1962). It would seem reasonable to hypothesize that the lighter the trance in which a visual-perceptual experience can be facilitated, the more the production can be guided by secondary (conscious or preconscious) processes, and, therefore, the easier it will be for the hypnocounselor in, for example, a university counseling center to interpret its meaning.

In contrast, fantasies and dreams reported during or following deep levels of hypnosis are much more likely to contain primary process concrete thinking and, therefore, require the sophisticated methods of dream interpretation developed by the psychoanalysts and thus require considerable clinical experience (Hill, Napayama, & Wonnell, 1998; Hill, Dimer, Sess, Hillyer, & Seemann, 1993). (Note: Clara Hill, noted for her research on dreams, is the former editor of the *Journal of Counseling Psychology*.)

Considerable research has been devoted to the comparison of "hypnotic dreams" with "sleep dreams" (Barber, 1962; Moss, 1967, 1970; Tart, 1964, 1965; Barrett, 1979, 1996, 2002). There have been a number of alternative interpretations offered by the different researchers. Some hold that hypnotic dreams and sleep dreams are extremely similar, whereas others conclude they are very different from one another. However, the research variable that was not controlled for in many studies is that of hypnotic trance depth. Walker (1984) reviewed numerous studies and concluded that hypnotic dreams were more like fantasy than nocturnal dreams. However, she also challenged the concept of "trance" itself. The controversy seems to reside in the extent to which images and fantasies reported in hypnosis have been subjected to psychodynamic distortion (Hill, Dimer, Sess, Hillyer, & Seemann, 1993), which psychoanalysts find in the manifest content of nocturnal dreams. E. R. Hilgard and Nowlis (1972) reported that some 63% of 172 subjects indicated that their hypnotic dreams were like real, night dreams. E. R. Hilgard (1986) considered the Thematic Apperception Test (TAT) themes and concluded that hypnotic dreams lay somewhere between night dreams and TAT themes. The most sophisticated research, discussed later in this chapter, was conducted by Deirdre Barrett, editor of the journal *Dreams*.

In an attempt to make the most sensible use of all of the data available for psychotherapeutic purposes, let us oversimplify a bit and recognize that imagery expressed as visual may constitute different points on a continuum, from images, through fantasies, to dreams, and then on to actual overt hallucinations, which represent diminishing levels of ego control but without clear dividing boundaries between them. The problem for us as therapists will be to decide at what level we will attempt to make our interpretation. Even as the "manifest" level of interpretation has been found to achieve significant meaning in true dreams, the psychoanalytic and symbolic level of translation has been shown to be of value in such ego creations as produced in stories and themes on the Thematic Apperception Test. What do we now know about the dreaming process itself?

Neurophysiological and Cognitive Basis of Dreaming

Hobson and McCarly (1977) were perhaps the first to propose a neurobiological basis of dreaming based on the activation synthesis hypothesis, which attributed the peculiar aspects of dream consciousness to the forebrain and its attempt to integrate chaotic signals arising from the brain stem. It took another decade to correlate specific cognitive facets of dreaming with the neurobiology of dreaming. Building on this research, Mamelak and Hobson (1989) theorized that aminergic demodulation of the brain increased the probability of spontaneous neuronal firing in the forebrain. This was thought to be a basis for the unpredictability or, if you will, infidelity of neuronal activation, which is related to discontinuities and incongruities in narrative, which are part and parcel of the bizarreness of dreams (Hobson, Hoffman, Helfand, & Kostner, 1987).

Before we let our discussion of the physiology of dreaming make an illogical leap to its separation from alert processes, as might be surmised from discussions of rapid eye movement (REM) sleep, let us state that the empirical evidence for the cognitive uniqueness of dreaming is contradictory, controversial, and to almost all researchers unconvincing at this point in time. The point, perhaps oversimplified, is that the results of most studies of dream-like mentations suggest that all the qualities of dreaming can be found in reports of conscious experience in waking and non-REM as well as REM sleep. Thus, let us accept that these findings are rather convincing in their implications for the use of psychoanalytic interpretations of dreams, given the link between consciousness and dreaming on a physiological basis. Although it may be an overextension of this data to see it as supporting the existence of repressed content, one might think that most researchers would agree that all of this data makes that a very likely conclusion, whether one chooses to use the words "repressed into unconscious" or not. As discussed by Kahn and Hobson (1993), there is already undeniable evidence of the qualitative distinctiveness of dreaming in the bizarreness subcategory of character discontinuity and incongruity. They note that "we know of no claim that the persons imaged by us in normal waking undergo character transformation either by transmogrification (as in the changes in the portrait of Dorian Gray) or by the condensation of two persons (or for that matter two sexes) into a single character."

The physiological basis for dreaming is now known to involve the combination of the withdrawal of aminergic inhibition with reciprocal cholinergic excitation. In dreaming, neuronal activation patterns switch discontinuously as a result of phasic bursts of acetylcholine, which activate otherwise quiescent neurons. Again, to perhaps oversimplify, for the purposes of this text let us note that all of this switching of neuronal firing patterns accounts for the discontinuous jumps among dream events. Indeed, even the earlier theory of Mamelak and Hobson (1989) postulated that the cholinergic pontogeniculoocipital (PGO) system is the basis for discontinuous dream narratives that we all have heard from our patients. This makes sense because there is considerable evidence that PGO activity is closely related to increased firing in the visual cortex and in the lateral geniculate bodies (LGBs) (Callaway, Lydic, Baghdoyan, & Hobson, 1988).

Given the reduction in activity of aminergic pontine reticular formation neurons, the excitability of the cells they inhibit increases, thus these REM turn-on cells (which are found in several brain stem nuclei) contribute to the REM sleep generator population. Perhaps one of the key systems that is disinhibited are those of the pontine reticular formation neurons themselves. The pontine formation neurons fire single spikes during waking, when we are involved in sensory motor integration (Callaway, Lydic, Baghdoyan, & Hobson, 1988) but discharge in clusters in REM sleep (for a review, see Hobson, 1989). But how does all of this complex activity produce images?

The most useful theory regarding the physiological basis for dreaming thus proposed and embraced by many is the "self-organization theory" of Kahn and Hobson (1993). Dream bizarreness can be defined as "highly unlikely elements in the dream narrative." These improbable events are typically associated with discontinuities in time, place, person, object, and action. They include abrupt, unaccounted-for changes in the dream narrative, which include, for example, the inaccurate matching of different characters, objects, or even scenes in the dream story line itself.

The numerous studies supporting differences between the nature of dream bizarreness and waking mentation have been evaluated and summarized by Kahn and Hobson (1993). Unfortunately, much of the work on dreams has been limited to analyzing reports gleaned from nocturnal dreams following spontaneous home-based awakenings. But then, this is often what we must deal with in the analytic context as well. Most of these reports reflect consciousness associated with both rapid eye movement and non-rapid eye movement sleep. Mamelak and Hobson (1989) reported having confirmed the laboratory-based assumption that 80% of reports exceeding 14 lines in length are obtained following arousal from REM (see also Strickgold, Pace-Shott, & Hobson, 1993). All of the empirical studies taken by Kahn and Hobson support the concept that dream bizarreness is clearly a result of a state-based cognitive process, which has its roots in REM sleep neurophysiological processes. Deep hypnotically induced dreams evoke REM similar to nocturnal dreams (Barrett, 1979)!

Perhaps the breakthrough gleaned from all of this data from both experimental as well as qualitative research is Kahn and Hobson's formulation accounting for the coherent aspects of a dream as attributed to the brain's capacity to self-organize (1993). Thus, we have direct implications for both psychoanalytic uses as well as hypnoanalytic uses of dreams because the external space/time information has been shown to be encoded in relatively orderly mental representations of a nature during waking that is absent during REM sleep. Their theory deals with this at the specific cellular level and the mechanisms involved. The theory accounts for the psychoanalytic conceptualization that the dreaming brain is a self-organizing system, thus there is sense to the apparent bizarreness and a basis for our interpretations.

Apparently, ordered connections between the unconscious and conscious processes become established only in the presence of noise. The implications of this insight from the data were regarded as profound by Kahn and Hobson (1993). Order out of randomness is seen as not only possible but essential, as it is a basis for triggering the emergence of organization. They note that "with respect to acceptance of the activation-synthesis theory of dreams, an appreciation of this dialectic between chaos and order might go a long way to easing the qualms of critics who have imagined an unintended and undesirable return to a 19th century pre-Freudian nonsense theory of dreaming." Thankfully, for our psychotherapeutic endeavors here, the data on cellular mechanisms supports rather than refutes the Freudian conceptualizations of representations from dreams and dream-like states.

The Psychoanalytic Theory of Dreams

Given a psychophysiological theory of dreaming, which now has numerous experimental studies supporting it, and because it lends itself to Freud's conceptualizations about dreams, and repressed and suppressed material, there should be renewed enthusiasm for the utility of dream interpretation in psychoanalysis, hypnoanalysis, and hypnocounseling (Emmerson, 2006) (see also the research by Clara Hill, editor of the *Journal of Counseling Psychology*, and her colleagues, 1993). Without the benefit of established neurophysiological underpinnings, Freud more than a half-century ago (1953b) described a dream as the guardian of sleep. He derived this at first from a study of his own dreams and formulated a theory of their formation.

An inner conflict arises between "instincts" and "ego" or "super-ego." The tension and anxiety it creates is repressed material trying to force its way into consciousness, which can be alleviated or dissipated through a kind of acting-out of the conflict in fantasy form, hence, the dream. This is consistent with Kahn and Hobson's (1993) finding regarding a requirement of chaos or noise leading to organization in the formation of dreams. However, because the material has been repressed below the level of consciousness, it is incapable of direct conscious expression (super-ego [*ueber es*]) and self-view (ego [*selbst*]) of the individual. It can emerge only if in disguised form. Freud termed the original material the "latent" content of the dream; the form in which it emerges is the manifest content. Manifest content is what we consciously remember and are only consciously aware of. The latent content that guides our behaviors remains out of conscious awareness.

The manifest dream was conceptualized as being made up of "the day's residues," by which Freud apparently meant the dreamer's experiences during the day prior to the dream. Albert Ellis, the father of cognitive psychotherapy who was first trained in psychoanalysis, had an almost identical view (Ellis, 1962; Ellis & Grieger, 1977). Potzl (Shevrin & Luborsky, 1974) presented subjects with very brief glimpses of material via a tachistoscope. Material from the scene, which was not noticed consciously at the time, appeared in their dreams later. This is consistent with Freud's formulation that preconscious impressions can be incorporated into manifest dream content, as well as Kahn and Hobson's (1993) organizational theory of dreams (see also Barrett, 1993; Hill, Napayama, & Wonnell, 1998). This inclusion of such material (often erroneously termed subliminal) into manifest dreams was replicated in additional experiments conducted by Fisher (1974).

Through such processes as symbolism, condensation, displacement, and substitution, "dreamwork" presents us with this manifest version of the original, which is more acceptable to the individual than the latent meaning (Heaton, Hill, Petersen, Rochlen, & Zach, 1998). The dream thus protects sleep by concealing latent meaning and revealing it only indirectly through the altered manifest version. The amount of defense change that is involved in the dreamwork of disguising its latent meaning is related to the anxiety attached to that meaning and to the motivational drive to express it. Obviously, if a certain meaning is very threatening to the conscious (perhaps better thought of as the person's self-image, what he or she likes to think of him- or herself as), we can expect much difference between the manifest dream and its latent meaning. On the other hand, if there is a strong drive to express this underlying meaning, the degree of disguise may be less but the patient will be under greater conflict. The task of the therapist then is to assist the patient in deciphering as well as interpreting the original (true) meaning. Thus revealing another piece of the "unconscious," dream interpretation, along with free association, became another basic technique of the analyst.

Freud's emphasis on "instinctual" demands was not shared by Alfred Adler (1963), who considered dreams as more of a problem-solving activity. Adler thought they could represent normal, everyday problems or, in a sense, as Ellis noted (personal communication to A.F.B., circa 1990), include "repetitions of the same irrational thinking that the person carried on through the day to justify their maladaptive behaviors." Adler did recognize that dreams also employ symbolic language, not only to solve problems, but also to rehearse solutions and prepare for translation of these solutions into more adaptive, overt behaviors. Elgan Baker (1981) went one step further, noting that dreams can be integrative in nature and thus facilitate the process of differentiating self from object representations.

Through experimentation, Moss (1961) showed that dream symbols constitute a language of "the sleeping mind," even if latent anxiety is not involved. This tends to vindicate the position that dreaming is at least to a certain extent a right-brain activity due to its reliance on images rather than words to communicate. Recognizing a person's regressive needs, Baker (1981) also noted that dream images in the adult may stand for "transitional objects," like dolls, teddy bears, and security blankets, which take the place of mothers or other original objects in the child's life that were lost through premature abandonment or had to be relinquished. In the dream, mental symbols take the place of more tangible symbols to which the child was originally attached. Filtering these out from the noise of the overall bizarre dream content can take considerable patience on the part of even the most experienced therapist. On the basis of Barrett's (1979) research showing that when deep hypnosis is employed, dream content most similar to nocturnal dreams is revealed, A.F.B. recommends efforts to maintain trance depth to produce more defense-free contents (see section on hypnotically induced dreams).

Interpreting Dreams

Numerous alternative systems of dream interpretation have been devised. The literature on the study of dreams is voluminous, beginning from records of the earliest civilizations to modern experimental studies. For those who wish a general acquaintance with the literature on dreaming, the following constitutes a tiny, yet representative, sample ranging from the anecdotal and theoretical to state-of-the-art research in the field (Barrett & Loeffler, 1979, 1988a, 1988b, 1991a, 1991b, 1992a, 1992b, 1992c, 1993a, 1993b, 1994, 1995a, 1995b, 1996, 2002; Dunn & Barrett, 1988; Zamore & Barrett, 1989; Gutheil, 1970; Heaton, Hill, Petersen, Rochlen, & Zack, 1998; Hill, Napayama, & Wonnell, 1998, Hall, 1953; Mahoney, 1976; Rossi, 1972; Rycroft, 1979; Ullman & Zimmerman, 1979; Wolman, 1979; Woods & Greenhouse, 1974).

A systematic four-step procedure was proposed by Means and a group of his colleagues (Means et al., 1986):

1. Collection and examination of dream images
2. Clarification of the affectual and kinesthetic components
3. Revivification of the dream elements and their associated affects
4. Integration of the dream meaning with the dreamer's past and present life experiences

The majority of early psychoanalytic writers (Federn, see Weiss, 1960; S. Freud, 1953c; Erich Fromm, 1951; Jung, 1958; Stekel, 1943c) devoted considerable attention to the study of dreams. Stekel advocated an intuitive approach to dream analysis. In contrast, Erika Fromm (French & Fromm, 1986) emphasized the activity of the ego and the problem-solving objectives of the dream. They advocated that the dream analyst must employ scientific objective exploration as well as intuition to arrive at valid interpretations. Nonetheless, there is essentially general agreement among all of the significant authors that dreams have personal meanings to the dreamer and that they represent communications from covert mental processes, which can often be interpreted to bring about increased understanding and insight. We will concentrate on techniques for interpreting dreams, inducing them, and therapeutically manipulating them as part of hypnoanalytic therapy, rather than make any attempt here to survey that enormous (and sometimes impenetrable) area of literature.

How to Interpret Dreams

In two experimentally controlled research investigations, counseling psychologist Clara Hill and her colleagues (Hill, Dimer, Sess, Hillyer, & Seemann, 1993; Hill, Napayama, & Wonnell, 1998) tested 60 undergraduate volunteers participating in three alternative conditions. She concluded that interpreting one's own dream led to greater depth and insight than interpreting another persons dream or interpreting one's own event. Although the experienced hypnoanalytic counselor or hypnoanalyst might consider the findings controversial because the level of experience and expertise of the outside interpreters is questionable in these studies, there is an important point for us to recognize. If there is too much activity on the part of the analyst, this will likely mobilize more resistance fromthe patient, thus delaying therapeutic progress. Alternatively, too much passivity on the part of the analyst allows the patient to proceed at such a "comfortable" rate as to prolong the treatment unnecessarily. We must achieve an appropriate balance if we are to achieve the most desirable result. As will be shown later in this chapter, dream interpretation in hypnoanalysis and in hypnoanalytic counseling is an even more active mode than in psychoanalysis but does not necessarily result in the classically predicted harm. Accordingly, our position is that we can generally apply more active techniques in working with dreams than the conventional or the conservative approaches have recommended. The following represents a general outline of techniques that you may wish to use in the exploration of a dream prior to using hypnosis:

I. Elicit and record the dream report
   A. You may ask the patient to write down his or her dreams or suggest that the dream that was forgotten before the therapy session should be allowed to remain in oblivion unless the patient's defenses permit it to be recalled spontaneously.
      1. If it seems desirable for the patient to write down a dream, he or she might be helped with the following suggestions:
         a. Keep a pencil and pad by the bed; write down the dream when you first awaken. Dreams tend to fade the longer you wait after waking up. The most significant parts of dream will be forgotten first.
         b. When you first awaken, do not jump immediately out of the bed; relax into a half-sleep state and revive the dreams of the night, reviewing them mentally. Then write them down at once.
      2. Should your patient arrive with his or her dreams unwritten, you may either listen to an oral presentation and analyze them or write the dream down for detailed consideration later.
         a. Even experienced therapists should have dreams written out either by the patient or by themselves. Consider this almost essential.
         b. It is sometimes warranted to ask the patient to report his or her dreams twice and note the changes in the reports in your chart notes.

II. Interpret the dream
   A. Initial questions you should usually ask:
      1. "When did you dream this?"

2. "Have you dreamed it before?" (Repetitive dreams are the most significant.)
3. "What happened during the day preceding the dream?" (This gives potential information as to whether or not there was a need for defensive reactions or alleviation of the need for defensive reactions during the prior day's demands.)
4. "What thoughts were on your mind when you went to sleep?"
5. "What problems were you concerned about during the preceding day?"
6. "What seems to be the main problem in your life at the present time?" (Obviously, do not ask this if you have just talked about it earlier in the session or if it has been obvious in the prior series of sessions.)
7. "Were you the hero or the victim in this dream?"
8. "Did you become involved actively in the dream, or were you like an observer, a perhaps passive observer?" (Alternatively, to maintain defenses, "Or was it perhaps as if you were watching a movie of the dream?")
9. "What do you think the dream might mean?" This question provides potential access to the kind of material Hill, Dimer, Sess, Hillyer, and Seemann (1993) felt was important.
10. "What are your associations to the dream? Go ahead, let your thoughts go and tell me everything that comes to mind, whether it seems important, relevant, or not; whatever comes to mind."

B. After the patient has exhausted the unguided and general associations, move to the more specific points "radially" (J. G. Watkins, 1978a):

1. "What about the large trunk that appeared in your dream?"
2. "Can you describe it in more detail?"
3. "Tell me everything that comes to mind in relation to the trunk."
4. "What do you remember about trunks?"
5. "What is a trunk?"
6. "What's a trunk for?"
7. "If I had come from a foreign country with little knowledge of the English language and asked you about the word *trunk*, and what it meant, what would you tell me?"
8. Ask for both the general and specific characteristics about each item in the dream ("specific radiality," A. Barabasz, in preparation). Hence, "You saw a bear in the dream. What kind of bear was it?"

     a. "Just what was the bear doing?"
     b. "How do you feel about bears?"
     c. "What would you say about a bear like this? Was he strong? Was he weak, masculine, feminine, passive, aggressive, cruel, cuddly?"

9. Dreams use a kind of paralogic, as explained by Kahn and Hobson's organizational theory (1993). Symbols tend to be equated with their true meanings over what might be considered a bridge in which the symbol and that which it represents have some part or element in common. Research has demonstrated (P. Kline, 1972) that Freud was not entirely wrong when he reported that long objects, like poles and swords, were masculine symbols and that openings and containers, such as boxes and houses, were feminine symbols. They commonly have those associations, but it would be an error for a therapist to generalize that all such objects do. It is enough to understand that this can still be the case. Perhaps it is more important to bear in mind that each person has uniquely individual meanings and through association these will, most often, eventually emerge.

    With sensitive intuition, the therapist may frequently determine the meaning of dream symbols in some patients, but without securing associations. Some people almost naturally seem to have an intuitive ability to sense unconscious communications and translate them into symbols, such as Stekel may have had. Reik (1948) called this "the third ear." Children often have it better than adults, indicating that our stress on objectivity, scientific validity, and logical argument during school has taught us to inhibit the sensitive and intuitive thought processes that a child possesses. As we age and become jaundiced in our relationships and educational experiences, this intuitive ability, which is the absolute hallmark of the most effective therapist or analyst, tends to get lost. In a misguided sense, it is even thought of by many as being a part of "growing up" (even a beneficial one). J.G.W. (1992) maintained that such therapeutic sensitivity, if still available in one's twenties, is amenable to retraining.

    Although dream interpretation was scorned as superficial and unscientific by many of his colleagues, Wilhelm Stekel was unquestionably recognized as a remarkably sensitive master of it. In addition to two volumes on it (1943c), Stekel published a series of detailed case studies on such topics as sadism and masochism (1939b), impotence in the male (1939a), sexual aberrations (1940), frigidity in women (1943a), peculiarities of behavior (1943b), and compulsion and doubt (1949). Stekel's remarkable two-volume works in each of these areas described many cases with innumerable dreams, which he had analyzed brilliantly.

Stekel hypothesized that the initial dream in an analysis constituted a kind of overview of the patient's entire neurosis. By that, he meant that at the end of analysis it was intended that the patient would understand its full meaning and the dynamic structure of his or her neurosis. Such a claim has not yet been experimentally tested but we can learn much through the study of his approach to dream analysis, in that it provides us with a structure to test the effectiveness of our own work.

Stekel's structure for the analysis of each case began with a description of the background and history of the patient and his or her presenting complaints, very much as one might do in a standard initial interview. Next he would report the patient's first dream, followed by his direct interpretation of it. The interpretation was essentially intuitive. He continued this pattern throughout each case by presenting the development of the analysis and several of the patient's dreams, and he followed this with his intuitive interpretations, which most any educated reader will recognize as both brilliant and logical if not easily subject to scientific verification. Somehow, Stekel seemed able to react with great sensitivity to the symbols and subtle unconscious communications in the dreams of his patients and thus fathom their meanings. In fact, he often bragged how, through his "direct" and intuitive analysis, he could shorten the time of treatment and achieve therapeutic results far more rapidly than his colleagues who were bound by the free-association approach, which was by its nature very slow.

We previously noted that, through intensive study and resonance with the analytic intuition of Theodore Reik (1948, 1956, 1957), therapists can sharpen their sensitivity at picking covert communications in the associations of their patients. Accordingly, we studied Stekel's recognized skills in dream interpretation in a similar fashion.

J.G.W. would read Stekel's description of the background of each case and then the patient's dream. At this point, he would lay Stekel's book down and write out his direct, "intuitive" interpretation of the dream. Next, J.G.W. would compare his interpretation point by point with Stekel's, noting identities, similarities, and differences. He would then take another of the dreams Stekel reported from the same case or from some of the 1,200 others Stekel published and do the same. In a sense, J.W.G. involved himself in a structured learning of Stekel's approach.

After practicing this exercise through several hundred dreams, J.G.W. found that his interpretations began approaching Stekel's more and more. Often they would be almost identical. This, of course, does not prove that either interpretation was correct. It does show, however, that J.G.W. was learning to respond to the same cues to which Stekel reacted, and in a similar way J.G.W. was incorporating Stekel's approach to dream interpretation. Subsequently, J.G.W. noticed that his abilities to "intuit" dream and projective fantasy meanings in his patients was enormously improved to their benefit. This was a kind of unconscious training for him, an extension of the skills acquired in his own analysis. Therapists can develop their analytic skills from reading, observing, and most importantly modeling other skilled practitioners, especially their mentor. Young analysts and hypnoanalytic counselors do it all the time in their "training analyses."

Hypnosis and Dreaming

The hypnotic modality allows us more leverage in the analysis of dreams that are normally created by the sleeping patient. Adding hypnosis to the technique of dream interpretation enhances rather than diminishes the value of the original psychoanalytic procedures. Free (S. Freud, 1953b), radial (J. G. Watkins, 1978a), and specific radial associations (A. Barabasz, in preparation) continue to be the desired approaches, and of course, nothing can substitute for the therapist's knowledge of symbol formation and the therapist's intuitive sensitivity; however, hypnosis adds a remarkable new dimension. Hypnosis permits us to initiate, intervene, and actually control dream activity to the benefit of the patient.

Given that dreaming tends to occur in the lightest stage of sleep (Stage I), this makes good sense as we conceptualize a progressive continuum in levels of consciousness from wide-awake alertness at one end to deep, almost coma-like at the other. Cognitive activities do not vanish. They gradually diminish. As the degree of awareness and mentation lessens, certain functions decrease faster than others. Thus, in classical psychoanalytic terms, the super-ego is the first casualty. As its vigilant function diminishes, the dream material that emerges is less subject to conscience and "parental" controls. Individuals dream vividly about activities that in the normal awake state would be taboo to them. Extramarital escapades, sadomasochism, and similar activities, which the person's super-ego attempts to inhibit and frequently prevents from being carried out in real life, begin to appear as primary. Sometimes very primitive impulses may become manifest. We can think of it this way: When the super-ego is away, the id will play.

The individual, in his or her development beginning from the fertilized egg to the development of the fetus to the mature adult, repeats the evolutionary history of the species (homo sapiens), or in more sophisticated terms, ontogeny recapitulates phylogeny.

The super-ego's socialized control system came late in the development of the human. Accordingly, because sleep, like hypnosis, is a "regression in the service of the ego" (A. Barabasz & Christensen, 2006; Erika Fromm, 1992; Gill & Brenman, 1959), we should expect the most recently formed psychological structures and processes to be the first to succumb as the regressive state begins to take over and more primitive ones appear. In deep sleep, curled up in the fetal position, and under the covers, we provide just one such example.

During the light sleep stage, there is much bodily movement such as tossing and turning, as well as the well-known REM eye movements that correlate strongly with the dreaming activity. Interestingly, if you conduct all-night EEGs on normal persons without known sleep disorders, you will find that a person typically dreams for about 90 minutes per night. If we interrupt a person's REM sleep every time EEGs show they enter REM to the point where they are dreaming, and then leave them alone the following night, almost invariably, the subject of our study will produce nearly 3 hours of dreaming the following night, as if trying to make up for lost dream time. Although A.F.B.'s labs at Washington State University and previously at Harvard Medical School and the University of Canterbury in New Zealand have incomplete data to warrant conclusions, it would appear that such correlational data promotes the speculation that humans' eagerness to make up for dream time means that dreaming may be in some way essential to survival as a normal adaptive individual. (There is further data from sleep labs that supports this but that discussion goes beyond the focus of this book.)

As sleep progresses to the deeper Stages II, III, and IV, both physical and mental activity becomes less and less. After the super-ego is inhibited, there is progressively less ego activity, and dreams are more likely to reflect very primitive motivations and processes. As the fantasies reach into this area, they are more and more likely to be forgotten when the dreamer awakens. This is partly because they occurred at a deeper level of consciousness and partly because, being more primitive, they are likely to differ, not only from the subject's accepted super-ego norms, but also from his or her self (ego perceptions). Thus, the ego would be the next to go, with the most primitive id processes, those that governed in earlier ontogenic and phylogenetic human development, being the last to manifest themselves before complete coma takes over. But how does this relate to hypnosis?

Reyher (see A. Barabasz, 1982) conceptualized the hypnotic state as the ascendancy of phylogenetically older and lower levels of neuro-cortical development. As A.F.B. demonstrated experimentally, Reyher's conceptualization was disproven as a physiological explanation of the hypnotic state in its entirety. However, it bears consideration for our present discussion when limited only to helping to provide a better understanding of certain hypnotic mechanisms as they relate to dreams and fantasies.

Given the process described above, let us recognize that something like this occurs in alcoholic intoxication. The drunk first loses social inhibitions. Depending on the underlying personality structure, he or she may make crude sexual passes, may be aggressively hostile, or may remain calm yet more talkative and open. With the ingestion of even more liquor, he or she becomes passive and loses physical coordination and becomes cognitively impaired. Finally, the drunkard "passes out" and enters a coma-like state of stupor, in which all semblance of consciousness and normal behavior disappears. As normal sleep becomes deeper, dreams take on a more concrete nature, reflecting primitive and earlier developing brain processes with less higher level cerebral activity (the ascendancy of phylogenetically older and lower levels of neuronal integration). This is also true with hypnosis when it is deepened from hypnoidal and lighter states to the profound somnambulistic trance and finally, in those rare cases, to that coma-like condition that Erickson (1952) reserved for the term "plenary trance."

Most people dream even when no dreams are reported. We seem to be made up of a group of dream rememberers and dream nonrememberers. This may be because the dreams required repression, hence, "forgetting," or because they were dreamed in such a deep state that they are no longer subject to recall or, more likely, a combination of both factors. To help break through these amnesias, hypnosis is the method that permits us to go back and "recover" or at least reconstruct these dreams.

The process can start at an initially simple level. With the patient as deeply hypnotized as possible, instruct him or her to go back, recover, and redream any dreams he or she may have had the previous night. Often we will find dreams now reported, and we have new material with which to work. This is most likely to occur during the initial stages of hypnoanalytic treatment. Most often, this process will reveal a dream that is consciously reported, only in the briefest form. A patient once brought the following:

"I dreamt last night that I was almost struck by a car." He was then hypnotized and the suggestion was made to "Go back to your dream of last night when you were almost struck by a car. It is happening again just as it did then."

The patient stated, "I am standing with a friend at the corner of Arthur and Beckworth. A red convertible driven by a blonde woman comes barreling around the corner and almost hits me. I jump back, fall down, and skin my knee. My friend says, 'Why doesn't that bitch look where she is going?'"

Notice the patient's amplification with increased detail. The working through of meanings related to a red convertible and the blonde, the friend, and his remark open up entirely new vistas to this person's treatment. The matter of whether or not the reconstruction was accurate with regard to what might have been dreamed is irrelevant. The gain is that the patient has provided new opportunities for exploration, which are freer from defenses than what might have been eventually secured through free association.

Hypnosis not only increases the opportunity to bring together dream reconstruction; we can also use it to suggestively create dreams, either by initiating the dream process or by inducing dreams about specific topics. In hypnosis, patients can be given the hypnotic suggestion that they will have dreams, or that they will dream about their relationship with their mother.

Once J.G.W. hypnotized his patient and suggested to her that she would dream about the treatment and her therapist. At their next meeting, she presented with the following:

I dreamed I was sitting on the lawn listening to a fatuous young man orating from a stump. He seemed to be very pleased with the sound of his own voice. [J.G.W. was alerted to her negative transference toward him and got the message to shut a bit more and listen instead of lecture.] J.G.W. noted, "As I behaved better, her therapy improved."

In another case, J.G.W. asked his patient for a prognosis dream after establishing a state of hypnosis. The next session came and the patient reported:

I dreamed that I went back to my old hometown. It was terribly run down. The streets had been neglected, the trees were dying, and nobody seemed to be in charge. Then I had another dream, in this one it seems that I went back again to the town 2 years later and there was much improvement. Somebody had cleaned up most of the garbage and planted new trees and flowers. I had the feeling that finally they had voted in a mayor who was going to do something. [J.G.W. reported feeling much better about the future course of therapy with this patient.]

As you can see, dreams are not always so difficult to interpret and secure meaning from them. Obviously, the two examples above are quite transparent, yet it is amazing to a therapist who asks the patient directly, "What do you think this dream means?" and get an answer like, "I don't know." If dreams are used frequently in therapy, patients become more skillful in interpreting them (Hill, Napayama, & Wonnell, 1998). But unlike the university students in Hill's research study, patients in therapy produce more and more sophisticated dreams, which are increasingly difficult to analyze. As the patients become educated, so also do their defenses. This is one reason why inexperienced therapists may be just as effective as experienced ones when working with inexperienced patients with relatively simplistic disorders. Given the development of a patient's defenses over the course of his or her pathology and in the course of his or her therapy, we should recognize that the effective therapist cannot exclusively use dreams as a single mode of therapy. Alternative hypnoanalytic and hypnocounseling procedures should be employed as well.

Some patients are simply not psychologically minded enough to decipher the dreams they report in therapy, especially if their intellectual abilities are quite modest. Erika Fromm and Kahn (1990) demonstrated that, after learning self-hypnosis, many intelligent and therapy-oriented patients are quite capable of inducing and interpreting their own hypnotic images and dreams. Again, Hill's success with university students deciphering their own dreams was with a preselected sample of individuals bright enough to obtain admission to a major university and inquisitive (Hill, Napayama, & Wonnell, 1998). Thus, her volunteers were likely brighter still than the average university student, given that they self-selected (via their volunteering behavior) into a study of such a demanding nature. Therefore, it's difficult to even begin to draw the conclusion that patients in general are all capable of interpreting their own dreams.

Psychoanalysts have raised the same question for decades regarding the screening of acceptable candidates for analysis. Some have proposed that patients should be at least above average in intelligence if they are to understand their neuroses. It is not always a matter of inadequate level of intelligence but can also be a correlate of a "working class, nine-to-five" mentality type of patient regardless of their IQ. Patient characteristics of the nine-to-five types include histories of putting in their time on the job during the "blue collar" working hours only, poor future planning (particularly in the long-range sphere), and a fantasy-laden notion of what the future may bring rather than a realistic one that would involve both intermediate and long-range goals. Such patients who occasionally seek therapy are likely to select themselves out of depth therapies rapidly, misunderstand them, and if they return to therapy at all, seek temporary quick-fix solutions via psychopharmacology or superficial cognitive approaches.

Another type of patient with adequate intellectual capacity as well as the ability to create a realistic goal structure with intermediate goals that they fulfill may compound their neurosis by their own above-average cognitive abilities. Consequently, the simplicity or complexity of a therapeutic approach must reflect the intellectual abilities of its creator (smart person-smart neuroses, dumb person-dumb neuroses), but the patient must always be bright enough to understand his or her own particular neurosis. Unfortunately, some individuals' neuroses are too smart for their analysts, and thus their defenses are never penetrated in treatment, whereas others (although perhaps of more-than-sufficient IQ) are simply too dumbed down by the values they took on in their upbringing. Thus, they maintain a maladaptive, simplistic, and fantasy-laden outlook on life. Such defenses can be as rigid as the personality structures of these nine-to-fivers. Nonetheless, if the patient presents for therapy, there is always a chance that therapeutic progress can be made.

Analyzing Dreams with Hypnosis

As Barrett (1995) explained, the greatest benefit of combining hypnosis with dreamwork lies in the fact that it greatly enhances the engagement of the primary process mode, which is underutilized in psychodynamic therapies as well as therapeutic counseling (see also Gruenewald, Fromm, & Oberlander, 1972). "By adding hypnosis to the important but already well-exercised secondary process we maximize the psyche's resources" (Barrett, p. 30). Logical thinking is employed ad nauseam in attempts to provide what amounts to band-aid cognitive therapy approaches. In nonhypnotic psychodynamic therapies, the logical thought, often in the form of intellectualization, supports defensive barriers to the curative effects of interpretation that might otherwise be wrought. Evoking primary process in dreamwork by hypnosis also can contribute significantly to what the rational mind has not achieved in a wide variety of therapies.

Hypnosis thus allows greater therapeutic effectiveness by bringing the combined effect of both modes of cognition. Virtually all of the techniques used in psychoanalysis, psychodynamically oriented therapy, and psycho dynamic counseling for interpreting dreams can be employed in hypnoanalysis. Just hypnotize the patient and apply them!

Because a patient is frequently able to decipher the meaning of a dream directly, especially when its latent meaning is little disguised, ask the patient what he or she thinks the dream means. Next, apply free and radial associations of the elements of the dreams, but this time with the patient in a state of hypnosis. Any or all of the questions suggested in the outline above can be applied in the hypnotic setting. Determine to what degree the manifest material has been distorted from its latent meaning to consider hypnotic depth. The greater the depth of hypnosis used, the greater the likelihood of distortion from its latent meaning. Our discussion of how to elicit the meanings of symbolic dream representations by the many dissociative and projective techniques at our disposal will be deferred to chapters 8, 9, and 10, where you can learn precisely how to apply the techniques.

It is also possible to intervene in dreams or at least into their reliving (reconstruction) of them. This approach is conducted without the use of hypnosis but rather by what Jungian analysts (see G. Adler, 1948) referred to as "active imagination." For example, let us say that our patient provides us with the recount of a dream as follows:

P: I was walking down the street of a strange town when I noticed a tall man. It was getting dark out and it made the man look dark, a dark man wearing a long dark cloak approaching me. I felt much fear and woke up in a cold sweat.

You might approach the interpretation of this recounted dream in the following manner:

Therapist: O.K., now close your eyes and let us visualize the dream. You are walking down the street in this strange town, and you are seeing a tall man, darkened by the approaching evening hour. You are frightened and you want to escape! However, I will walk with you, there is no need to be afraid, I am with you and I am strong and powerful [thus, you are strengthening or adding to the patient's ego strength by your relationship with the patient]. Now walk up to him and look at his face, look right into his face. Who does he look like? Have you ever seen him before? Where? [Continue questioning to establish who or what "the man" represents.]

P.:   [Replies to your questions.]

T.:   Ask him who he is. Say, "What is your name?"

The example above and the incident described represent one way a Jungian analyst might practice "active imagination." To be sure, patients with higher levels of hypnotizability will no doubt, in many but certainly not all cases, achieve some level of hypnotic trance with your very first suggestion (Nash, 2005). Nonetheless, the situation is not introduced to the patient as a hypnotic one in any sense. It can be just as effective either way at that level.

The same active intervention can be applied with the patient in a light or even a deep hypnotic state. Again, let us not think of hypnosis as being a completely different treatment modality from the psychoanalytic approach of the therapist or counselor, but rather that at times it can provide considerably greater effectiveness and flexibility, and the altered state of consciousness in which to apply analytic procedures one might use without it.

Freud rejected hypnosis, most likely because he had fears of the powerful reactions it could evoke (M. V. Kline, 1958) (see Barabasz & Watkins, 2005, for further references to this conceptualization). Unfortunately, Freud wrote down his rejection as a kind of dictum for other analysts, which many of them have followed quite religiously and without question for decades. Otherwise, they might well today be integrating hypnotic procedures with their regular psychoanalytic techniques to great and positive effect with their patients. The polished words of the great innovators, whether they be right or wrong, carry enormous weight with their followers.

In the next chapter on projective hypnoanalysis, these fantasy and dream intervention procedures will be explained in detail and at sufficient length to put them to use in practice. However, for the present, the working through of a particular dream may be of use as well as interest.

A patient of J.G.W. presented the following dream:

P.:   I was walking down a city street when I saw a large colonial mansion. It was on fire. I was trying to put out the fire but not succeeding very well.

[The patient was hypnotized, told to return to that dream, and when he could see the burning house to lift his index finger on his left hand. The finger lifts.]

J.G.W.:   Now, while you are watching the burning house, time is going to reverse until you see the house just before it begins to burn. Let your finger lift when you can see it that way. [The finger lifts.] Describe the house.

P.:   It's white and has two large pillars, one on each side of the door.

J.G.W.:   Go up to the door. Let the finger lift when you get there. [The finger lifts.]

J.G.W.:   Fine, open the door and go in.
P.:   The door is locked! I can't open it. [The patient manifests his resistance.]
J.G.W.:   Perhaps if you looked around you might find a key which would open it. [The patient squirms in the chair and moves his head about.]
P.:   I don't see any key. [More resistance.]
J.G.W.:   There is a doormat there, have you looked under it?
P.:   Yes, there does seem to be a key there. [Resistance is lessened partly because we are now trying to only find the key, which is a primary process concrete thinking function, and are not keeping in the foreground of consciousness the goal of opening the door.]
J.G.W.:   Insert the key into the door lock. [Notice the symbolic communication of "finding the key"].
P.:   [Begrudgingly and with consternation in his voice] Well, it's hard to turn it.
J.G.W.:   Keep trying.
P.:   Yes, I have opened it now.
J.G.W.:   Go in. What do you see?
P.:   Just a long hallway. [Matter of factly, yet with a veiled tone of hostility in the patient's voice as the recognition of the breaking down of resistance is processed at an intermediate level.]
J.G.W.:   Go down the hall until you come to a door that is slightly open. [We make it "slightly" open so as not to challenge the patient's defenses too directly. Thus, he can still resist going into that room.]
J.G.W.:   What is in the room?
P.:   Nothing.
J.G.W.:   Keep looking. Maybe there is some furniture there.
P.:   There is a rocking chair in the center of the room.
J.G.W.:   What does rocking chair remind you of?
P.:   My mother had a rocking chair, she used to hold me and rock me in it before putting me to bed.

The associations have now led us through resistance from the burning house to the mother. We will not pursue the inquiry further, except to note that eventually he was able to see his mother rocking in the chair.

We do not accept Freud's belief as to the universality of the Oedipus complex in all male neuroses. Nonetheless, it does occur at times and this happened to be one of those times. The patient's sexual impotence did represent his sexual tie to his mother, and his passivity covered up his "burning" desire for her. In classical psychoanalytic symbolism, houses often represent women, who represent the first "house in which we live." Mothers are large compared to children, hence "a mansion." They are not sexual (the house is white, symbolizing virginity or untouchability), and like all women they have an entrance between two pillars (legs). Once we get through the initial resistance, the meaning of the dream becomes clear. Unfortunately, though, the patient was not yet ready for its complete interpretation. Direct confrontation, at this point, with his erotic feelings for his mother might well have scared him away from treatment. With more working through, J.G.W secured from the dream the direction treatment had to take. What we have done is to apply Jungian "active imagination" as the method of choice, yet we have intervened in the dream using hypnosis to decipher it. The advantages of hypnosis in these types of cases seem obvious.

Hypnotic Dreams

The research comparing nocturnal dreams and hypnotically induced dreams reveals that the physiological correlates of hypnotically induced dreams resemble the waking relaxed state rather than any stage of sleep (Barrett, 1979; Brady & Rosner, 1966; Tart, 1964). However, contrary to the waking relaxed state, hypnotic dreams show rapid eye movements as found in nocturnal sleep during certain dream themes (Brady & Rosner; Schiff, Bunney, & Freedman, 1961). More important to psychotherapy is Barrett's finding that the contents of hypnotically induced dreams during deep trance states were found to be very similar to the same subject's nocturnal dreams. Furthermore, they clearly differed from waking daydreams on a wide variety of characteristics including length, emotional themes, characters, plot settings, and the amount of distortion. Subjects in medium hypnotic depths showed dream contents that fell between their nocturnal dreams and their daydreams. Thus, one of the key issues to consider in dreamwork with hypnosis is the issue of establishing trance depths consistent with psychotherapeutic goals (see also A. Barabasz & Christensen, 2006).

Once the hypnotic state has been established with your patient, he or she can be asked to "dream" about some general or specific problem while in the trance state and to report it immediately thereafter. Because such dreams are not the same those that occur in nocturnal sleep, some therapists prefer to use the term "to image" instead of "to dream" in describing the phenomena, as well as in their instructions to their patients. It may make little difference, but to us it seems that to most people, "dreaming" has a special connotation quite different from "simply" imagining. We feel it is probably better to use the word "dream" in our hypnotic suggestions. We have no specific dream study data from controlled experimental research to support this contention. However, we do know from experimentally controlled EEG research that the wording of hypnotic suggestions can be crucial (A. Barabasz, 2000; A. Barabasz, M. Barabasz, Jensen, Calvin, Trevisan, & Warner, 1999; D. Spiegel, 2003; H. Spiegel & D. Spiegel, 2004).

A "dream" reported by a lightly hypnotized patient has much more character of a conscious daydream than that of a true nocturnal dream. However, hypnotic dreams more closely resemble nocturnal dreams that are reported several days after the dream event took place (Wright, 1987). Hence, such dreams are more subject to defensive amnesia, as well as the mastering of a myriad of other defenses, than those described immediately after awakening. Furthermore, you will also observe that the deeper the hypnotic state, the more likely it will be that the production will manifest the defensive elaborations that separate an overt dream report from its latent meaning, while at the same time often obtaining revelations of meaningful repressed material, albeit at a symbolic level. Adopting Osgood and Luria's semantic differential (1954) approach, which uses bipolar adjectives with seven numeric choices between them, Moss (1970) demonstrated experimentally that the symbols elicited in hypnotic dreams, although differing from those in nocturnal dreams, nevertheless have real meaning and relate to significant conflicts within the dreamer, both overt and covert ones.

Hypnosis can also be used to induce a sequence of dreams related to a specific therapeutic problem (Sacerdote, 1967b). Each hypnotically elicited dream is intended to build upon the previous one. Although not so attributed, the technique reflects B. F. Skinner's successive approximations method of behavioral shaping to approximate the true essence of the underlying conflict.

It is long been known that hypnosis is not the same as sleep (for a superb review, see Evans, 1979b). Nonetheless, Sacerdote (1967) felt that hypnotic dreaming was more productive if hypnosis was induced by using the word "sleep," because most people expect to "dream" when they are asleep. This point of view had such an impact that the inductions developed for the Stanford Hypnotic Susceptibility Scales of Weitzenhoffer and E. R. Hilgard (1959, 1962) included the word "sleep" repetitively despite having but 1 of the 12 test items relating to a "dream." For decades now, the "sleep" instructions in the induction of hypnosis have been almost entirely abandoned. However, the instruction "sleep and have a dream" may simply be used after hypnosis is induced, such as in item number 2 of the Stanford Hypnotic Clinical Scale (Morgan & J. R. Hilgard, 1975). Similarly, that model suggestion can be employed for dream inducement. The process of building upon dreams sequentially remains just as valid a technique today as it was when an approximation of that approach, predating Sacerdote, was recommended by Gill and Menninger (1947). They would ask the patient to dream a second dream to help explain the first one if the first one was not clearly explicable and interpretable. A.F.B. continues to be astonished as to how remarkably well such a seemingly simple approach can be in revealing meanings that lead to interpretations.

A wide variety of hypnotherapeutic techniques can be combined with the use of hypnotic dreams. Jerome Schneck (1974) found that hypnotically induced nightmares were essentially the equivalent of normal nocturnal nightmares. Thus, Regardie (1950) traced the development of conflicts by studying hypnotic dreams through the use of age regression techniques. The majority of hypnotized subjects are closer to their own unconscious; therefore, it is not all that surprising that they may be better able than conscious individuals to decipher the meaning of dreams other than their own. The only published example we have been able to find regarding this hypnotically pervasive concept was reported more than half a century ago by Erickson and Kubie (1941). They described a hypnotized participant who apparently was able to interpret the automatic writings of another participant. It would be interesting to conduct an experiment to determine whether or not the analyst who is able to enter a light hypnotic (hypnoidal) state might produce better communications, finding his or her own intuitive sensitivity to the dream to be enhanced.

Dreams and psychotic hallucinations present us with concrete ideation. It has been suggested the dreams represent a psychosis experienced in sleep, or that psychosis is a dream when we are awake. Because hypnosis serves as a modality for intervening in dreams, it should not be surprising that some prominent therapist-researchers (personal communication to A.F.B. from Frederick Evans, 1992) have employed it to intervene in the mental processes of psychotics and to facilitate their treatment.

A classic case reported by Joan Murray Jobsis (Scagnelli, 1977) was a confrontation with a schizophrenic patient who was terrified of losing ego control both to the therapist "without" and to the fantasies "within." She taught him to use autohypnosis to control his own states of consciousness. She then developed with him a procedure by which he could manage and "control" his hallucinated "monsters" and other frightening phantasmagoria through hypnotic dreaming. As he practiced this creator control technique, he reportedly began to master his psychotic ideation and to learn to distinguish subject from object representations. Within only 14 months of therapy, he had reintegrated and formed a stable self-identity, probably for the first time in his life. The patient learned how not to be frightened and helpless at his own unconscious because he had learned that his former hallucinations had changed into normal dreaming, which he felt he could control. J.G.W. (1992a) noted that this technique shows enormous promise in working with psychotics. The prominent journals focusing on clinical and experimental hypnosis would likely be interested in any case or research data that is forthcoming from therapists using the technique with their patients.

Summary

Hypnosis facilitates the techniques used by analytically oriented therapists and counselors for deciphering dreams, images, fantasies, and hallucinations. These are visual creations that may communicate preconscious and unconscious processes. Dreams as well as hallucinations, although subjectively created, are experienced as if they are external objects. The most recent theoretical understandings of the neurophysiology of dream phenomena relates well with what is known about the hypnotic process. A wide variety of hypnotherapeutic techniques can be used for the initiation of dreams, interpreting them, and intervening in them for both diagnostic and therapeutic purposes. Hypnotic dreams differ from sleep dreams by being closer to conscious fantasies but may at least approximate the concrete thinking characteristic of sleep dreams during deeper states of hypnosis. Dreams are known to occur during Stage I rapid eye movement light sleep. Yet, REM has not yet been shown to represent scanning of some sort of internal visual field. In A.F.B.'s opinion, it is doubtful that it ever will, given that REM-type EEGs have been shown to exist even in fish that were born without eyes, taken from the dark great depths of the oceans. The psychoanalytic theory of dreams holds that through "dreamwork," the original latent dream is transferred into the manifest dream experienced by the dreamer.

There is evidence that dreams can be interpreted by associations using the methodology described in this chapter or by some of the most experienced and sensitive therapists "intuitively." In hypnosis, dreams may be reported that are not consciously remembered. Another method is to hypnotically suggest the dream and then interpret that dream. Sometimes dreams can be initiated through hypnosis that focuses on prognosis for the treatment, which will be useful to the therapist. Jung's "active imagination" approach can also be used with hypnosis to facilitate its effects. It involves the therapist's direct intervention into the dream process where dreams are suggested to help. There is at least one brilliant clinical example that shows that dreams can be suggested to help a psychotic patient establish stable object representations. Clearly, more clinical research is needed to further our understandings of how best to use dream interpretation to our patients' greatest benefit.

Nonetheless, the increased access to unconscious processes afforded by the hypnotic modality in the study of dreams makes hypnosis a worthy addition.

8
Projective Hypnoanalysis

"You can't trust anybody these days." Although there is some truth to the assertion that many are not trustworthy, the claim that nobody is reveals more about the honesty of the speaker than the situation. Projection is a common psychological defense whereby an individual imputes to someone or something in the outside world aspects of his or her own self. The very honest person tends to be more trusting of others, often to his or her own detriment. A (pathological) individual loaded with repressed hatred may present a smiling face (outwardly appropriate affect) full of jealousy and envy but insist that he or she is the victim of somebody else's vendetta or, in a more global sense, an "unfair" world. It is a common defense to protect the integrity of one's personality when it is filled with desperate elements. In severe cases, projection eventually develops into a psychotic paranoid reaction. The unique way that one perceives the world can tell much about one's own (maladaptive) personality because different people perceive events so differently (J. G. Watkins, 1992a, p. 121).

Projective Hypnoanalytic Technique

Recognizing the tendency of humans to externalize or "project" their own motivations, attitudes, and feelings onto their perceptions lends itself to exploration by a set of psychological test instruments and diagnostic devices referred to as "projective techniques." The use of these instruments by a skilled diagnostician makes it possible to disclose facets of patients' functioning that neither the patient nor the therapist may be aware of at a conscious level. These instruments offer a modality that can reveal that which has been concealed. The Rorschach Inkblot Test, when reliably scored by the Exner system, can disclose structural aspects of an individual's personality including the nature of his or her defenses, the impending possibility of a psychotic breakdown, the degree to which the patient can control emotions, the extent of inner fantasy (spontaneous dissociation), and his or her compulsiveness, as well as many other traits. Other projective tests, such as the Thematic Apperception Test (TAT) and the Make-A-Picture Story (MAPS) Test (Schneidman, 1947), can probe inner psychodynamic processes and reveal attitudes toward parents or toward the self, or even the current state of the transference relationship with the therapist or significant others.

When these projective tests became available more than half a century ago, they seemed to hold such promise that they were used for purposes well beyond those conceptualized by their creators. For example, Orne (1951) used the Rorschach to evaluate hypnotic age regression. Because age regression is incomplete and more topographic than temporal, tests such as the Rorschach, which at the time lacked reliable scoring, were inadequate in detecting complete regression. Indeed, the test was never designed to measure the nature of age regression produced by hypnosis (see A. Barabasz & Christensen, 2006).

Using a test with appropriate psychometric properties designed to test a developmentally fixed stage of focal point dependency and inversion perception, A. Barabasz and Christensen (2006) experimentally demonstrated that hypnotic age regression, tailored ego-syntonically with the hypnotizable research participants, produced responses characteristic of children aged 5 that could not be role-played.

Rorschach (1949) produced what has become the most widely studied of the procedures. He produced 10 cards made up of colored inkblots (like clouds), which were all vague, unstructured stimuli. Participants' responses to the cards showed that different people saw them in very different ways. Unlike the Rorschach, the TAT consists of pictures that are shown to the participant, who is then asked to make up stories about them. As a teenage undergraduate, A.F.B. extended the procedure to determine future temporal orientation among delinquents and nondelinquents, as well as successful and unsuccessful university students' photographs, similar to that with which such individuals would come into contact (A. Barabasz, 1970c). The participants in A.F.B.'s studies revealed their temporal orientations. Delinquents and unsuccessful college students, for example, were more present oriented than their better-adjusted contemporaries. The principle behind all of these projective techniques is to present the research subject or patient with vague unstructured stimuli, and then encourage a response to structure them according to the person's own, unique personality needs.

In contrast to "objective" personality tests, projective tests are based on an entirely different concept. In the "objective test," each item is rendered as specific and succinct as possible, so that the probability of the subject misinterpreting it will be minimized. In the projective tests, we intentionally make each stimulus vague so that our patient can "misinterpret" it in his or her own individual way. Projective techniques are intended to tap the more preconscious and unconscious aspects of a personality. Hence, projective tests are more valuable in psychoanalytic or hypnoanalytic therapy; however, many therapists use both objective as well as projective tests because they yield different aspects of personality functioning.

In an effort to combine the three most significant approaches for gaining access to unconscious process (psychoanalysis, hypnosis, and projective) techniques, J.G.W. (1952) coined the term "projective hypnoanalysis." J.G.W.

hoped, by combining all three into an integrated therapeutic methodology, to develop a more powerful therapeutic approach that might be superior to any of the three alone. Unfortunately, this initial effort, while successful in combining several powerful probing techniques, did not give the attention to transference and other relationship factors, which we now recognize to be of critical importance (A. Barabasz & J. G. Watkins, 2005). However, as J.G.W. pointed out even earlier (1949), technique plus relationship is better than either alone.

This chapter is intended both to illustrate, using a "classic case" (considered one of the first examples of hypnoanalysis) treated by J.G. Watkins, and to elaborate and expand upon the work of many authors in the field, (Watkins, 1949). All of these approaches attempt to combine projective, dissociative, and fantasy procedures (Barrett, 1992a; Erikson, 1967; Brenman & Gill, 1947; M. V. Kline, 1967; Wolberg, 1945; Schneck, 1965). Hypnotically induced drama has been tried (Moreno, 1946; Moreno & Enneis, 1950; Shaw, 1978). Cognitive-behavioral therapists and researchers have also rediscovered the value of projective covert fantasies in facilitating behavior change reconceptualized outside of psychoanalytic theory (Cauttella & Bennett, 1981; Ellis & Grieger, 1977; Meichenbaum, 1977). Numerous other terminologies have been used to describe the very same therapeutic foci, such as guided fantasy, guided imagery, and most recently eye movement desensitization reprocessing (EMDR) (Shapiro, 2001).

Combining the procedures described in the chapters on abreaction, hypnography, hypnoplasty, dreams and fantasies, ego-state therapy, and the dissociated handwriting technique (which will be described in later chapters), we will illustrate the integrated procedure of projective hypnoanalysis below. This chapter marks a departure from the emphasis on techniques in the earlier chapters of Barabasz & Watkins (2005) by placing more attention on both relationship and transference factors. Following are excerpts from a case of projective hypnoanalysis (J. G. Watkins, 1949). Included in this case are projective test instruments, Jungian "active imagination," dissociated handwriting, dream interpretation, symbolic communication, projective forecast of conflict resolution; and evidence for the validity of a parent "insight" via the resolution of neurotic dreams.

Entrenched Phobia: Treatment by Projective Hypnoanalysis

The patient referred to as "patient X" was a young Army lieutenant who suffered from a constant feeling that someone was out to get him. He experienced this as a "fear of the dark" continuously for 3 years before seeking treatment. He was seen for 65 sessions over a period of 10 months. No claim is made that patient X was "fully analyzed." However, the treatment did represent an exploration in considerable depth and an insightful resolution of his conflicts and symptoms, as well as a measurable and substantial growth in his personal maturity.

The case is considered classic not only in that it represents the first example of projective hypnoanalysis, but also because it was J.G.W.'s first example of interaction of internal ego states that he had ever recognized (J. G. Watkins, 1952). As such, it initiated the genesis of J.G.W.'s extended study of dissociated entities, which developed many decades later into the formulation of both the theory and technique of ego-state therapy (see Chapter 10).

Session of October 26

In an effort to obtain clues as to the psychodynamic underpinnings relating to his fear symptom, the Thematic Apperception Test was administered early in his treatment. His responses to two of the cards are presented below, to be compared with responses offered to the same cards by two distinct ego states within the patient that emerged later in treatment. From the patient's alternating behavior styles, he had borderline multiple personality (DID), although J.G.W. did not so recognize at the time. In A.F.B.'s experience, early recognition of DID personalities can often be as elusive as early recognition of the borderline personality disorder as defined by the *Diagnostic and statistical manual IV-TR*. Clinicians and, in particular, counselors tend to underdiagnose these individuals as merely suffering from some sort of yet-to-be-identified neurosis.

TAT Picture Number 11   (A weird prehistoric scene)

> X: We have had an earthly disturbance—earthquakes and landslides. Can't make out this object in the extreme front. The object in the left is blended into the background. It could be an animal. I can see webbed feet. It could be a delusion. These are animals here [patient points]. They are round. It may even be prehistoric times. It may be years ago. It looks like dinosaurs. I can't see much else in this picture.

TAT Picture Number 12 M   (A young man reclining on a couch; older man leaning over him with hands in front of the young man's face)

> X: Well, we have here a boy. He is a young man. He is lying on his couch. He is the son of this man, the old man, and he has just come back home and has laid down to rest. He has slept too long, and his father is trying to wake him. The boy hasn't seen his father for many years, and this is first trip away from his job. He wanted to come home to tell his father that he was going to get married and invite his father to go with him back home. The older man had lived in that community for years and years. He finally decided that the boy should go home alone, and at a later date return to pay a visit to his father, which he does. He gets married and has a little boy and is very happy. The father gets old and dies. The young man lives happily ever after.
>
> J.W.G. note: In TAT picture No. 11, the patient reacts with anxiety and confusion, wishes it away by saying, "It could be a delusion," and

is obviously upset by the long-necked dinosaur-like animal resembling a penis in the foreground.

In TAT picture No. 12 M, the patient portrays the reconciliation of a long-absent son with his father; his decision to embark on a heterosexual commitment, "marriage"; and the father's willingness to accept his independence and maturity. Then he predicts his own future as a happy adult.

A.F.B. note: Predicting "happily ever after" is characteristic of a scared child's defenses, note lack of intermediate goal structure to achieve "happily ever after." The response is not characteristic of a "young man" but rather an adolescent. A more mature response would show some content as to how one would reach a "reasonably contented life."

Under hypnosis, two underlying entities were revealed: George, a rather psychopathic ego state, and Melvin, a weak but high super-egoed personality (overcontrolled personality). George was strong, tough, rough, promiscuous, and little concerned with those around him and their needs. In contrast, Melvin was high principled but ineffective. Both Melvin and George were hypnotically activated and given the TAT test cards within the evocation of their separate entities. Their personality differences are quite noticeable from the responses to the same two cards as previously given to the conscious patient.

Session of December 4

TAT Picture Number 11

Melvin:	These are prehistoric times. There is a giant lizard at the left. Right over here is some animals. Naturally, the giant lizard is trying to get at them. He isn't able to get the animals, however, because they run out over the road, and escaped.
George: *[in a very angry tone of voice]*	There is nothing in this picture! Why do you want to show me something like this? It is ridiculous! Anyone who would draw pictures like this must have their head in the fog. What the hell! This looks like a lizard. It's a stupid picture! I can't see anything about it. (George throws the picture down on the floor.)

J.W.G. note: Melvin perceives a threat by the lizard who is "naturally trying to get at" the smaller animals, which escape by running away. George sees no threat but rejects the entire picture. As you can see, George is, in fact, far more threatened than Melvin, and he must reject the whole concept of threat by not revealing anything about it. He rejects the entire picture and the therapist for asking him to respond to it by virtue of the tone in his voice and the slamming down of the picture on the floor.

A.F.B. note: There are also similarities between Melvin and George in that both sets of responses share the characteristic of brief exclamatory sentences, suggesting to this therapist evidence of the borderline nature of this dissociative disorder rather than the complete demarcation between personalities, as is characteristic of a full-blown multiple.

TAT Picture Number 11 M

Melvin: This is a sickly boy, he has been supporting his father and working very hard. He comes home at night. The old man doesn't like it because he has to work so hard. He is sickly too. One day the boy flops on the couch. The old man walks over to him and tries to soothe him. He wants to help the boy along. This is an intelligent boy, but he is working at a job that he is not fitted for, so the old man gets dressed and goes to the factory to talk to the foreman. He then gives the boy the right kind of job. The boy is very happy and successful and gets promotions and raises in pay.

George: This is a clubhouse. The boy is traveling across the country. He has a few hundred dollars sewed in his shirt but he doesn't want to spend it. The damn fool ought to know not to keep it there. The old man sees the boy and figures he might keep it on him because he looks good. He goes over and takes the money out of the shirt. The old man beats it. The boy wakes up and is broke. He goes to the police, but the police don't believe his story. They won't back him up. Instead, they throw him in jail for 3 days as a vagrant. He wants to get back at the police but he can't do it, and when finally they take him off to the city limits, he goes away beaten and broken. He wants to do to others what they did to him.

J.W.G. note: To Melvin, father figures are kindly and solve his problems. To George, father figures are menacing. To Melvin, stories have happy endings; to George, they end tragically. To Melvin, heroes are hard-working, honorable people supporting a loving father, to George, they are bums or hoboes with a bitter, cynical view toward life. In the conscious response of this patient to this card, the hero reconciles with the father, but not too closely, then becomes mature, marries, builds a happy life. In the hypnotically activated Melvin ego state, there is a caring father and a sickly, martyr son who doesn't leave the parental home, a typical neurotic solution. But in the hypnotically activated George ego state, the solution is quite psychopathic. The hero is the victim of uncaring fathers: first the old thief, then the cruel police. He then becomes cynical and uncaring toward others. Much of the patient's past career has been like George, but obviously Melvin, the super-ego part of his personality, who wishes by hard work to gain the approval of and be dependent upon a loving father, has been condemning his way of life. And thus there is inner conflict.

Mr. Y and His Knife

Next, various projective hypnoanalytic techniques were employed to investigate the interactions between the main personality and its two ego states.

Session of January 14

George, Melvin, and X (the Conscious Patient) Hold a Conference   Patient X reported the reappearance of night fears. He knew he was not asleep, but felt he could not open his eyes. They kept sticking together. He had been unable to sleep the entire night. He experienced several dreams, but no matter how hard he tried, he could not recall any of them. After considerable resistance, he was finally hypnotized. Once in trance, he could easily recall all the dreams that he could not remember in the conscious state.

J.G.W.:	Would you tell me what it was you dreamed last night?
X:	I dreamed I was talking to a man who was eating peaches.
J.G.W.:	Peaches [a simple reflection]. What about peaches?
X:	Wheelbarrow man; the man was eating peaches out of a wheelbarrow, and he had eaten all of them.

J.W.G. note: Patient X's real name is closely associated with peaches. A "man" is orally destroying him. He notes that J.G.W. queried first with a selective reflection on "peaches," a very typical and often effective method used by therapists who wish to keep their interactions with the patient nondirective. Failing to achieve an immediate response, which is more likely to be less ridden with defenses, J.G.W. immediately asks, "What about peaches?"

The way you approach cases during hypnotic inquiry of dream content can simply reflect your usual mode of interacting with patients: directive, nondirective, or somewhere in between. Nondirective approaches will usually take longer and in this particular case would have allowed the potential mustering of a defensive posture. In other situations, the direct question, by virtue of its challenge, can also muster a defensive response.

Wheelbarrow? Patient X refused to associate this but immediately launched into another dream. This is another form of resistance as the primary defensive posture at that particular moment.

X:	There was a big black bird flying through the air. I tried to catch the bird, but I couldn't.
J.G.W.:	Who did this bird represent?
X:	He was Mr. Y, some kind of enveloping power.

J.W.G. note: The patient actually used the term "Mr. Y" to represent his phobia and, hence, "the man" who would stab him in the dark with a knife. A.F.B. notes that the use of the word "enveloping" suggests the patient is defenseless in the face of such an attack.

A Conversation with the Hands

There were no other associations that could be secured, so J.G.W. tried to dissociate the hand (see Barabasz & Watkins, 2005 and Chapter 8 in this volume). This technique can involve hypnotically anesthetizing and paralyzing the writing hand, which is then asked or told to answer questions. Because "the hand" is no longer part of the patient, hence, no longer under the patient's conscious control, it is now "free" to reveal "secrets" or otherwise bypass ego defense mechanisms and super-ego inhibitions.

In this instance, both hands were dissociated (an unusual technique), and deep hypnosis was used to connect the underlying ego states as follows:

J.G.W.: Your right hand is losing all sense of feeling and movement. It is no longer under your control. Now, it is under the control of George—the George personality. George has control. It will write whatever George wants to say. [This was accomplished by rubbing the hand and using hypnotic suggestions to hallucinate the hand away from the wrist. The same procedure was used for the other hand.] Your left hand is now no longer under your control. It will write only for Melvin. In a moment I shall wake you up. You and I will continue our discussion, but you will not have any control over either of your hands. George will write with the right hand, and Melvin will write with the left hand. They will make their own comments independently of you or of each other.

In using this two-handed technique, A.F.B. recommends that the appropriate hand for each personality entity be touched as well as noting right or left. Remember that hypnosis involves primary process thinking: a regression. Many children do not know their left from their right without evoking considerable secondary process thinking, which is rather precisely contraindicated with hypnotic interventions in general.

The patient was seated at a desk, pencils placed in each hand, and sheets of paper conveniently arranged. He was then realerted from hypnosis. He seemed a bit surprised and stared in a puzzled manner at the two hands over which he now had no control. (A.F.B. recommends some sort of reassurance at the first sign of puzzlement or dismay simply by saying quietly and confidently, "That's O.K., the hands can write.")

The George Hand: Where is X? [Referring to the entire patient]
J.G.W.: X can speak with his mouth. You are not in trance now. You are wide awake. You and I can talk as usual. Only your hands are not under your control. [The hands are dissociated from George via posthypnotic suggestion.]

	The two hands will write for George and for Melvin; do you think maybe George might be able to interpret some of your dreams further?
The George Hand:	THE MAN IS EATING ALL THE GOOD THINGS THAT BELONG TO X. [As you will recall from the previous dream of a man eating peaches out of a wheelbarrow.]
J.G.W.:	What about the man in the dream?
The George Hand:	THE MAN IS [the hand filled in a small place with black pencil lines and then continued writing] DARKNESS, BLACK, BLACK. [Resistance even by a "dissociated hand."]
A.F.B. note:	*Just as age regressions are incomplete, so can dissociations of bodily parts. This is consistent with Orne's (1959) concept of "trance logic" (see Barabasz & Watkins, 2005).*
The Melvin Hand:	[This hand drew a picture of a peach, labeled it as a "peach," and then it wrote]: WHY DOES X FEAR?
The George Hand:	BECAUSE HE IS AFRAID OF HIMSELF. [The threat is from within.]
The Melvin Hand:	DOESN'T HE HAVE WHAT EVERYBODY ELSE HAS?
The George Hand:	X IS A NORMAL, SENSIBLE MAN WITH NATURAL INCLINATIONS FOR THE PROPER METHODS OF LIFE. FRUSTRATION AND INFERIORITY COMPLEX WILL NOT HELP HIM.
J.G.W.:	Do you notice the significance of the dream, choosing peaches to symbolize your various abilities and possibilities? It is associated to your name, isn't it? What relation do you think all of this has with your feelings of guilt?
X:	THE NUMBNESS IS GOING AWAY OUT OF THE MELVIN HAND. I THINK IT'S GONE ENTIRELY NOW. IT FEELS PERFECTLY NORMAL. [X lifted his hand, opening and closing his fingers.]
J.G.W.:	Is the George Hand still numb?
X:	YES, IT IS.
	While this was going on, the George hand apparently, still dissociated, started doodling on the top of the sheet of paper that had been placed in front of him at the beginning of the session. The hand first made an eight and two zeros, then a picture of a house, an old pattern, some circular scribbling, a picture of a funny old man, and a circle. (See Figure 8.1.)
J.G.W.:	I think maybe George might tell us more about the guilt feelings.

J.G.W. directly pushes the client toward a breakthrough.

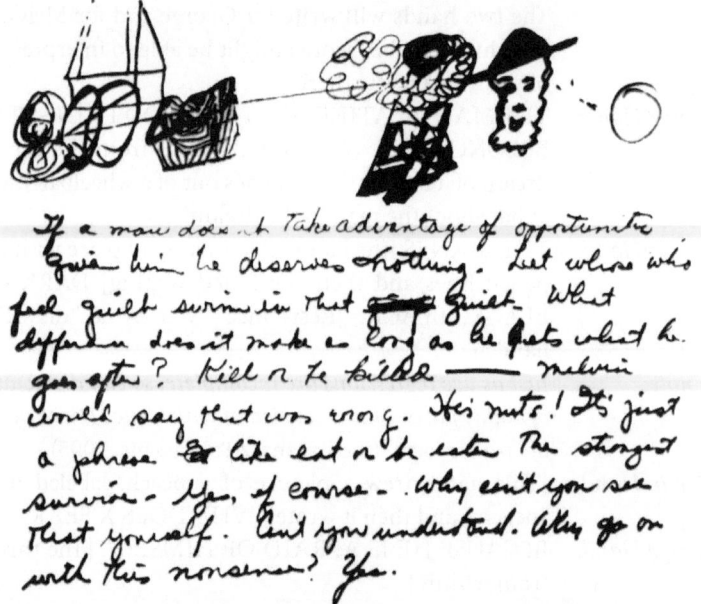

Figure 8.1

The George Hand: IF A MAN DOESN'T TAKE ADVANTAGE OF OPPOR-
TUNITIES GIVEN HIM HE DESERVES NOTHING!
LET THOSE WHO FEEL GUILT SWIM IN THAT
GUILT. WHAT DIFFERENCE DOES IT MAKE AS
LONG AS HE GETS WHAT HE GOES AFTER? KILL
OR BE KILLED—MELVIN WOULD SAY THAT WAS
WRONG. HE'S NUTS! ITS JUST A PHRASE LIKE EAT
OR BE EATEN. THE STRONGEST SURVIVE. YES, OF
COURSE—WHY CAN'T YOU SEE THAT YOURSELF.
CAN'T YOU UNDERSTAND? WHY GO ON WITH
THIS NONSENSE? YES. [Both X and J.G.W. stared at the
hand in astonishment.]

J.G.W.: Is George angry?
The George Hand: YES!

   J.G.W. then reassociates the George hand by a nonverbal communication
of rubbing it until feeling and movement were restored. After "the hand" had
been connected again to X, J.G.W. and patient X began discussing news events
of the day.

J.G.W.: X, look what your hand is doing.
X [Glancing over]: What about it?

J.G.W.:   Doesn't it seem a bit odd that it is making all that doodling on the paper? Does that mean anything? Can you think of anything in associating to those figures?

X tried but could not associate to any of them. The patient was now placed on the cot, and a deep trance induced.

J.G.W.:   You will open your eyes while staying asleep and look at these funny pictures that you drew. What do they make you think of?

Patient X slowly opened his eyes and gazed at the pictures.

X: Nothing. I can't think of anything.

A.F.B. note: Doubtful to this therapist that hypnosis was successfully induced. J.G.W.'s enthusiasm in the immediate interchanges above perhaps mustered defenses by asking several questions in a row followed by X's recognition that he could not associate in any way to them. Perhaps greater effort in inducing hypnosis immediately following that may have produced more here-and-now responsiveness to the pictures rather than the defensive reaction of "Nothing. I can't think of anything."

J.G.W.:   Tonight you will have another dream. This will indicate still further the nature of your guilt feelings.
X: I think it's a good idea. I don't want to forget the dream. I am going to take a paper and pencil to bed with me.
J.G.W.:   Do you think you could associate any more ideas in connection with the two dreams you told me? What about the bird—you said something about an enveloping power?
X: I don't see anything about the bird now. I remember something, though, that happened the other day. I was up walking in the dark, and suddenly I had the feeling that Mr. Y was there, but Mr. Y *no longer had his knife.*
J.G.W.:   Mr. Y has lost his knife.

A.F.B. note: J.G.W.'s recognition of the resistance caused by the directive nature of his series of questions above changes his therapeutic tactic to a nondirective simple reflection.

At this moment, the patient became very agitated. With raised pitch of voice filled with emotion, he repeated:

X: Mr. Y has lost his knife. Why didn't you tell me this before? Mr. Y has lost his knife.

A.F.B. note: There is possible confusion here given the primary level at which the patient is reacting in hypnosis. It is as if J.G.W. had suggested Mr. Y losing his knife and X's hostility portrays this.

J.G.W.:   Why has Mr. Y lost his knife?

A.F.B. note: J.G.W. keeps it simple, stays on track, and focuses on the potential for insight rather than being sidetracked by the patient's affect.

Suddenly, X sat up on the cot with his eyes wide open, emerging instantly from what was thought to be deep hypnosis.

X: I've got the most wonderful feeling, the most wonderful feeling I have had for a long time. Mr. Y has lost his knife. Now I can handle that guy. I feel as if a great weight has been lifted from my shoulder. I'd like to find a dark place right now. I want to try it out. I am sure I am not going to have any more fears.

A.F.B. note: Contrary to Irving Kirsch's emphasis on the notion that expectations account for change via hypnosis and therapy (Kirsch & Council, 1989), J.G.W. with complete confidence in his hypnoanalytic approach to this case does just the opposite.

J.G.W.:   Better not be too optimistic. You've had feelings something like this before.

X: Never like this before. This is important. Mr. Y has lost his knife.

A.F.B. note: J.G.W.' s confidence is not misplaced; what he has done here is managed to obtain further determination that genuine insight, not mere cognitive change, has occurred.

J.G.W.:   Do you think perhaps this means that part of your fear is gone? Maybe it represents a partial gain in insight because you now realize that guilt feelings are the basis for your fear. Recognition of this point may have reduced the fear symbolically by causing Mr. Y to lose his knife, thus making him a less fearsome creature.

J.G.W. note: We should always greet new insight with positive but cautious acceptance. I am fishing in uncharted waters here, breaking in new ground, exploring a new world.

A.F.B. note: The reader should remember that J.G.W. is now conversing with patient X out of hypnosis and therefore calls upon the full involvement of the patient's secondary process.

X: Yes, maybe that's true. Maybe that's what caused it. I only know that I am happy—that I am not afraid.

A.F.B. note: This is a crucial point in that the patient has achieved "happiness" before in the very immediate sense, short term, simply by withdrawing from a situation rather than facing it. The question arises here: Has this been a cognitive change only, or has genuine insight been achieved that results in personality reconstruction and a more adaptive satisfying long-term lifestyle?

X: I can handle this guy! This is the most important thing that has happened to me in the whole analysis! MR. Y HAS LOST HIS KNIFE.

    J.G.W. note: Has patient X now lost his "castration fears"? And if so, why? He has accepted for the first time that his external fear is related to an unconscious sense of guilt, repressed into Melvin and denied by George with psychopathic-like behavior.

Whether complete insight was achieved is not known, but what is certain is that treatment proceeded much more rapidly after that session.

Sessions of January 16, 17, and 21: Dreams of Fear and Frustration

Several dreams were now hypnotically initiated in an attempt to learn more about Mr. Y. Hypnosis was induced and evidence of deepening was obtained:

J.G.W.:   I am going to count up to ten, when I do you will dream again about Mr. Y. One, two, three, … ten.

Patient X began to twitch all over. It began with anxiety exhibited by tremors and breathing in a labored manner. This continued for about a minute. He then relaxed; then it began again and would disappear once more after a minute or two. Finally, he began to talk.

X: I was standing in a big place or field—like a desert. In front of me were a dozen different lanes or roads.

    A.F.B. note: The level of bizarreness and incongruities point to the more abstract symbolism characteristic of that elicited via a deeper level of hypnosis.

X: I wanted to go on one of them in front of me but there were a dozen different lanes or roads. I wanted to get some drinking water because I was getting right thirsty. I started down the one on the extreme left and had gone about 10 paces, then suddenly a fierce animal appeared in front of me. He had bared his teeth and grimaced at me. I turned back. Then I tried each one of the roads, and each time there was the animal and he showed me his fangs and he wouldn't let me through; so I came back and lay down on the ground. I was very, very thirsty, but I didn't really care. I couldn't go on. That was all.

J.G.W.:   I think maybe you can add more to this dream.

    A.F.B. note: It seems that at some level of communication, J.G.W. recognizes the level of fear the patient is experiencing and attempts to attenuate it by reminding him that this is a "dream."

J.G.W.:   Do you want to go back and finish it?

    A.F.B. note: Again, J.G.W. in this case keeps it very tentative, nondirective, and entirely under the patient's control.

J.G.W.:   You can describe it as it is happening.

    A.F.B. note: A bit more directive but again protective in the sense that by the use of "describe it as it's happening," he allows the patient to use a defensive level as if viewing it from the outside—dissociating from the fear-producing stimulus.

X: I am very thirsty but there is a little girl coming toward me. She is taking me by the hand. She is taking me out of the woods, but I can't stop her. Nothing can stop her, but there is no animal and we come to a light spring, and I kneel down to drink. I look in and I see the face of the animal. I look again, and only the little girl looks down. The animal is gone. I drink, and the little girl is gone now, but I don't care because I can go on by myself now, the water is so very, very good.

    J.G.W. note: Is he to be rescued from Mr. Y by a little girl, e.g., accepting femininity and immaturity? Is this the only solution to his problem? Or is the little girl a symbol of his own femininity, his "animal"?

J.G.W.:   What does the little girl make you think of?
X: She is the helping hand.
J.G.W.:   What do you mean by the helping hand? [Recall that X had previously referred to his mother as "the guiding hand."]
X: It's you and others. Someone to guide me. She is just a little baby. What a little girl should do, I should be able to do. She needs to be led herself.

    A.F.B. note: Is this dependency the problem?

    J.G.W. note: The little girl represents "femininity", not "dependency."

J.G.W.:   Can you think of anything else about her?
X: No, she just means the helping hand. Oh, I see a beautiful horse, a beautiful animal. He is that black horse again, isn't he? [Referring to a previous dream not discussed here.]

J.G.W.:   Yes, he is. All right, you are going to catch him and ride him. He is coal black. There is no body on him.

> *J.G.W. note: This is an attempt to see if X can "master" and control Mr. Y by hypnotic suggestion.*
>
> *A.F.B. note: This is to a certain extent a fairly universal theme that you will see in a wide variety of DID patients and particularly borderline DID patients. You may recognize a similar theme in the lyrics to "The chestnut mare," a classic song by the Byrds: "I'm gonna catch that horse if I can." In the song, the horse is only "mastered" for a short while and flees by leaping off a mountain into a pool of water, and the quest for mastery is renewed.*

X: I don't think I can catch him. I am trying to catch him. I have got hold of his nose, but he keeps moving away, and in a circle, running away. Now he is gone. I would just rather watch a horse like that. I knew I shouldn't try to ride that horse. He was very beautiful. [Patient X turned his head reproachfully toward J.G.W.] You said to ride him.

J.G.W.:   I am going to count up to ten once more and you will have another dream regarding Mr. Y. One, two, three, … ten.

X: [*After X had dreamed for 5 minutes without speaking, he began to talk.*] I was at a party, a Halloween party. Everybody was there. I knew them even though they had their faces covered with masks. A girl came up to me and took me by the hand. She was in a mask, and she said, "Follow me," and then led me downstairs off into a little wood. And then she said, "Do you know who I am?" I said, "I don't know." She said, "Don't you want to find out?" Then she said, "Catch me." And she ran into the woods. She was quick, and I couldn't catch her, I heard her laughing and laughing. I wanted to catch her. I wanted to stop her, but I couldn't catch her. You were driving me on to catch her. Something tells me I can't catch her. I wish that I could. I could hold her hand. She is playing tag with me.

J.G.W.:   Are you afraid of her?

> *A.F.B. note: In classic form, J.G.W. cuts to the quick by posing a direct question. If a more nondirective style is more consonant with your therapeutic mode, you could pose the same incisive point by simply making it more tentative such as, "I wonder if you're a little bit afraid of her" or "Is it that you may be afraid of her?" The result is likely to be the same.*

X: No, she isn't sinister, but she makes me very nervous and excited by her actions. I wasn't afraid of her. I could have left her alone if I wanted to. I didn't even have to follow her down. She is only toying with me now because you are here to help me. [Patient X was now realerted from hypnosis. He could add nothing more to his description of the dreams.]

In the next session, "dissociated hand writing" was again employed, as were other projective techniques including a tautophone (verbal summator) (Skinner, 1939; Trussell, 1939; Shakow & Rosenzweig, 1949). The tautophone was originally developed as a test instrument. Garbled sounds were played to the research participant, and he or she was asked what "the voices were saying." J.G.W. employed the tautophone with patient X as a technique to determine whether or not patient X could hear "unconscious" communications in the voices.

Once the patient had been hypnotized, and his right hand dissociated, he was asked to listen to a tape, which was played backwards, and to tell what the voices were saying. He showed resistance, would not write at first, and insisted that he heard only jumbled stimuli. The dissociated hand displayed a lot of negativism, making wavy motions up and down. But then it started to write. (see Figure 8.2.)

The George Hand: I DO–[I DON'T KNOW].
J.G.W.:   Of course you know.
The George Hand: JUMBLE, JUMBLE.

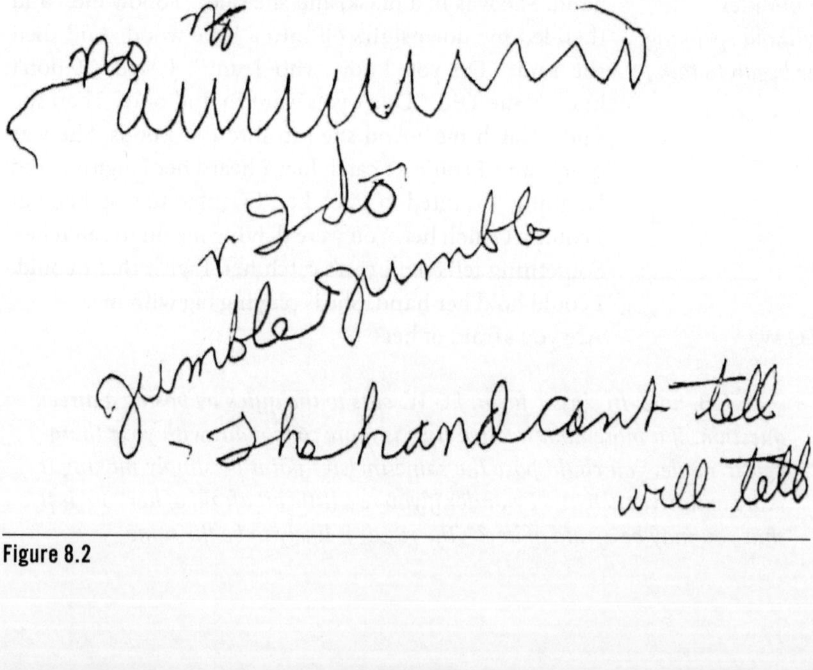

Figure 8.2

J.G.W.:	That's right. But what do these jumble voices say? They say something.
The George Hand:	THE HAND CAN'T TELL. X WILL TELL!

> *J.G.W. note: The tautophone procedure does not in itself produce the voices hoped for, but did stimulate another round of significant material to emerge.*
>
> *A.F.B. note: Individual differences in hypnotic as well as nonhypnotic responding are paramount, J.G.W.'s exploration of the use of the tautophone approach may well have worked as intended with another patient.*

X:	It sounded pretty badly jumbled, but I do have a dream, which the voice has made me think of. There is a horse. It is the same horse again, and he has a beautiful saddle and bridle this time. Everybody is trying to get on the horse, and the horse wouldn't let anybody get on. He just stood there. I got one foot up, but couldn't get up on top. The reason I couldn't get up was because I had roots in the ground.
J.G.W.:	Do you think maybe the hand could explain better your inability to mount the horse?
X:	What do you want to let the hand write for? I don't want the hand to write, why can't I say it myself?

> *J.G.W. note: Apparently X is afraid that the hand will reveal something he doesn't want to become aware of. Hostile remarks like this continued for some time. Finally, the hand began to write. (see Figure 8.3.)*
>
> *A.F.B. note: Note the increased level of sophistication in mounting defenses, as J.G.W. gets closer to the underlying conflicts.*

The George Hand:	RESULTS ARE MEASURED BY DEEDS.
J.G.W.:	How do you mean that?
The George Hand:	HE WHO STEALS MY PURSE STEALS TRASH, BUT HE WHO STEALS FROM ME MY GOOD NAME LEAVES NOTHING.
J.G.W.:	Who has stolen X's good name?

> *A.F.B. note: This could also be done less directively and in a less challenging tone by simply reflecting back "good name" or "stolen good name."*

The George Hand:	YOU—BUT, WHAT?
X [Covering his head with his hands]:	I am not going to talk anymore.

> *A.F.B. note: Once again challenge has produced a dramatic mustering of resistance.*

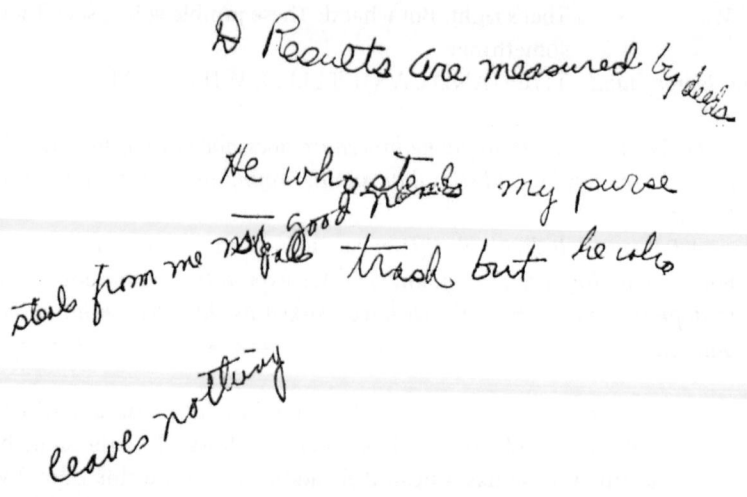

① Results are measured by deeds.

He who steals my purse steals from me not good trash but he who leaves nothing

Figure 8.3

The George Hand: LET HIM. I HAVE NO MORE TO ADD.

   A.F.B. note: The dissociation of the hand is either incomplete or we are achieving a permeability among the personalities so they can begin to share thoughts without such rigid barriers. In the present case, it was fostered via the patient's desperate need to rally the most defensive posture possible. It is remarkable to this therapist to see that the challenge by J.G.W. that initially produced greater resistance had the overall effect of breaking down barriers between unconscious and conscious processes to a certain extent.

J.G.W.:	What do you mean by "let him"?
The George Hand:	LA CASA ES NEGRA Y MUCHO SENORS [Translation: The house is black and many men]. (see Figure 8.4.)

At this point, the hand became quite rebellious and refused to write for some time. Eventually it was induced to hold the pencil again.

J.G.W. [Challenging the patient again]:	I think the hand can reveal more.
The George Hand:	NO. THE HAND IS OUT.
J.G.W.:	You mean the feeling has returned to the hand?

   A.F.B. note: J.G.W. employs the counseling technique of "deliberate misinterpretation" to irritate the patient into further responding.

The George Hand:	YES–NO.
J.G.W.:	What do you mean by that?

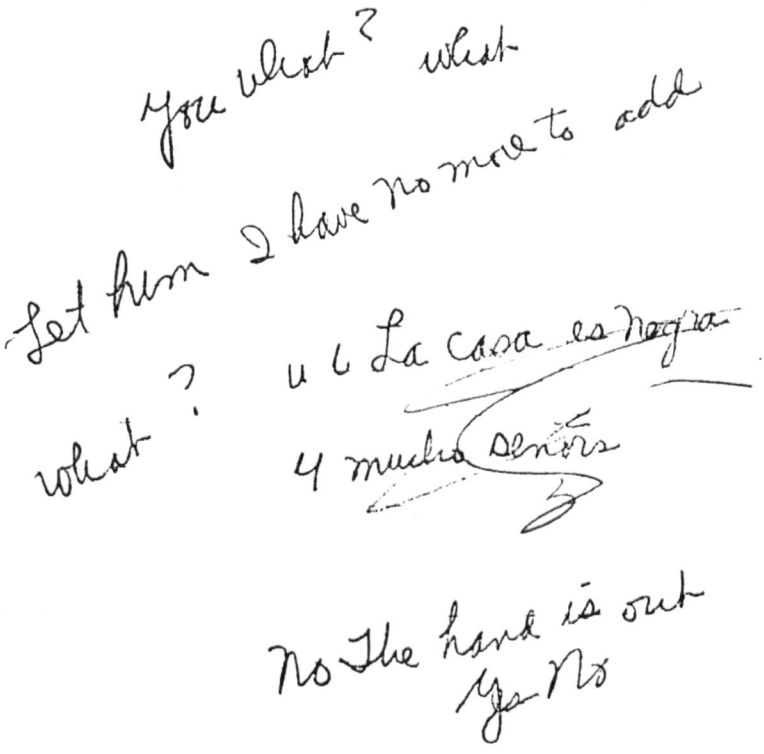

Figure 8.4

The George Hand: NO ORGANS TO FORM WORDS.

> *A.F.B. note: A greater degree of abstraction may be shared by virtue of the depth of hypnosis as well as the fortress of resistances the patient is attempting to build.*

J.G.W.:   You mean that the hand is incapable of further writing?

> *A.F.B. note: Again a deliberate misinterpretation lead, which irritates the patient intentionally.*
>
> *J.G.W. note: The hand first wrote "no" and then "yes," finally scratching it out. Then the patient became very angry. He started pouting like a small boy. He threw the pencil away. He threw the hand away. J.G.W. put the pencil six times back in the hand before the hand would grip it and continue writing.*
>
> *A.F.B. note: When you're on to something and you know it, persist. As a therapist, you have the strength of character to do so.*

The George Hand: I HELP X TO RECOVER. MR. Y SAYS YOU ARE BAD FOR HIM. (see Figure 8.5.)

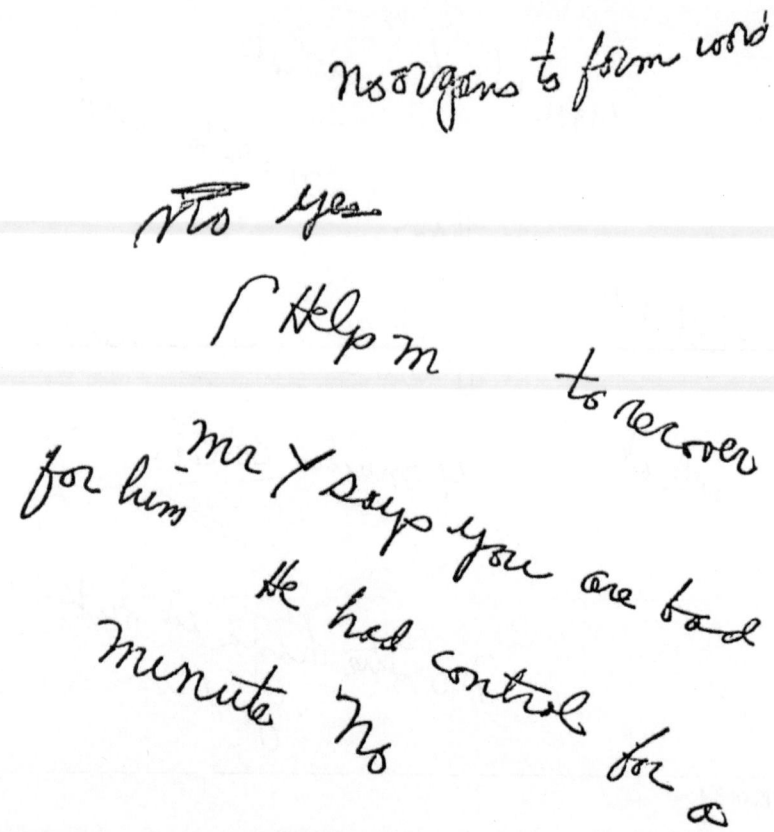

Figure 8.5

The patient physically appeared to show a relief and loss of tension, which pervaded his entire body. He then continued writing.]

The George Hand: HE HAD CONTROL FOR A MINUTE.

  A.F.B./J.G.W. note: This is an example of a brief change of the dominant (executive) ego state.

J.G.W.:   Can you tell me more about Mr. Y?
The George Hand: HE IS MY DARK PAST.
J.G.W.:   Can you explain more about this?

  A.F.B. note: Asking "can you" invites the potential of refusal; this therapist prefers to simply state, "You can explain more about this" or "Tell me more."

The George Hand: NOT ENOUGH CONFIDENCE IN ME, X.
J.G.W.:   What do you mean by this?

A.F.B. note: J.G.W. allows the patient no wiggle room for resistance, thus the patient once more becomes irritable, yet the hand finally starts scribbling again.

The George Hand:	YOU KNOW HOW. HE HAS FALSE TEETH. HE IS A COWARD.
J.G.W.:	Does that mean that Mr. Y represents that part of you which is cowardly?
The George Hand:	YES.
J.G.W.:	In what way are you cowardly? What are you afraid of?
The George Hand:	NO MAN, BUT VARIOUS DAILY ENCOUNTERS.
J.G.W.:	Do you think that the fear of Mr. Y has anything to do with your wife or marital difficulties?

A.F.B. note: This interpretation goes well beyond the patient's comments, hence, risks considerable resistance yet may well save an enormous amount of therapy time. I recommend avoiding that far of an extension until you gain considerable experience and confidence with this form of therapeutic intervention.

[At this point, the patient became very anxious and tense. The hand did not want to write. It threw the pencil away a number of times. Finally, the patient was induced to hold the pencil again, but the hand would not write this time.]

J.G.W.:   I am going to count up to five and when I say five you will have to write. One, two, three, four, five.

A.F.B. note: The counting might imply some sort of release from the hypnotic situation, yet there is no such release but instead a directive to write the numbers 1 through 5.

The George Hand: NO. MR. Y IS A BUG, WHO PLANTS EVIL THOUGHTS IN CONNECTION WITH SEX. (see Figure 8.6.)

A.F.B. note: J.G.W. replies with a silence lead and says nothing to directively stimulate a further response. It is difficult for a patient to maintain integrative defensive postures with the alternation of therapeutic intervention styles.

The George Hand   X IS SATISFIED.
[After a pause with nothing said, the hand again continued writing.]:

At this point, feeling and movement began to return to the hand, whereupon it was reassociated to the body. The session was continued verbally.

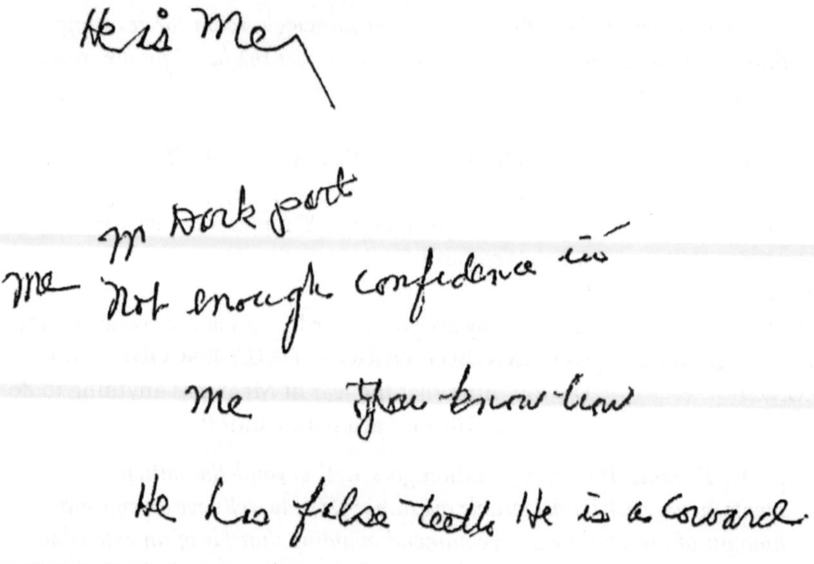

He is me

me   m Dark part
      Not enough confidence in

      me   You know how

      He has false teeth He is a Coward.

Figure 8.6

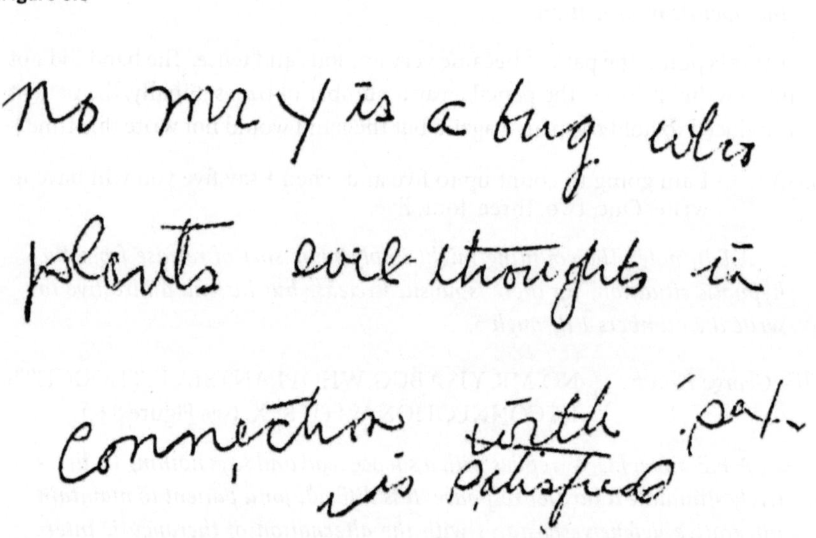

No mr Y is a bug who

plants evil thoughts in

connection with sex.
            is Satisfied

Figure 8.7

J.G.W.:   You can discuss the matter now without using your hand. The hand
           wrote something about sex. What does this mean?
X: This means desires for another woman. [He then added, concern-
           ing Mr. Y, "He's the guy that put the bug where it shouldn't be"; X is
           afraid of losing his potency.]
J.G.W.:   Why?

X: Well, look at the life I have lived—continuous sex relations with women. Don't you think it would take away some of my strength—from my ability?

J.G.W. note: In psychoanalytic theory, Don Juans have latent homo-sexual impulses, which they repress and deny by having affairs with many women.

[X was then asked why he had had 2 weeks of resistance. Exact quote unavailable.]

X: You know, Mr. Y was cornered. We were so close to his home. He was flanked on all sides. If he went forward, he ran into you. If he went to the right, he ran into you. If he went to the left, he ran into you; so he didn't have any place to go except to come back on me, and that is what made me all excited, anxious, and tense. He's right over the crest of the next hill. He hasn't got much ammunition left. I am going to get hold of him and drag him out.

At this point X, still in hypnosis, began to ramble about many apparently inconsequential matters. He discussed the recent fire department handling of an auditorium fire. Then he commented about Mr. Byrnes's talk on the "English loan." For about 15 minutes he continued in this manner.

J.G.W. note: When you ease up on pressure, very revealing material will emerge.

J.G.W. [He seemed childlike at this point, so this was suggested]:   Let's play a new game.
X   [Patient X picked it up instantly.]: That's a good idea. It'll break the monotony.
J.G.W.:   When I count up to 13 there will suddenly pop into your mind the number of days it will take until we finally uncover the last of Mr. Y and get him out of his lair.
X: Make it 14.
J.G.W.:   All right, 1, 2, … 13, 14.
X[Responding instantly]: 21.

While J.G.W. was counting up to 14, the patient was making a number of rather odd-looking passes with his hands in the air. He seemed very interested in the number that had emerged.

A.F.B. note: The patient is operating at a childlike primary process level and may indeed be playing a game and producing number 21 just for fun; it may be entirely meaningless. Nonetheless, J.G.W. now has a "number of days" produced by the patient to facilitate the uncovering of Mr. Y. My point is that the number 21 may or may not have meaning, but it can be used as a therapeutic tactic.

X: That's a lot of fun. Let's play that game again.

J.G.W.:   All right. I am going to count up to eleven, and some important word about what will happen to Mr. Y will emerge, only the word will be scrambled. The word will be in scrambled form. One, two, three, … eleven.

X [Reeled off the following lettersinstantly]:   R-E-M-B-A-E-C-O-G-Y. I know what that word is, it's "remember." I am going to remember some thing, which issignificant and will have something to do with Mr. Y. [Spontaneously, he appeared to become fully alerted from hypnosis.]

A.F.B. note: Although there is little risk to pursuing the material in this way, it might be a "blind alley" for the majority of therapists.

J.G.W. [Opening his appointment book, which had a page for each day; he started slowly counting pages.]:   One, two, three, ….

At first, X didn't understand. Then he opened his eyes in apparent amazement and smiled. Finally, when number twenty-one was reached, the therapist drew a large circle around March 7.

X: So that's the day we're going to beat Mr. Y. I remember now. I told you it would be 21 days, didn't I?

After about 10 minutes the session came to an end, and the patient started to leave the office. When he reached the door, he turned around and looked back.

X: By the way, how are you coming with your book?

J.G.W.:   Oh, I get to do a little work on it from time to time.

X: How many chapters are in it?

J.G.W.:   There will be 33 [the number planned at that time].

X: I thought you said there were 21.

J.G.W. [Laughing]: There aren't 21 chapters in my book. There are 21 chapters in your book, and remember, the last one is 21. Isn't that right?

A.F.B. note: As you may have noticed, when X appeared self-realerted from trance, J.G.W. did, in fact, make no effort to ensure, as is usually the practice, that the patient been fully realerted and was indeed out of hypnosis. Here, even with the passage of over 10 minutes, J.G.W. is likely looking for clues to full realertness before releasing the patient, but at the same time takes advantage of specifically and concretely restating the issue of 21 as being the concluding chapter in the patient's book and looking for confirmation from the patient. Whether the effect is a carryover hypnotic effect from residual trance or simply a waking reminder to a fully alerted and conscious patient X need not be determined.

[Patient X laughingly agreed.]

Session of February 28: A Turkey and an Eagle

First, X was induced into light hypnosis, again after considerable resistance.

J.G.W.:   I am going to count up to nine and something will pop into your mind that is significant. One, two, three, … nine.

X: Barnyard fowl.

J.G.W.:   What do you mean, "barnyard fowl"?

X: Well, this means chickens, pigs, and hogs.

X was unable to provide further associations, but after J.G.W. used a "silence lead" for an unspecified period of time, he began talking again.

X: There was a turkey, which got the idea in my mind, a relatively large turkey at that.

J.G.W.:   What about the turkey?

> *A.B.F. note: J.G.W. prepares the ground for a radial inquiry.*

X: Well, the turkey has got big feathers like a peacock or something who is strutting.

J.G.W.:   Who is it that struts?

> *A.F.B. note: Carefully, J.G.W. here states, "Who is it?" rather than merely reflecting "strutting." He is attempting the accelerated therapeutic progress. If you are uncomfortable with taking the risk of so directive an approach, the same goal would probably be reached in a bit more time simply by using nondirective reflections drawn from the patient's last statement, simply a repetition of "somebody strutting."*

X: Well, that's myself. I put on a big front.

A.F.B. note: Apparent insight, at least at a cognitive level.

J.G.W.:   Now, X, I want you to make the fingertips of your two hands touch each other. That's fine. Now each one of those fingers represents a root of Mr. Y. Pretty soon you are going to have a tingling feeling at the tips of one of those pairs of fingers. [X lay quietly on the cot; again, J.G.W. doesn't push the issue and simply uses a silence lead by saying nothing.]

X: It's the third finger.

J.G.W.:   All right. Remove all the fingers except the third fingers, keep the tips of them together. Now right between those fingertips a word is going to form, it will have raised letters on it, like the kind the blind feel [braille]. This word will slowly emerge, and you're going to be able to spell it out.

X [Starts spelling immediately]:   P-R-O-A-N-T-I-R-A-N-S-U-B-S-T-A-N-C-H-I-I-O-N-I-S-T

J.G.W. [Greatly surprised]:   Do you think you could spell it again? [Correct spelling is pro-antitransubstantiationalist.]

X [The patient spelled it again, exactly the same way as he did before, even with the double "i".]:   I read it years ago. Proantiransubstantionalist. It was way back in the Civil War, history, and it was about a man who had a certain kind of social standing. They gave that name to him. He was a man that had a pro and con against certain elements. He had two different kinds of standing at the same time.

> A.B.F. note: The patient's recognition of his bisexuality is emerging at a near conscious level, given the light hypnotic state that this session is conducted in. Tempting as it may be to simply reveal this interpretation to the patient in hopes of some sort of therapeutic breakthrough, there is substantial risk of resistance and retrenchment into the unconscious. Be patient.

J.G.W.:   What do you think the word means?

> A.F.B. note: As you can see from the patient's statement, the patient explained the meaning of the word; however, J.G.W., recognizing the symbolic nature of the patient's statement, does not accept the meaning given by the patient, but inquires further.

J.G.W.:   What do you think the word means?

X [Still with resistance]:   It means absolutely nothing; [pause] maybe it might apply to me, because it goes two ways at the same time.

J.G.W.:   You can concentrate real hard on those two fingers. Let's see if another word doesn't begin to squeeze in between them.

X [Pause]:   A-L-L-E-V-I-A-T-E. You know what "alleviate" means? It means to alleviate my symptoms!

J.G.W.:   Right between your two fingers will run a ticker tape.

> A.F.B. note: You will recall that this session is one conducted by J.G.W. in the late 1940s with an Army lieutenant; at the time, a method of transmitting information from one site to the other involved sending a signal to a kind of abbreviated typing machine where the abbreviations (for example, stock quotes) could be transmitted across country in very close proximity to the fluctuations in the actual value of the stock. It was

just a tape about ½ an inch or so wide, which ran continuously through a typing machine with a limited number of characters and symbols, which were used as abbreviations.

J.G.W.:   It will have raised words on it. You will able to spell the words.

A.F.B. note: Remember that J.G.W. said the words would be like the kind the blind feel (braille).

X: H-O-M-O-B-I-O-L-O-G-I-C-A-L-H-O-M-O [He then spelled] P-R-E-S-S-I-V-E.

J.G.W.:   There's no word "pressive," maybe you mean "oppressive"?

A.F.B. note: Here J.G.W. attempts a simple interpretation that does not lead very far beyond the material presented.

X [Becoming very playful]:   I'm a radio station—tick, tick, tick.

A.F.B. note: Again we are on the ticker tape. Back in those times, radio stations would often receive news from the national and international press via ticker tape.

X: P-R-O-C-L-I-V-I-T-E.

A.F.B. note: Another misspelling.

J.G.W. [Using a simple selective reflection counseling lead]:   "Proclivity"? What does that mean? I am going to count up to seven. When I say "seven," an idea telling you what proclivity means will pop into your head. One, two, three, … seven.

X: Of all the things in the world, proclivity is you—proclivity Watkins. You have a proclivity for pulling things out of me. [Pause] Do I have to hold these fingers together anymore? You know I can't open my eyes. I've been trying to.

J.G.W. [Attempting another projective technique]:   In front of you there is a great fire. You can see it. It is a great picture on fire.

J.G.W. note: The patient immediately seized on this unstructured stimulus and started fashioning a concept with it.

X: Yes, I see this very, very clear. It stands out like the wings of a bird— an eagle. The eagle is getting larger and larger. He is just standing there like a statue. What does the eagle mean?

J.G.W.:   I am going to count up to five, and when I say "five," an association will come to your mind which will tell you something about what the eagle means. One, two, three, four, five!

X: Huh, when you said "five," the bird disappeared.

J.G.W.:   Let's try another angle. Answer yes or no quickly. Now regarding this bird, is it—you?

X: No.

J.G.W.:   Is it—Melvin?

X: No.

J.G.W.:   Is it—George?

X: No.

J.G.W.:   Is it—Mr. Y?

X: No.

J.G.W.:   Is it—me?

X: No.

        [J.G.W. recognizes that the rapid probing technique has mustered additional resistance rather than facilitating a breakthrough. He changes his tactic once again.]

J.G.W.:   This time I am going to count up to seven, when I say "seven," a scrambled word will come to your mind.

     A.F.B. note: Providing the "out" of using a scrambled word allows the patient to maintain thinly veiled resistance.

X: H-E-R-A-E-T-C. But I can't interpret it.

J.G.W.:   All right. I am going to count to seven once more. This time you will be able to spell the word in a little better form. One, two, three, … seven.

X: I knew you were going to analyze it. I told you so. Well, here it goes. C-H-E-R-T-E-A.

J.G.W.:   Does that mean "cheater"?

X: No. It means "teacher."

J.G.W.:   Tell me what the word "teacher" brings to mind.

X: Well, the teacher struck me. Ms. Jordan was her name. The boy in front of me whispered something. She came over and slapped me because he was a pet of hers. I then threw a bottle of ink all over her, all over her white blouse. She took me up immediately to the principal, and the principal, after finding out what was wrong, censured her instead of me.

J.G.W.:   Yes, but I don't see what all this has to do with an eagle.

X: Don't you see? An eagle is a leader, a teacher. You know, I am going to be a teacher. I want to be an eagle that can fly and not have a broken leg. That means I need education and support because my own wings, my own education, are broken.

J.G.W.:   What about that long word, "proantiransubstanchionist"?

     A.F.B. note: Recall that the word goes back to the Civil War, referring to someone holding conflicting views of reality and commitment, thereby having divided loyalties.

X: What's that got to do with …? [Pause]

X: Don't you see that it is a big long word? That is the front that I have to have. I always put up a big impressive front. [Recall that X had spelled out the word "pressive."] That's the kind of guy I am.

[He further integrated these concepts. He recognized that he wanted to be an eagle, a leader, but he felt that he was more of a turkey, a showoff, just someone with a big impressive front, but nothing to back it up.]

A War for Survival

As can sometimes often be the case after a major therapeutic breakthrough in the development of insight, the next week brought a tremendous period of resistance. As the last of the 21 days began to pass, and the significant date of March 7 approached, patient X became more and more tense, more nervous. His fears at night became stronger. Following the session of February 28, he did not report fears at night. He conjured one excuse and rationalization after another not to come for therapy. It was obvious that a terrific battle was going on within him. He had set up the date of March 7 for the final uncovering, yet deep down inside, Mr. Y was waging a tremendous conflict to remain hidden in patient X's unconscious.

On March 6, patient X entered the office appearing tired and haggard. His eyes showed lack of sleep. He was nervous, tense, and jittery, and his face was covered with an apparent deep depression.

X: We've been on the wrong track. I know there is no use of going any further. We are never going to find the solution to my problem. I am going to just have to live with it, I guess, for the rest of my life.

   J.G.W. note: Mr. Y was obviously pleading to have the treatment called off at this point.

The Masquerade Is Ended

A decisive battle had been going on now with the patient for 2 weeks. His nights were spent helplessly tossing around the bed. The few moments of sleep were filled with vague forms of fear dreams and fantasies. Patient X's headaches appeared often. At times, tremors shook his body. He had avoided the therapist like poison. March 7 was approaching and Mr. Y, cornered, was fighting like a wild beast.

Session of March 7

Patient X opened the door, came in, and sat down. For a few moments he said nothing. The expression on his face was a mixture of anguished apprehension and stoical fortitude. Finally, he spoke.

X: There are dreams I meant to tell you about, but I can't think of them now.

[X was asked to lie down on the cot and suggestions to induce hypnosis were started. Recognizing his state of agitation, J.G.W. had felt severe misgivings as to the possibility of actually inducing hypnosis at this time. These were not groundless. Indeed, after the session was finished, patient X himself said, "When I came in I didn't think you'd be able to hypnotize me today."]

> A.F.B. note: As you will recall, there have been several instances where the patient was highly resistant to hypnosis during the course of therapy thus far.

[After about 15 minutes, patient X's right hand began to slowly rise into the air and he touched his head, the prearranged signal that had been used in each hypnotic session to indicate to J.G.W. and to the patient himself that a deep degree of trance had finally been reached.]

J.G.W.:	X, you are in a cave, a dark cave [symbolic of the "unconscious"]. There are steps leading down the cave, not into darkness, but into a light, which is ahead. You are going to go out at this very bright light. [J.G.W. counts the steps as the patient walks toward the light.]
X [Describing his dream]:	It's all shining. There is big, open, hollow tunnel. Light is in one section, there is nothing in the tunnel. There is only an old tunnel. [Growling belligerently] You got me to come down here!
J.G.W. [Attempting another projective tack]:	Maybe there are some pictures on the walls of this tunnel. Look around and see.
X:	Yes, it has markings. Someone chiseled them on the stone. I am trying to see what they say. These markings were written years and years ago. [Patient X is conveying that whatever happened, happened a long time ago in his life.] Oh, the light is going out.

> A.F.B. note: Once again, just as there is a breakthrough coming with regard to insight, the resistance is again mustered.

J.G.W.:	You're very strong now, much stronger than you used to be. You can put the light on again, you can "will" the light on. I am going to count up to 10, and as I do you'll be able to "will" the light back on: 1, 2, 3, … 10.
X [Smiling]:	Yes, the light is back on again. Let me turn it on and off again.

> A.F.B. note: First asserting that he has control, next testing it.

X: I want to see if it will work. I wonder if I could make colored lights too.

A.F.B. note: Further attempts to confirm control of the situation.

J.G.W. [Allowing a few moments to elapse while the patient "turned the light on and off again"; the patient shows a change of affect by smiling in apparent satisfaction.]: What do you see?

X: It is so light now, the wall is turning all white. There are nurses and doctors around me. I see myself as a boy. It is at St. A---'s Hospital. I had my tonsils taken out; there's nothing to it, but across from me is a boy who is blind. I wonder where he is now. My mother just brought me ice cream. This throat feeling is hard to go down, but it does in time. [X clears his throat repeatedly and begins to speak in a hoarse whispering voice, describing his feelings.]

> *J.G.W. note: Much symbolic communication is apparent here. He is reminded of a childhood surgery because he is faced now with "psychological" surgery on an immature self.*
> *A.F.B. note: So much of the "reliving" that goes on in therapy where obstacles are overcome makes it possible for patients to "grow up" and mature psychologically so that they can function as adaptively as possible in their adult bodies.*
> *J.G.W. note: "The boy" has been blind—psychologically. He is now about to see, but it is painful to speak about what he is to reveal. He has oral pain. His throat hurts.*

J.G.W.: See if you can look again at the messages on the wall.

X [Completely ignoring J.G.W.'s request, simply continues]: I see myself being taken out of a hospital. I sit around the house. Her boyfriends come in to see me now. Naturally, they think I am brave. The only time I've been in the hospital for an operation.

> *J.G.W. note: The session today, like the tonsil operation in his childhood, calls for "bravery."*
> *A.F.B. note: The patient recognizes at a conscious level that he must be and can be brave enough to deal with an unpleasant insight.*

J.G.W.: How old are you?

X: Ten years old.

J.G.W.: I am going to count up to ten and something will come over your mind that is very important, very, very important! One, two, three, ... ten.

X: You don't have to make it gel. I see now.

J.G.W. note: X is at last ready for the insight.

X: There is a bully. His name was George. Huh! Did I ever tell you about him before? He was much older. I used to go out to the railroad yards and jump on the trestle. I was the only one who was brave enough to do it. If I missed, there would be no telling where I would have fallen to. He said he wanted me to come up there with him, and we were in a boxcar. He took his peter out. He wanted me to do something—to kiss him there. Then he said, "Do it or I'll beat you up," and he rushed at me. It was a railroad car filled with sawdust, and I got terribly mad and beat him and beat him, kicked him until he cried and hollered, and then I came to my senses and I left. He got out, 'cause I saw him later. I whipped him terribly. He was much bigger than I was. How could I do that? There was some kind of revulsion in me, something terrible. I felt a lot better afterwards. Imagine me beating George. It would be like beating Joe Lewis.

A.B.F. note: A famous boxer of that era.

X: I was still afraid of him, though, even afterwards.

At last, we have the missing link, the handle on the last door, the fear of Mr. Y with his knife, the great emphasis on athletic prowess, manhood, and leadership. We have an explanation of the basis for his need to have many, many sexual affairs with women, the enormous rage and superhuman strength in beating this older boy, and now finally, the tremendous blinding fear of this childhood incident, which had been so repressed and apparently forgotten. They all ended up to what patient X was afraid of to face within himself, the existence of which his whole life had been one constant striving to deny. Almost instantly, innumerable pieces of the jigsaw puzzle fitted together, and the pattern they made that was now so obvious was latent homosexuality. Patient X had developed a major life-changing insight.

Remember once again that this patient was treated half a century ago at a time when even fewer people were educated. In those days when J.G.W. treated this case, homosexuality was a diagnosable disorder. It did not have the acceptance it has today. Homosexuals were treated with the utmost derision. Being called one was one of the most powerful insults a person could sling, and boys were taught that being a homosexual was about the most terrible thing that could ever happen to them. Glimmers of the past remain today with gang beating of homosexuals still occurring occasionally. But then, to be known as a homosexual was to be known as a social pariah of sorts, to be avoided by "decent" people. In those times, to be a homosexual meant in the popular view to be a woman, to be castrated (clitorectomy). At the time, Eastern cultural practices of female castration, which is still carried on today, were certainly known to a few. Castration invariably referred to the castration of males.

Bizarre attitudes such as these were stonily held in both the era and the culture in which X was raised. It is, therefore, no surprise that he fought so hard with "revulsion" against the older and stronger homosexual perpetrator. But though when he won the fight with George, he did not realize that the invitation to homosexual gratification had attracted him and left him with unconscious desires that required all of the resistance and defenses he could mobilize, not just to avoid carrying them out, but merely to avoid recognizing that he might want to. This is revealed in his almost apparently casually made remark that he was "still afraid of George." What he meant, as revealed from his unconscious, was that he was afraid of his own impulses.

To be constructive, insight must reach deep down within the patient. Could this understanding be initiated in X without creating a panic? Could this concept, obviously so terrible to X as to have warped his whole life, be integrated into his understanding? J.G.W. continued the session:

J.G.W.: This older boy, you said you felt fear toward him?

X: Yes, it was intense.

J.G.W.: What kind of feeling was it?

X: I never knew what it meant, it just came from within. Since that time I have thought a lot about that boy. I wanted to tell you about him, but somehow I forgot to.

A.F.B. note: "Forgot to," a now feeble defense from the patient's resistance.

J.G.W.: Did you ever have any other experiences involving homosexuals?

X: I have seen so many men approach me. I can tell them when I first see them. I know them right and left. I know what they eat, drink, and sleep, I've had enough of them as friends, but my relations with them have always been platonic. I can sure spot them a million miles away. [X mused a bit to himself and then continued.] How do you think I can tell them? My brother is the same way. Isn't it funny that I can spot them? Doesn't affect me, though.

A.B.F. note: The defensive structure remains despite the breakdown of resistances in the development of insight; however, this is likely merely a from of cognitive preservation; old habits die hard.

X: [I] Don't get angry with them anymore.

A.F.B. note: The patient maintains the semblance of the denial defense structure that he has been using for his entire prior life.

X: I just believe they are sort of sick. I knew a girl, and she was a lesbian, a very good friend of mine; only she got angry at me when I started to go with a girl she had a crush on. We had that kind of a relationship.

I wouldn't let a man do that to me, but a woman, yes. I got to enjoy it quite a bit.

J.G.W. note: Oral sex.

A.F.B. note: As foreshadowed by J.G.W. earlier, the intimidation by George as a child and demands for oral sex, although strongly repudiated at the time, left him with a wonderment about the pleasures of such behavior, contrary to the norm of heterosexual relationships. Oral sex in the present case, although given by the female, in fact met the homosexual needs that were seeded by the conflict with George. However, to be clear in this specific case it met homosexual needs due to the patient's past. Oral sex by itself should not be equated with such a latent need; it most often is not.

J.G.W. explained to the patient that there was a certain amount of homosexuality in latent form in all of us, that there was nothing wrong about having a female component, that it does take a form of actual homosexual relations in most cases, but that many persons are afraid to face it in themselves. At one point, when the discussion centered around homosexual relations, X remarked, "I wonder what it would feel like to do it."

J.G.W. now refocused the discussion on a return to the waves of anger that overcomes many men on being approached by a homosexual, including the frequent great desire to strike or injure the person.

X: You know, that's me. Yes, that's me [and then X began to smile].

A.F.B. note: The patient recognizes his insight at the emotional feeling level not just the cognitive-intellectual one.

J.G.W. next called X's attention to the fact that overt actual expressions of homosexual tendencies were regarded by the ancient Greek society as an acceptable form of sexual expression. X was told that all he needed to do was to recognize this, that he, like many other men in the world, had this feminine component within him, and that once he recognized it and ceased fighting it, he would no longer fear it.

A.F.B. note: The reader will recall that J.G.W. first published this case in 1949 and, indeed, the patient was an Army lieutenant. This was decades before the diagnosis of homosexuality as a clinical disorder was removed from diagnostic criteria of mental disorders. J.G.W. then was decades ahead of his contemporaries.

J.G.W.:   How did this manifest itself in you?
X: You know, Mr. Y, ... Mr. Y with his big knife, ... the knife is like a penis.

A.F.B. note: The development of insight is reaffirmed as the patient becomes more confident and is willing to bring to consciousness other aspects of these symbols and even begin to interpret them himself in the safety and presence of J.G.W.

J.G.W. note: At this point X's tension in his body began to dissipate.

X: The darkness has faded away. Everything is becoming light.

A.F.B. note: The reader will recall the light at the end of the tunnel that was introduced by J.G.W. in an earlier session.

J.G.W.:   By the way, X, do you know what day today is?

X: Oh, yes, it's March 7, isn't it? This is the day you said Mr. Y would be uncovered.

J.G.W.:   I didn't say it. You said it. Now, I am going to describe a dream to you, and you can finish the dream. You can see yourself out in a field, and there is a big black horse in this field.

A.F.B. note: J.G.W. safeguards against the reintellectualization of the insights and reaffirms it was the patient's proclamation of the number 21 that led to the March 7 date in an earlier session.

X [In instant reply]:   Like a flash I am on top of that horse, I am galloping off, galloping off. I can ride it, I can handle it.

J.G.W. note: "I can handle my impulses."

J.G.W.:   Now I want you to see another dream. You are at a masquerade. Everyone has on masks. You know them all except one young woman. She runs downstairs with a mask on. You chase after her, and she says, "If you want to see who I am, catch me first." Now go ahead and finish the dream.

X [Jumped in his seat, writhed, fidgeted, and wrinkled his forehead, and then at last replied]:   I've caught her. I am removing the mask. Huh—that's me, I am the woman.

J.G.W. note: X's feminine component is finally unmasked.

J.G.W. [Once again suggesting another dream]:   You're on a desert again. There are many roads leading out in all directions. You are very thirsty. What happens?

A.F.B. note: Again J.G.W. brings back prior symbolized material from earlier sessions to help ensure insight is fostered from all that has been introduced by the patient, that there are no "loose ends."

X: I am walking down the road. There is no wolf anymore. He is gone. Now, all the many roads merge into one, there is a clear straight road.

A.B.F. note: A clear path in life at last.

X: There are roses around the road.

A.F.B. note: X now confidently recognizes that his insights will allow him to interact with the outside world adaptively; hence, there are roses along the road.

J.G.W.:   You can walk down this road. Tell me what you see. Is there a house?

A.F.B. note: The reader will recall the house that was "flanked" by J.G.W. in an earlier session.

X: Yes. Only now the house has changed. It has been painted white. Now it has solid, brick foundations under it. It is well built. It is now changed from the shaky foundations to solid ones.
J.G.W.:   You know what the house means, don't you?
X: Yes, it means me!
J.G.W.:   That's right. And now you will no longer fear the old traces of homosexuality because you understand them.

A.F.B. note: The patient accepts them as part of himself.

J.G.W.:   You don't have to repress them any longer. You realize you can have a female component within, like other males, only you are not afraid of it anymore. [Pause] You have nothing more to hide from yourself. Mr. Y is gone. Melvin and George are gone now, too. They merged into one person. That's you. They will not need to fight each other any more.

A.F.B. note: Dissociation, although not overt to the point of creating true multiple personalities (DIDs), did separate X into at least two covert ego states that alternated in governing his feelings and behavior. Was the psychopathic "George" personality an introject of George, the big boy who had intimidated him and tried to force him into giving oral sex, hence, an identification with the aggressor?

J.G.W.:   I am going to count up to five, and when I do, you will wake up, you will feel good, and you will remember distinctly everything we have discussed. One, two, three, four, five.

A.F.B. note: As discussed in Barabasz & Watkins (2005), perhaps a better realerting approach is to count down to take the patient out of hypnosis, five, four, three, two, one, because counting up has been used exclusively in the induction procedures as a method of deepening and taking a person down into hypnosis; in the present case, it is of no significance. However, it is a good habit to get into to keep the counting in and counting out differentiated because patients at the primary process level take things at a very literal level.

X [Opening his eyes and smiling]:   Isn't it fun, I don't feel wild exhilaration, I just feel a calm sense of satisfaction, a feeling of relief as if a burden has gone.

At this point it would appear that the case was nearly ready for termination, and J.G.W. looked forward to "closing this chart" so the patient could be "discharged to civilian life." At this point, the process of what counselors refer to as summary clarification was ready to take place. J.G.W. rediscussed in the conscious state all the material that had been processed. The plan was to go over the patient's entire treatment with him.

As discussed in Chapters 1 and 2, the meaning of "true insight" was discussed. It is not always easy to determine whether a patient has achieved it or only an "intellectual insight," often to impress the therapist during a period of positive transference. This critical difference must be tested if we are to determine whether or not the patient's personality has been repaired. One of the best ways we have found to test this is to feed back to the patient neurotic, uncompleted dreams that may have arisen during the course of his or her analysis. It will be recalled that J.G.W. tried earlier to get the patient to "ride the black horse" and to "catch the masked girl." The patient could not do that initially. Then, after a reconstruction "reliving" of the traumatic seduction incident by the older boy George when the patient was a youngster and after securing some meaning into it all, the patient was able to ride the horse. He could also catch and unmask the teasing girl, which he, in fact, recognized was his own feminine part of himself. When closure can be brought to such neurotic dreams, we have more support for our hypothesis that the "insight" is genuine, true progress has been accomplished, and the patient's personality has been, at least in part, reconstructed to make him or her a happier, healthier, more adaptive individual for the rest of his or her life.]

One More Battle

Moses and Aaron once looked over a hill and saw the Promised Land of Canaan, but it was only a glimpse. The Children of Israel wandered in the wilderness for years before they were permitted to enjoy that Promised Land. Sometimes insight is like that. The cause is unearthed, the patient sees, the patient understands. It looks all too clear. Then, as we saw repeatedly in the course of the case above, the fog of resistance closes down again, the clouds congeal, the light is obscured. The explanations–interpretations are again rejected. Mr. Y still had one more round of fight left in him. As explained in A.F.B.'s note, the patient has had a lifetime of practice repetitions of maladaptive responding and a history through therapy of repeated evocations of sometimes profound levels of resistance. The habit is far more engrained than even the greatest revelations or interpretations that resulted in true insight.

Patient X again came to see J.G.W. 4 days after the breakthrough session of March 7. He described the tortures through which he had been going. J.G.W. gave him reassurance and again pointed out the necessity of understanding and accepting, not rejecting. X was now involved in that stage that psychoanalysts have termed "working through." X left slightly reassured, which is usually the best we can hope for in such cases, but the death agonies of Mr. Y continued for 7 more days.

Finally, on March 18, his anxieties had subsided somewhat, and he returned. Reassurance was again given, plus further discussion as to the meanings behind the material uncovered. It was apparent that he left the session feeling much better.

The therapy hour on March 19 was devoted to an exhaustive review of the entire treatment. This was not merely the hypnocounseling "summary clarification," recounting in simplified and limited form such as, "We talked about [this], we talked about [that], and then we concluded [this]," but rather a word-by-word, line-by-line, event-by-event discussion of the material from the patient's chart notes that had been meticulously maintained by J.G.W. To carry out this part of the procedure effectively, it involves placing all the pieces in a pattern where they could make sense to the patient as interpreted in the light of the uncovered key information, which was the latent homosexual component that patient X had been desperately trying to conceal from himself for so many years.

At last, so many things now made some sense. As you will recall from the session of February 28 when the patient's dissociated hand wrote, "H-O-M-O-B-I-O-L-O-G-I-C-A-L-H-O-M-O" and the delving of the word, "P-R-O-A-N-T-I-R-A-N-S-U-B-S-T-A-N-C-H-I-I-O-N-I-S-T," an unusual Civil War term referring to a person with two different kinds of social standing, representing in this patient's unconscious heterosexual and homosexual. At another time, the patient dreamed of being chased from behind with a "big nickel-plated engine," a male genital symbol. The patient's ability to "know" homosexuals "left and right" plus "what they eat, drink, and sleep" attests to the patient's underlying resonance with them. Indeed, make no mistake, it is resonance rather than rejection at this level of expression, yet still deeply repressed. There were many more such items that arose in therapy but which we have not mentioned in this brief account of X's treatment.

In X's session of March 26, he reported sleeping well for 5 days; except for a slight uneasiness, he felt little disturbed. There were no more nightmares. He was not awakened at night, and concerning his fear of the dark, he said, "I just forgot it."

Clearly, we had not yet had evidence of any sort of "complete analysis." Nonetheless, certain strata of the patient's unconscious mind had clearly been penetrated, and that is the time the therapist must recognize that such penetration does not imply the accomplishment of therapeutic change as yet. It is a basis for therapeutic change but only that and will take the patient nowhere without further guidance from your expertise. The existence of latent homosexual impulses and the fear of the patient's feminine component with considerable "castration anxiety" were revealed. He apparently derived insight into these and mastered his fears. The evidence is his mastery of this dark side as expressed by loss of the symptom of fear of the dark.

Obviously, we must ask ourselves why these homosexual fears originated. What were the childhood fantasies that occurred in this patient's psychosexual development? How did his Melvin and George ego state split off? Although there are many other questions that could be asked, we had reached a point where the treatment could be stabilized. It was time for X to go home, to leave the security of the military hospital environment and return to civilian life. J.G.W. had time for just one more meeting with X.

Session of March 28

X: You know, I had a dream recently. I saw a baby. It was dying. It did die. Its heart protruded, making the skin extend. I saw it suffering, and then it was dead.

A.F.B. note: Is this the patient's repressed representation of the death of his own neurotic immaturity?

J.G.W. [Taking the patient back to the field]: There is the black horse again.

X: It is very wild. It is running away from me. He comes back, he runs away, he comes back, he circles me, [Pause] and he stops. I get in the saddle. Now I am on top of him. He is a wild animal, he throws me off. I am getting on again. He jumps over fences and throws me off again. I get on again. We are running down the road. He takes off into the air. I can ride him! And now he disappears. He is just a flash in the distance.

J.G.W. note: "I can master my neurosis."

J.G.W.: You will have a dream now that will indicate your future. Will you be riding the horse in the future?

J.G.W.: [The patient sat quietly for 5 minutes but wiggled his fingers.] Have you finished your dream?

X: Yes, first I saw an Army barracks like we have here. Suddenly one of them began to change into a house, a nice house. It had a small fence around it; outside the house was a horse. I started to go to the field, playing polo. I can't imagine why, riding him.

J.G.W. [Reassuringly]: You can ride your horse!

X: All right. You are now at a masquerade ball, there is a girl there who has a mask on.

J.G.W.:   She probably needs to keep her face covered because her face is horrible, my face.

X [Laughing]:   That's a good joke.

A.F.B. note: The introduction of humor here is a very clever move on J.G.W.'s part; it conveys to the patient his confidence in the patient's ability to overcome what little remains. Both patient and therapist have nearly completed their journey and success is assured.

J.G.W.:   Who is this girl?

X [Replying instantly]:   I don't want to chase her. I know who she is.

J.G.W.:   Are you afraid of her?

X: No, of course not, I am not afraid of her. [The patient began to rub his eyes.] I am getting awake.

J.G.W.:   What happened to George and Melvin?

X: I don't know, they've taken long trips … gone away, and they're not coming back. Poor Melvin. [The patient appeared to muse for a moment and then stated] If they had combined their best traits in one person, what a person.

J.G.W.:   Maybe they have.

A.F.B. note: This is not only a hopeful comment by J.G.W. but a very important therapeutic tactic. Personality entities, or ego states, do not want to be killed off; they have a contribution that is positive as well as psychopathological. The psychopathology has been dealt with, so in stating, "Maybe they have," J.G.W. protects the patient from reoccurrence or the re-emergence of the old maladaptive personalities and makes a hopeful comment that now unpathologized ones, as recognized by the patient with his statement "what a person," will be available to contribute to all that conscious X can be.

X: I want to get back to civilian life and start driving, the old push, the old force, like I used to have. If I were cleaning streets, I'd have the cleanest streets in the block. Mr. Y will be just a bad memory. [Patient X opened his eyes and smiled.]

Summary

Before being discharged from the hospital, patient X had the Rorschach test administered again. Unfortunately, the test was not conducted under optimum conditions; hence, the total number of responses was low. However, the results were indicative of normal personality function, with little evidence of neurotic maladjustment. Ego strength was good and regard for reality as well as contact with reality was high. His intellectual approach to problems was now appropriate, rather than pathological, as had been the case for many years. Mild depressive features were noted, as well as some residual anxiety. X was now able to exhibit sensitivity to emotional stimuli from his environment, but his capacity for emotional identification with others was still not fully mature and stabilized. There were no longer indications of severe psychopathology. His general Rorschach pattern now was that of a reasonably normal and adaptive personality.

Afternote by J.G.W.: *What are my reactions to this case today (2007), 60 years after treating and publishing it (J.G. Watkins, 1949)?*

I was a daring young beaver then fascinated with exploring the unconscious, and, in projective hypnoanalysis I was testing the limits (J.G. Watkins, 1960). I had not yet learned all the precautions I was taught later. It could have ended disastrously, but it didn't, and for that time was unusually successful. In some 65 sessions, it covered ground that traditional psychoanalysts in those days treated for hundreds of hours.

In the army at the Welch Convalescent Hospital (J. G. Watkins, 1949), we were flooded with PTSD patients from the Anzio beachhead and the Italian campaign (J.G. Watkins, 2000). I had been taking personal analysis with an aggressive training analyst who had moved to the U.S. from Berlin. His aggressiveness excited me, and encouraged me to be more directive in my therapy with the combat veterans; it also frightened me. My later analyst, Eduardo Weiss, former president of the Italian Psychoanalytic Association (who was analyzed by Federn and trained by Freud), remarked that "the Prussian analyst says "YOU ARE RESISTING," but the Italian analyst says, "Oh! I am so sorry; I did not understand you."

In developing "projective hypnoanalysis" I reasoned that the great length of traditional analytic treatment (several hundreds of hours, often over many years) was because of its few techniques—free association, dream interpretation, analysis of the transference—and that if we added dissociated handwriting projective techniques plus hypnosis, we could reach unconscious levels sooner. So what lessons can we learn from the case of Patient X?

First, that the aggressive confronting and interpretation of resistance may not be as dangerous as traditionally thought. The ego will not go psychotic, but will simply change its manner of defense or withdraw. It will protect itself. Second, that we can be more aggressive if we will resonate intensely with the patient, e.g., holding the patient's trust. I learned more about resonance (see Chapter 12) from Helen Watkins, who learned hypnosis from me, then went on to become a "concert artist" therapist, and a master of the technique of resonance.

I have thought about this case much over the years. It influenced my life as an "experimental" therapist, and spurred me to the discovery and development of many innovative hypnoanalytic techniques.

9
Dissociative Hypnoanalysis

Trauma can be understood as the experience of being made into an object, a thing. One suddenly becomes the victim of someone else's rage, whether expressed as overt anger or as a clever manipulation, of bad luck, or of nature's indifference; e.g., a lightning-strike disaster kills one child (Dollinger, 1985). The essence of traumatic stress is the experience of helplessness and loss of control rather than fear or pain. One young man whose leg was so badly broken in a motorcycle accident that it was eventually amputated had initially managed to save his life by walking off the freeway where he was lying, without conscious experience of pain, by engaging his imagination such that he was at a mountain lake fishing with his father. He used his concentration (self-hypnosis) on this imaginary scene to detach himself from the immediate experience of terror, pain, and helplessness. Many rape victims report floating above their body, feeling sorry for the person being assaulted below them (H. Spiegel & D. Spiegel, 2004, p. 424).

During dissociation, certain behaviors and experiences seem to be split off from others. In psychoanalytic terms, there is a division in the ego that separates it into two or more different states. A personality construct that has been correlated with hypnotizability is ego receptivity. It taps openness to social input such as that which might be brought about by the therapist that is designed to alter inner experience. Ego receptivity has been shown to be significantly related to absorption (Tellegen & Atkinson, 1974) and together they account for variability of hypnotizability (Goodman & Holroyd, 1992). H. Spiegel and D. Spiegel (2004, p. 148) explained that such receptivity is a different construct from self-monitoring such as occurs in social interactions (Snyder, 1995). Kirsch (1991) hypothesized that the social role-playing (role enactment) explanation, if true, would show that self-monitoring would be associated with higher hypnotizability. This was disproved by Bachner-Melman and Ebstein (2002). Clearly, the cart cannot be made to go ahead of the horse.

If the dissociation is severe enough, we have multiple personality disorder (MPD) (dissociative identity disorders), in which each of these entities, at least initially, is oblivious of the existence of the other.

I was called in March, 1979, to hypnotically interview Kenneth Bianchi, a mild appearing young man accused of murdering two coeds in Bellingham, Washington. He claimed amnesia about the event. With great difficulty he was hypnotized, whereupon a dissociated alter, "Steve," emerged.

Steve not only claimed "credit" for the murders, but also revealed himself as the Los Angeles Hillside Strangler by bragging about all the girls he had killed, as well as those that is cousin Angelo Buono had killed. During a later session in which Steve was activated indirectly without a formal hypnotic induction, Steve and Ken were given Rorschachs separately, with results that were totally different from each other, as were their handwritings, manners, use of the language, etc.

The prosecution's position was that Bianchi had faked both hypnosis and multiple personality, and had confessed to ten additional murders to establish an insanity defense. In view of the fact that Ken had repeatedly maintained he wasn't "crazy" and had finally agreed to plead insanity only at the insistence of his attorney, this position was not very compelling. The controversy about this case has been debated in print (Orne et al., 1984a; Watkins, 1984).

I mention such a case because, in the criticisms of hypnotic hypermnesia and regression the fact that people can lie under hypnosis is emphasized, and it is assumed that subjects will always try to use hypnosis to "prove" that they weren't really guilty. My experience has been quite the contrary. Hypnotized individuals often reveal their guilt, while consciously maintaining otherwise. Like a naïve child, they blurt out a self-incriminating truth. Hypnosis is a regression, and regressed subjects think more concretely—like a child. Hypnosis is also a focused concentration and a restriction of the experiential field. Accordingly, the pre-censoring cautions that might warn the defendant being interviewed not to say something that could later be incriminating may not be operating very well.

These different personalities, as in the case presented in the previous chapter, may take turns being "executive" (see Barabasz & Watkins, 2005, pp. 72–75). During the period when personality A is functioning, personality B is dormant, asleep, or "unconscious." When personality B appears, it is amnesic to the period during which personality A was active (J. G. Watkins, 1984).

Dissociation, whether involved to the point of DID or not, affects memory in ways that are analogous to the key elements of hypnosis compared to memory processing: encoding, storage, and retrieval (H. Spiegel et al., 2000, D. Spiegel, 1998). Dissociation also isolates memories through a process of separating them from common associative networks such as may be involved in repressive mechanisms. Amnesic barriers that have common links between dissociation and hypnosis include evidence that hypnotically induced amnesia for autobiographical information is similar to functional amnesia (Barnier, 2002; E. R. Hilgard, 1977; Kihlstrom, 1987; Kihlstrom & Hoyt, 1990). H. Spiegel and D. Spiegel (2004) noted that Whalen and Nash (1996) found an essentially nonsignificant correlation between a standardized measure of hypnotizability and dissociation in a laboratory study but also recognized that there is an important distinction between pathological dissociation as found in our patients and adaptive, normally functioning individuals (Barrett, 1992a). The relationship between trauma dissociation and hypnotizability is strongest in clinical populations (D. Spiegel, 1988). The operational conclusion is that the involuntariness of clinical trauma can mobilize a strong spontaneous hypnotic response, which is not necessarily evidenced in less stressful dissociative or formal hypnotic situations. D. Spiegel also directly dealt with the criticism that somehow expectancy and waking suggestion play an important part in apparent dissociative phenomena (Kirsch & Lynn, 1998). D. Spiegel noted that although social context may contribute to the subjective experience, it cannot account for the variance associated with hypnotizability as a trait, which is robust (E. R. Hilgard, 1965; Piccone, Hilgard, & Zimbardo, 1989). There remains little legitimate evidence to support the social context phenomena conclusion that suggestion can produce a full-blown dissociative disorder (Brown et al. 2000).

E. R. Hilgard's attraction to dissociation became apparent in the early years of his work on hypnosis (1965). He found the term "dissociation," particularly "partial dissociation," to be more useful than regression as an interpretation of hypnotic phenomena (pp. 392–393, 395–396). Hilgard's Stanford Laboratory of Hypnosis Research was involved in numerous experimental studies that revealed less pervasive types of dissociation, such as those found in routine hypnosis and illustrated by Milton Erickson in Hilgard's lab (see Barabasz & Watkins, 2005, p. 53, for this dramatic example).

Our focus on dissociative hypnotic techniques in Barabasz & Watkins (2005) was concerned primarily with direct hypnotic suggestion approaches in the many remarkable, as well as routine, uses of hypnosis for the alleviation of pain. Our focus here will be on its use as a key to dealing with serious pathologies. We will explain the use of dissociation as a diagnostic tool, as well as its use in the treatment of dissociative identity disorder and less severe forms of DID, such as presented by the borderline DID patient described in a prior chapter. We consider hypnosis itself as form of dissociative behavior (E. R. Hilgard, 1977). It is also a modality for creating, manipulating, and terminating dissociations. There are numerous dissociative procedures that can be used within the hypnotic modality for the diagnosis and treatment of many disorders, but the modality is almost a sine qua non in the treatment of amnesias and dissociative identity disorders. We will consider those hypnotic techniques that can be used through hypnoanalysis, as well as ways in which they can be employed in dealing with spontaneous (natural) dissociations such as those encountered as amnesias and dissociative identity disorders. H. Spiegel and D. Spiegel (2004) emphasized, as do most theorists, that there is no absolute dividing line between nonhypnotic and hypnotic alterations in consciousness. Dissociated experiences, where one's usual pan-awareness of the surrounding world is suspended, occur naturally.

Dissociative Diagnostic Procedure

Interviews with patients, observations of their behavior, and case histories including reports of "time out" provide a basis for inferring the presence of dissociation. The Perceptual Alteration Scale (Sanders, 1986) is a useful objective instrument. In virtually all cases, the presence of some sort of dramatic dissociation can be traced to early trauma or inner conflict.

Inner conflict within the neurotic disorders is caused by the impact of two contradictory elements on each other. Thus, a sexual desire for a friend's wife or husband may conflict with a conscious need to be regarded as a "moral" person. Anxiety and other symptoms may result. The sex drive may be fully repressed, but the person is completely unaware of it. Such repressions are widespread, as there is no evolutionary evidence to suggest that humans or any other animals are monogamous by nature. Quite the opposite is the universal norm. Moralities are entirely a matter of social learning and context. Once inculcated by the individual, they provide the basis for a wide variety of neurotic conflicts.

Psychoanalysis attempts to receive communications that reveal to the analyst unconscious motivations when they are still beyond awareness to the patient. The psychoanalytic techniques of free association, dream analysis, and transference are employed to "wrest" from the unconscious of the patient the "secret" impulses, which underlie this conflict. How does the therapist get the patient to "reveal" such unconscious secrets, while at the same time permitting him or her to "conceal" them from their own awareness?

Anxiety arises because the two elements of the conflict are both "on stage" at the same time. The fictitious patient may be partially aware of a sexual attraction to his friend's wife but be unwilling to let such a recognition reach full comprehension. He cannot verbalize the conflict because to do so would be to reveal to himself, as well as to his analyst, its true nature. If we could just devise a way whereby his "unconscious" self could inform us of the hidden desire while his "conscious" ego is still kept in the dark about it, then we would have preknowledge of the conflict and could plan our therapeutic strategy accordingly. We recognize that the information so derived may be withheld from the patient until he or she is strong enough, prepared enough, and willing to deal with this insight. One such procedure is dissociated handwriting.

Using Dissociated Handwriting

Dissociated handwriting can provide clues to the patient's underlying conflicts. The recommended procedure to initiate dissociated handwriting is as follows:

1. Measure the patient's hypnotizability using one of the standardized tests that includes dissociative items, such as the Hypnotic Induction Profile (HIP) (H. Spiegel & D. Spiegel, 2004), the Stanford Hypnotic Clinical Scale (SHCS) (Morgan & J. R. Hilgard, 1975), or the Stanford Hypnotic Susceptibility Scale: Form C (SHSS: C) (Weitzenhoffer & E. R. Hilgard, 1962). The testing procedure will provide clues as to how to best hypnotize the patient for the more demanding task of dissociated handwriting, verify or disprove your clinical evaluation regarding the dissociation that you had inferred from your interviews with the patient, and provide clues as to resistances to hypnosis you might encounter.

2. Hypnotize the patient with an induction tailored to your assessment of his or her capabilities.

3. Suggest anesthesia in his or her writing hand. "Your hand is becoming stiff and paralyzed. It is getting completely numb, so that it has no feeling in it. It is no longer part of you. It is separated from your body at the wrist." If the patient is highly hypnotizable and able to enter a fairly deep state, he or she can then be told: "Open your eyes and look at your hand, you will see it is just floating in space and that it is no longer connected to your body at the wrist. Notice that because it is no longer part of you, you have no control over it, you cannot make it move, and you cannot stop it from moving if it wishes to do so. You are now free to close your eyes or to keep them open and watch the movements of the hand over which you have no control."

   Removing feeling from a person's hand is to change it from "subject," hence, part of the person, "the me," into "object," a "not me." "Not me's" are outside our self and are not subject to our volitional control or censorship. They do what they want and say what they want, even if this means revealing secrets we prefer to conceal from ourselves or others. Now if the patient's eyes close, it probably means that he or she does not want to read what might be written. Accept this defense at the time and recognize that it is telling you there is a lack of readiness about what may be revealed. Alternatively, if the patient keeps his or her eyes open, it may mean that either he or she is prepared to become informed about the message, or he or she is so deeply dissociated he or she will not be able to remember what may be seen upon being realerted from hypnosis.

4. Put a pencil in the patient's hand and a paper under it. Suggest the following: "That hand is like another little person. It knows many

things, perhaps things you do not know about yourself. It will begin to write and say whatever it needs to." Your relationship with the patient must be established on firm ground, and all of this must be done with absolute inner confidence that "you know it will work." Quite often the hand does not move at all initially. It just holds the pencil and is still. This is a typical reaction that can "reveal secrets" that the patient does not want to uncover. This stillness of the hand is only a symptom of resistance if the preconditions noted above have been met. The movements of the hand must be removed still further from conscious observation and control. The Hand may need to be warmed up into action on innocuous material.

5. Proceed as follows: "The hand seems to be moving a little, just a little, maybe it wants to move up or down. Its movements are so slight you may not even notice them at first, but they will become greater in time." Note here that we are implying the typical first step in initiating the hypnotic state by stating things in the future tense. Be patient, your patience must be perceived as essentially infinite. Watch carefully and encourage some slight movement, any movement in the hand. Reinforce any movement whatsoever, whether it involves writing or not and take your time. This can be regarded as the period when the hand is gradually becoming increasingly dissociated from volitional controls.

6. Once the hand has begun to move, say, "Perhaps the hand will draw a letter, any letter?" This is the next stage of the "warming-up period," which may take some time as well, but with perseverance by the therapist a letter usually appears. It may be printed or it may be in cursive handwriting. When it appears, simply continue, "Good! Now maybe the hand will write another letter. Fine. Now another. And another."

In a little while, the "letters" begin to form words. Communication begins; sometimes the words are negative, such as "I don't want to write." Or in the more hostile pathological defense, "It's none of your business." In one case, the hand made scribbling marks and then wrote, "jumble, jumble, jumble," as described in the previous chapter with patient X. All of this is part of the warming-up period. Resistance, when permitted expression, will tend to wear out, and that which is being resisted comes to the fore. This is quite in line with the often-noted psychoanalytic response that when one side of a conflict is expressed, in time the other side will become manifest. For example, when an angry spouse is encouraged to ventilate his or her hostile feelings and disparaging comments about the other, there comes a time when the person says, "Well, he or she isn't always bad. Sometimes he or she is nice." That is why we wear out resistance by encouraging its expression. This is also particularly useful in Ego State Therapy when dealing with a malevolent, usually covert, ego state.

Treat responses from the hand in the same way. When using the dissociated handwriting technique, we are concerned with getting communications about inner conflicts through the censorship of the ego. The analytic use of dissociated revelation does not eliminate resistances or their appropriate handling, but it does make it easier to secure pertinent information about a patient's conflicts.

Dissociated handwriting takes much time. Clearly, this is a drawback, given all the time required for warm-up periods and afterwards. Furthermore, if the patient's eyes are closed, the pencil will frequently run off the edge of the paper. You will have to adjust the hand on the paper continuously and put new sheets of paper under it. Finally, remember that it takes a deeper level of hypnotic involvement to get such involuntary, dissociated movements. If the patient is quite passive, and the hand does not move no matter how much effort you put forth, "hallucinated" dissociated handwriting might be a better choice.

Hallucinated Dissociated Handwriting

A deep level of hypnotic involvement is required to attain success with suggested motor movements. Thus, we may choose to keep the responses entirely out of the patient's field of perception. Obviously, the patient must still be able to talk while hypnotized. Initiate the procedure as follows:

"You are walking down a street. Can you see the cars passing by? There is a school up ahead; you are going into it. You proceed to a very special class and sit down. You can learn some very important things here. As you sit at the desk you look around the room. Can you describe how it is furnished?"

The above initiation is intended to help the patient fantasize images. The following suggestions are also indirectly imbedded: "You are going to the school to learn. This is a very special school; hence, you will learn something very important to you. Confirm to me that you are really there in this situation; just raise a finger to let me know that." These hypnotic suggestions are both dissociative and projective. We now can focus more closely on what we seek.

"Notice the whiteboard in the front of the room just ahead. If you look at it carefully you will see a hand with a marker in it. The hand is writing something. Tell me what it is writing."

This is often the dissociated handwriting technique of choice. It taps into the same material that we probably would have revealed if we had actually dissociated the hand physically and then asked "projective" questions. The hallucinated hand may have to be warmed up and urged in the same way that the patient's physical hand required in the more classical dissociated handwriting technique. In fact, the two techniques may be combined if the patient can actually write with a dissociated hand. He or she may be instructed to read what is written on the board and then told the hand will copy the writing. In fact, here it is less important to refer to that hand; because the hand is copying what has already been written on the board, it can even be referred to as "your" hand if this is helpful in initiating the writing response. There are innumerable variations that are possible as we seek to get revelation of unconscious material and wish to place distance between what the patient is communicating and what he or she understands and is aware of concerning those communications.

The ideomotor technique of finger raising can also be used as a variation of the dissociated hand technique (see Barabasz & Watkins, 2005, chapter 10, p. 250; Cheek, 1962; Cheek & LeCron, 1968; Ewin, 2003). The technique has the advantage of asking for only minimal movements, merely lifting a finger rather than moving a hand. It can also be used frequently in a formal hypnotic induction and thus may involve a lesser degree of dissociation. This latter observation has not yet been tested empirically and would make the basis for an excellent controlled experiment. The technique, however, is limited because questions must be answered with a "yes" or a "no" answer (and possibly an "I don't know" or "I don't want to answer" option). To carry it out successfully, you will have to have a very good idea of what the patient's repressed material is all about. It also means that you can lead yourself down frequent blind alleys if your clinical hypotheses are off-target. The patient will answer your questions with ideomotor responding but you may be going further and further from the unconscious material underlying this conflict.

Many moderate as well as more highly hypnotizable participants have spontaneous dissociative abilities. Communication may be established through "automatic writing," which has a considerable history of study (Messerschmidt, 1927–1928). It is simply a script that is spontaneously produced involuntarily and, in some instances, without conscious awareness. Although it is quite similar to "dissociated handwriting," we prefer to reserve that term for writing by a hand that has been specifically dissociated hypnotically by the therapist. Automatic writing occurs spontaneously and without prior hypnotic induction. There are some remarkable early examples of these phenomena, such as the "spirit" writings of various "mediums." Many experiments and observations have been made about these phenomena (E. R. Hilgard, 1986; Cardeña (in press).

Automatic writing was found first by Meuhl to help her patients unearth hidden conflict, obtain access to early childhood thought forms (primary process), discover latent talents, and reorganize their personalities more effectively. Meuhl would place her patients' writing arms in a sling so that they would be suspended about an inch over a table. She would sit behind them and whisper questions into their ears. Sometimes she had them read so their conscious mind was distracted. She reported that often the first communications were simply wavy lines or single letters. By repeating what they had written (simple reflection), she found that letters began to form into words. The operative technique here is to repeat what they had written, very much like we discussed earlier. Repeating the letters as they were formed would, in fact, eventually turn into the formation of full words. Sometimes communications were in a code that was difficult to decipher. Some of the time, she used hypnosis, which would then make her procedure almost identical to "dissociated handwriting." Meuhl noted that the communications could be divided into two general classes: fantasy and actual recall. Some subjects who were predisposed to doodling wrote naturally without using the sling, whereas others required the free movement offered by the hand and arm being lifted off the desk. Her observations and uses of the technique were very carefully recorded, and you have enough of the essence of it here so that you may try it as well. Arranging the sling can be cumbersome, and you may simply prefer the dissociated writing technique, using hypnosis to facilitate the response.

Our preference is to use hypnosis; however, J.G.W. reported that one patient brought in "automatic messages" that he wrote while in the school library in a state that he described as sitting in a kind of fog. J.G.W. interpreted the writing as a spontaneous appearance of a child ego state because the kinds of things he wrote included statements like "You good daddy. You take care of me. I love you." This discovery of the patient's child ego state was found to be a significant element in his problem, which was dealt with effectively using ego-state therapy, as will be discussed in Chapter 10.

Creative therapists will be the most successful with many of these patients. Therefore, your flexibility and ability to use a variety of different approaches combined with acceptance of whatever covert communications the patient may offer you will best facilitate therapy. Some patients communicate best through projective techniques, whereas others communicate best through dissociative procedures. If you offer a combination of both, it is very likely that you will obtain greater knowledge of the patient's repressed conflicts in the shortest possible time. Your flexibility and acceptance of the patient's spontaneous responses are the keys.

Treating Dissociative Reactions

Dissociative reactions are not limited to dissociative identity disorder, borderline dissociative identity disorder, and post traumatic stress disorder (PTSD). The *Diagnostic and statistical manual IV-TR* (American Psychiatric Association, 2000) includes a new diagnostic category, acute stress disorder (ASD), which has prominent dissociative symptoms including intrusion, avoidance, and hyperarousal symptoms, in recognition of the frequency and predictive importance of acute dissociative reactions to trauma. The same sorts of problems we encounter in attempting to deal with repressed conflicts are evident in the attempts to deal with trauma-related memories. Appropriate treatment of ASD patients currently emphasizes grief counseling as well as an exploration of the traumatic experience. However, the majority of those patients are reluctant to talk about the stress-inducing events. In those cases, direct hypnotic suggestion can be used to help the patient maintain control and mastery over the trauma-related dissociative symptoms to reinitiate their surface functioning at, for example, work, while therapy takes place at the deeper levels that we are focusing on here. All of these mental disorders, primarily amnesia and dissociative identity disorder, are the result of spontaneous and uncontrolled dissociation. Clearly the hypnotic modality is the treatment of choice for such disorders. While A.F.B. served as chair of the Examining Board of Psychology for the state of Washington in 1998, the board at one point considered the fact that it may be unethical for a therapist to treat such disorders without a formal training in hypnosis.

Amnesia

Disassociation always involves a failure in the usual integration of identity, memory, and even consciousness (American Psychiatric Association, 2000). Although all but the few remaining psychologists of the socio-cognitive persuasion now recognize that a certain degree of dissociation occurs in everyday life, this phenomena was probably first elaborated upon by Herbert Spiegel (H. Spiegel & Shainess, 1963). Both J.G.W. (1992a) as well as Spiegel and Koopman (1994) noted that pathological segregations of mental contents involve enhanced difficulty of episodic memories that would normally be available to consciousness. The memory storage process is clearly affected by dissociative phenomena, as is the potential for retrieving critical memories, although they may have been stored. Amnesia just seems to happen. Assuming that the amnesia has not been produced by the physical injury of brain trauma or some other organic cause, we can best conceptualize it as a result of an unconscious conflict that protects the patient from the awareness of unpleasant consequences, such as in the example given at the very beginning of this chapter or derogatory self-motivations.

As Tulring (1983) explained, amnesia is best thought of as occurring when information that is potentially available is not currently accessible. The problem is one of retrieval. H. Spiegel and D. Spiegel (2004) pointed out that some kinds of functional memory disorders may be related to organizational and storage deficits. As we suggested in Barabasz & Watkins (2005), sometimes memory traces are simply never recorded in the first place or are lost. The brain does not have some sort of audio/video recording system. We might say that a person's amnesia caused by protective unconscious conflicts essentially "commits amnesia." This is essentially the same phenomena that was originally thought of and classified as a type of "hysteria" (Janet, 1889; see also Kihlstrom & Evans, 1979). Even more than a century ago, such "hysterical" reactions were considered to be quite amenable to hypnotherapy. However, they can be quite resistant to hypnosis if they are based on the patient's need to conceal certain conflicts from conscious awareness. If the patient sees hypnosis as an approach that threatens to break that defensive structure down, logically expect such resistance. This was precisely the case with a patient with the pseudonym "Richard Billings," who developed amnesia for his entire life after suffering from combat fatigue (J. G. Watkins, 1949).

Richard stared blankly at the floor. He wandered about the hospital in a daze and appeared not only to forget all of his prior life but his wife, child, and parents and even his own name. No responses, whatsoever, could be evoked during psychological testing of intellectual abilities or projective techniques such as the Rorschach. He did, however, provide a single declarative response to Jung's verbal association test (1958), "Mine [evil] act." This single response suggested to J.G.W. an underlying enormous guilt. J.G.W.'s repeated attempts to hypnotize him failed. Interviews even with the use of sodium amytal (popularly known as truth serum) also failed to provide any information. Richard moved directly from light relaxation, into heavier narcosis, into a deep sleep without response to any suggestion that was offered.

He was sent home in the hope that familiar surroundings might trigger some return of his memory, but alas, he did not even recognize the town or any of his family members. This is an example of profound amnesia and is characteristic of many patients who flee their surrounds in a fugue state (Mullin, 1960; A. Barabasz, 1980a). Such patients assume new identities and maintain the changed identity at another location that has no reminders whatsoever of the earlier lives that they led. J.G.W. was desperate. He resorted to a powerful motivation to try to induce hypnosis. He used fear.

J.G.W.:   Richard, you went home on furlough, and you still were not able to regain your memory. Now you've come back to the hospital. You'll have to stay here until you get your memory back. If, after treating you here, we still cannot bring your memory back, it may be necessary to use very drastic methods. You may have heard that people sometimes recover their memories if they are taken back to the place where they lost them. If there is no other way to get this memory back, it may be necessary for us to send you back into Germany, back into the combat zone, into battle, in order that you get your memory back where you lost it. We hope this won't be necessary, but we have been thinking about it.

Now just imagine the effect of this intervention on a neurotic patient who has broken down under stress, who escaped from it all by adopting the defensive posture of profound amnesia. Of course, such things are not done with neuropsychiatric patients; nevertheless, the implied threat was there. We had no intention of sending him back. The battle had been won, but more than half a century ago men in the Army were accustomed to the idea that almost anything might happen, and thus a tremendous fear was evoked in Richard, a fear that could be strong enough to break through this amnesic barrier. Even then, the ethics of such a maneuver were certainly debatable, but at the time it was perceived that the problem was such that we had a need to rescue the patient from himself and send him home. It was hoped that reality would reward a more normal adjustment.

In the next induction attempt, J.G.W. used a postural-sway technique, which was successful (see Barabasz & Watkins, 2005, Chapter 6, p. 149–154). Richard went into hypnosis, which was then progressively deepened. The ability to hypnotize him was in itself a breakthrough for this patient. J.G.W. reported spending almost an hour regressing him to various periods in his life, from preschool up to his marriage and entrance into the Army. He then relived his trip across the Atlantic and then his transportation to the battle-front in France. Richard was next brought up to the actual combat scene that preceded his breakdown, and he abreactivly relived it. His emotional pain and stress was obvious. He began to writhe and twitch.

R.B.: They're shooting, they're shooting all kinds of shells. It's just hell. I am scared to death, but I have got to go on, I have got to go on. Hey, they've got our range now, look out! That one was really close. I can hardly hear myself think. They're all too damned close! They've hit everyone on both sides of me. Huh—that's funny. I don't know much. Everything has gone black. All in a daze now. I am in a dream. I can see myself going back to the hospital, hospital, … .

We had no information to suggest such underlying dynamics of the patient's profound amnesia other than the need to escape from what was obviously an intolerable combat situation. J.G.W. had hoped to do more analytic explora-tion but the requirements at the time, that men be discharged from service in the Army as soon as possible, mandated his premature release. He had him relive his presenting symptom, amnesia, by a rather desperate pressure tac-tic involving evoked fear. Richard worked through the apparent precipitation trauma but J.G.W. never knew much about his personality structure.

J.G.W. wrote follow-up letters to many of his former patients to try to check up on their postdischarge adjustment. Several months later, J.G.W. received the following note: "Dear sir: My husband received your letter some time ago but refused to answer it." Obviously, Richard was not about to forgive J.G.W. for dragging him back to reality, a more-than-reasonable passive-aggressive resistance. The letter went on, "So I will. He is just fine, has no trouble at all. Maybe a few headaches when he first returned, but that is all. I think drinking was mostly the cause of them. You see, my husband is mean, very, very mean. Those who are good have to suffer. He went to a specialist, the doctor found nothing wrong with him. His mother tells me that he is just as well as he ever was before he entered the Army." The letter was signed by Richard's wife.

Would the patient, his family, and society have been better served if we had let the amnesia remain intact? He could have spent his days in a veteran's hospital facility, and his family would have received a pension.

Much later, J.G.W. was afforded the opportunity to relieve amnesia in the more classical hypnoanalytic fashion by uncovering the underlying psychodynamics, working through to a more permanent and happy resolution. The technique is illustrative in that it teaches a number of techniques that can be used in dealing with functional amnesias.

Will [After walking into J.G.W.'s office]:   You do hypnosis?

J.G.W.:   Well, yes, sometimes.

W.:   This memory [pointing to his head], it's all gone. I was in a motor-cycle accident, but I don't remember being in it. I've also got a plate in my head. [He then rubbed the left side of his skull.] My head got bashed in here quite a bit.

Given that this was a left parietal injury, it is not surprising that he also manifested considerable aphasia. He understood everything said to him, but could not think of or speak many specific words. Will had much medical treatment and failed efforts at rehabilitation. No other neurological studies were then contemplated, and he had been written off as a stabilized, organic "vegetable."

J.G.W.'s new graduate class in hypnotherapy had just started at the University of Montana. Will agreed to being treated while a video camera monitored the therapy session for viewing by the class in another room. This was the first of 10 sessions, during which his amnesia was resolved and a satisfactory work and life adjustment established. In view of the severe known organic pathology, no such outcome was envisioned at the time. The presenting disorder was not functional but organic; hence, we should not expect a hypnoanalytic/hypnotherapeutic technique to overcome the brain damage. But Will was motivated and very cooperative.

J.G.W.:   Will, have you been able to work since the accident?

W.:   I haven't had a job. No.

He then went on to describe how he existed on a small pension, didn't go out to see movies or go out with friends, and just sat around at home. He then gloomily said, "A real dull life."

Thirty-five minutes were spent in hypnotizing Will and regressing him to a time prior to his accident 2 years earlier when he was in the Navy.

J.G.W.:   Will, you are forgetting all about what year it is and how old you are. You are going back to a time when you were in the Navy. You're on a ship. What can you see?

W.:   Water.

    J.G.W. note: His first memory.

    A.F.B. note: Recognize this could merely be a confabulation; obviously,
a ship would in all likelihood be in the water.

J.G.W.:   You are talking to a friend. What is he saying? [A projective
        technique]

W.:   "Hey, Mac, how's the guns holding up?" [A gunner's mate, Will then
        described an interaction with his buddy in some detail—an exercise
        in "warming-up" reconstructed memory.]

From this point, J.G.W. proceeded with the patient's visit to San Francisco, where he recalled the bar wouldn't serve him a drink because of his age, which is unlikely to be a confabulated memory. He then described his "liberty" in Sydney, Australia. He described the "pretty thing" over the harbor but because of his aphasia couldn't use the word "bridge" until it was called to his attention. J.G.W. attempted to stimulate recall first but then followed up when it was not successful with attempts at securing recognition.

J.G.W.:   Did you go to a nightclub? Meet any girls?

W.:   Oh, yes. There were plenty of girls. [Will grinned.]

The grin in the above recall brought on a marked change in his previously flat affect. His once listless features became more animated. He spontaneously remembered going to Saigon (now Ho Chi Minh City) then to Hong Kong; he described the floating restaurants and the Tiger Balm gardens. Next, he recalled his travels to Honolulu. He waxed eloquent over the fact that they could "surf, and surf, and surf."

Will was next regressed to the age of 7, where he without pause named his teacher and a number of his classmates in the second grade, and after that to the fifth grade at age 10, where he also named his teacher. This suggested to J.G.W. that the patient was not mentally retarded (recall that the IQ test could not be administered with any success) and that he had progressed through school apparently normally. A.F.B. believes it is important to note that J.G.W.'s technique of going back to an earlier grade first is precisely opposite to that which we usually use in experimental situations, where it is assumed we can go back to grades nearer to the patient's present age first and progressively work backward in the age regress periods. In cases of amnesia, just the opposite, demonstrated by J.G.W., is the procedure of choice, as the earlier memories are more likely to remain intact.

Other events in his life were reconstructed and relived at home, with playmates, and in high school; he spontaneously described his graduation.

J.G.W. had sampled a wide number of times and events in the patient's life that he had successfully reconstructed. The amnesia had been breeched on a broad front. He was then asked the following:

J.G.W.: Will, when I count up to five would you be willing to become alert and remember everything we have talked about, your service in the Navy, San Diego, San Francisco, Sydney, Australia, Hong Kong, Honolulu, your school days in the second and fifth grades, your friends and playmates, and your graduation? Would you be willing to remember all these things?

   A.F.B. comment: Always the psychotherapist, J.G.W. allows for pathological resistance potential to maintain a resonate relationship with the
patient. Resonate relationships will be discussed in chapters 10, 11, and 12.

W. [Without hesitation]: Yes!
J.G.W.: O.K., you can remember all these things and you can remember a lot more.
W. [Emerging from hypnosis in astonishment and
with the utmost excitement]: Egad! I can remember. I really can remember! Egad!

Will then proceeded to recount the many details that had been reconstructed while in hypnosis. He also expanded his memory greatly and described many, many other events in his life. The amnesic barriers had been broken. However, it had all been through direct hypnotic suggestion. The question arises as to whether there could be other psychodynamic reasons that were involved in this symptom besides the known brain trauma. The comparative ease with which J.G.W.'s intervention succeeded suggests all the more that much of the amnesia was due to some form of repression rather than the organic brain trauma and damage it involved. Will left the session with apparent happiness, and this was just his second session.

W. [At the beginning of the fourth session]: I got my driver's license.
J.G.W. [Startled, but reverting to the counseling
technique of simple reflection in his disbelief]: You got your driver's license?

Will hadn't driven a car for over 2 years, but after only three sessions of directive hypnotherapy, he had apparently not only reconstructed much of his memory but his helplessness and dependent behavior had also disappeared. On his own, he had gone out, volunteered for the driver's license test, and passed it. He also demonstrated remarkable perseverance in that he had failed the driving test twice in a row before passing it. J.G.W. noted that he had never seen such a profound apparent recovery in so short a time. These things rarely happen to a psychotherapist. J.G.W. could not get over it, but kept returning and obsessively asking the same questions about his recovery. The videotapes of the sessions thus far were reviewed over and over again. Will's aphasia remained, but not the amnesia nor the passive, defeatist attitudes of his immediate past.

In Will's fourth session, J.G.W. rehypnotized him. In the third session, Will had been told that his accident occurred when returning home from attending the funeral of a buddy, who was killed in a motorcycle accident 3 days before. Will was now regressed to the funeral.

J.G.W.:   You are at the funeral, Will. What is happening?

A.F.B. note: While placement at the funeral is highly directive, J.G.W. keeps the range of potential responses entirely open within that circumscribed event.

W.:   My buddies are there. It's quiet. There's a body in a funeral case in front. We are all praying for him.

A.F.B. note: Word substitutions are often common adaptations/ defenses for those suffering with aphasia; here he substitutes the word "case" for "casket."

J.G.W.:   You're feeling just like you did at the funeral.

J.G.W. note: An affect bridge.
A.F.B. note: J.G.W. is trying to set the stage for an abreaction by evoking the patient's emotion at the time.

J.G.W.:   You are thinking out loud. What are you thinking?
W.:   My god! Why in the hell do I have this motorcycle? Get rid of the damn thing or it will be my death, too.
J.G.W. [*This time using a simple reflection/reflection of feeling with the tone of voice*]:   Get rid of the damn cycle or it will be your death.

There is no further emotional abreaction; Will simply ruminates more about the situation at the funeral.

J.G.W.:   We're at the end of the funeral. What happens next?
W.:   We're going to bury him. He's being buried. There goes Ivan. There goes Ivan.
J.G.W.:   What are you thinking, Will?
W.:   I wish I could be in his place.
J.G.W.:   Why?

W. [*Apparently unable or refusing via resistance to answer*]: We're going home now.

J.G.W.: Where is your cycle?

W.: Just off the burying ground. [Spontaneously, Will re-enacts getting on his bike, holds his hand in front of him as if on the handlebars. He sadly talks about Ivan. When asked, he indicates what street he is on. Then, suddenly, he comes up behind a truck, which is stopped.]

W.: Damned truck! [Will pulls out into the left lane to pass the truck impulsively and faces another truck coming the other way and manifests extreme anxiety.]

J.G.W.: What's the matter?

W.: I am having an accident.

J.G.W.: Look out! Look out!

> *A.F.B. note: Perhaps in hopes of precipitating an abreactive resolution of the trauma situation, J.G.W. attempts to keep the patient in contact with the trauma of the accident. Will, instead, suddenly slumps back into his chair and is totally silent. (This is not a defense. He was knocked unconscious by the collision.) Resistance is difficult to overcome. Psychotherapists must be both patient and unwilling to give up therapeutic efforts and the provision of a safe environment for the patient.*

J.G.W. [*After pausing for a while*]: Good morning, Will. How are you feeling today? [Talking to Will as if he was visiting him in the hospital.]

W.: I wasn't even paying any mind. The accident shouldn't have happened.

J.G.W. engages in a series of counseling assurance/reassurance leads before asking Will if he would be willing to remember the entire incident clearly when J.G.W. alerted him. Will agreed. He was then counted out of trance.

W.: Egad! I had a dream about the accident. It's so firm.

Will proceeds to describe the accident and ended up noting that the next thing he remembered is waking up in the hospital. The many details of his early life were again reviewed as well. J.G.W. then rehypnotizes Will:

W.: Who's going to like me now?

J.G.W.: Why?

W.: Who's gonna like me, a dumb nut?

J.G.W.: So you think you're a dumb nut?

W.: No. That's just the way I act.

J.G.W. [Using a simple hypnocounseling way? approach here]:   Do you always
         have to act that
W.:   No! No! I don't have to act that way [anymore].

Will appears almost jubilant at grasping this point. He laughed with animation at his new insight. He is then realerted from hypnosis with the posthypnotic reminder that "it will stick in your mind that you don't have to act that way (anymore)."

In the sixth session, Will expressed further information. He was hypnotized and asked to dream about a situation. He then revealed that the motorcycle gang was also a homosexual gang. He had had heterosexual experiences and was deeply disturbed over his membership in this gang. He recalled he had been arrested just before the accident in a gay bar and was about to come before a judge the next Monday. In hypnosis he said, "They're going to hang me." Ivan's funeral was the previous Saturday. What was really at play here was that Will urgently needed relief from his punishing guilt. He was again hypnotized and this time asked to "go to sleep, and have a dream" about his problem. In a few minutes, Will reported he was dreaming about the motorcycle gang and their activities. I asked him how he felt about them, and he replied that at first he thought that what they were doing was "all right." Later, as the session continued, he revealed that he'd felt differently and said that for 3 months prior to his accident, he was "mixed up" and had a "feeling of disgust inside me." J.G.W. then began to use the Socratic counseling technique of probing, a rapid firing of questions but with the advantage of hypnosis. J.G.W. pursued the possibility that Will was suffering from considerable guilt at the time of his accident. Then Will revealed the accident was not an act of carelessness but an impulsive subconscious drive to relieve himself of overwhelming guilt.

J.G.W.:   When Ivan was killed, what were your thoughts?
W.:   I thought, look, if you get killed what the hell would your mother do?
J.G.W.:   Why did you think you might be killed?
W.:   Well … [Pause. Will was resistantly evasive.]
J.G.W.:   Was Ivan killed by chance, bad luck, or for some necessary reason?

   A.F.B. note: Risky, but clever, J.G.W. leads well beyond the content of the patient's comments.

W.:   I think there was a reason.
J.G.W.:   Because he was bad?
W.:   Yeah. That was probably it.
J.G.W.:   Do you think that if people are bad they get punished?
W.:   Yes, I do.

J.G.W.:	Was Ivan punished?
W.:	Yeah.
J.G.W.:	And how was he punished?
W.:	He had an accident.
J.G.W.:	Do you think that people who are bad might get punished by accidents?
W.:	Uh huh.
J.G.W.:	Then how about you?
W.:	I had an accident.
J.G.W.:	What does that mean?
W.:	It means I am bad.

A.F.B. note: A cognitive restructuring approach to this would be to challenge the non sequitur the patient has just revealed. The result would likely be intellectual insight if the process were carried out well. This is far too incomplete for the hypnoanalytic approach, which seeks true resolution, so J.G.W. continues.

J.G.W.:	Do you think that maybe if a person has one accident that pays enough for being bad?
W.:	Yeah.
J.G.W.:	They don't have to pay anymore. They've paid it off?
W.:	Right. [Pause.] That's right! [Will's affect changed; he seemed to be beaming as if coming to life.]
J.G.W.:	Then the slate's clean! You're not bad anymore!

A.F.B. note: J.G.W.'s tone here obviously would have been as a statement of fact rather than a questioning reflection of feeling. Recognize the very sharp contrast between the incisive analytic approach here versus the more superficial alternative cognitive restructuring one that would so often be used in such a case.

W. [Like a sudden burst of sunshine during a gloomy day, sheer joy swept over Will's face.]:	Yeah. Well, that's all right.
J.G.W.:	After a person's paid off his debt, he's free to be anything he wants. It's a fresh start!
W. [Exploding into almost a paroxysm of ecstasy]:	Egad! A brand new start. This dumb nut, not to realize that—egad!
J.G.W.:	And he doesn't have to stay home, does he?

A.F.B. note: Reconstructively, J.G.W. fosters independence.

W.:	That's right!
J.G.W.:	And he doesn't have to be, as you say, "a dumb nut" anymore?

A.F.B. note: Although J.G.W. has emphasized this twice before, including a posthypnotic suggestion, it is wise when a person has a lifetime habit or near-lifetime habit to reaffirm the point.

W.:   Oh, for crying out loud. Oh geez, I've been such a fool all of this time.

A.F.B. note: Many people remain like "such a fool" for much of their lives and never learn to function adaptively; Will's cooperation and trust in this therapeutic relationship has paid dividends that will last him a lifetime.

J.G.W.:   You have been punishing yourself.
W.:   Yes, and there really isn't any need. Oh, for crying out loud.

J.G.W. note: These expressions of surprise, amazement, and insight continued for some time. Will became deeply involved in reorganizing his self-perception at a feeling as well as intellectual level. It is important to recognize the emotion throughout all of these revelations rather than mere intellectualization and agreement with something offered up by the therapist.

J.G.W.:   Would you like to open your eyes, remember all these things, and think them through?

A.F.B. note: Cautiously J.G.W. allows for possibility of the reemergence of defensive resistances and at the same time tests whether or not these will still be regnant.

J.G.W.:   If you want to be a free man now, you can. Everything has been paid off.

A.F.B. note: J.G.W. reaffirms the patient's insights.

W. [*Emerging from hypnosis in a universe of magnified joyful expression*]:
Oh God, doctor!
W. [*Describing the change in his feelings*]:   It's as if a great weight was lifted off me."

J.G.W. went on to note that Vocational Rehabilitation had contacted him, renewing its offer to retrain Will and to help him get a job. Beaming with confidence anew, on that high note, Will left.

When a repression is at last lifted, or a dissociation reassociated, there is often a feeling of exhilaration. This phenomenon has been observed and recorded frequently by psychoanalysts. It represents a freeing of repressive energies that are at long last available for other ego activities. The patient has discovered a new-found wealth of energy. An enormous amount of both psychic energy and physical energy is required to maintain conflictual material in the unconscious.

Once released, previously repressed material seems quite familiar, as it is reassimilated back into the ego. Wilhelm Stekel (1943c) recognized that after having recovered (reconstructed) a previously forgotten (repressed) episode in their lives, patients would remark, "I guess I always knew that. I just didn't pay attention to it." The same thing occurs when a dissociative identity disordered patient reintegrates a personality alter. It is no longer an object, but a subject (self) representation. Accordingly, it is expressed as self. "Rhonda" (J. G. Watkins & Johnson, 1982), when asked several years later about "Mary," her previously tormenting alter, said simply, "She was me."

Counselors who have heretofore limited their practices to the person-centered orientation may well have occasionally experienced a similar phenomenon when a patient has, at long last, resolved an issue and concludes something on the order of "I guess I figured this out all by my self, didn't I? I really didn't need you. This was just a good place to come and talk." There seems to be an almost immediate reintegration of the new awareness, as it becomes part of the conscious ego. These phenomena are seldom, if ever, experienced in the realm of therapy that is limited to the cognitive behavioral domain, where the situation has been superficially reframed at an intellectual level so the person can assume an approximation of normal functioning. Putting a cast on a broken leg may allow one to walk on crutches, but to function fully, the healing has to take place at a deeper level—internally.

Will was again hypnotized in his eighth session, where we once again relived the accident. This time, he reported that at the last minute he had specifically (intentionally) turned his bike into the truck, not away from it.

After just 10 sessions, Will felt no need to return to therapy with J.G.W. but rather than terminating in the usual sense, we left the continuation of therapy entirely open. Careful follow-ups were continued over a period of the next 6 years. Will reported no more difficulty, other than continued residual elements of his aphasia (due to the physical brain trauma). There was no evidence of his regressing to previous maladaptive functioning. He became entirely self-supporting, having found a job and holding on to it. At last contact, he was leading a normal life.

Much was learned from this case:

1. Just because a patient has severe, known brain damage (even when manifested by aphasia and a plate in his skull), it does not mean that other symptoms, including amnesia, are irreversible and untreatable. Persistence is the key; we should not give up. Psychotherapy sometimes works with surprising results.
2. Although amnesia can sometimes be relieved by hypnosis when the proper hypnotic suggestions are used, deeper and more analytic

probing is likely essential if the gains are to be maintained over time and be translated into continued better adjustments to life. Notice the differences between the cases of Richard and Will. Contrary to the usual order in Will's case, the eliciting and working through of his repressions followed the suggestive elimination of his main symptoms rather than preceding them. Had we been content (as would be the norm in the hurried practices of most therapists, who are under the gun of short-term treatment by third-party payers) with the elimination of the amnesia after the second hour, we in all probability would have missed the opportunity to help him reach a new, significant, and permanent life adjustment, leading to an essentially normal self-supporting life. Hypnoanalysis resulted in considerably more improvement than could have been effected by suggestive hypnotherapy or alternative approaches such as cognitive behavior therapy.

Amnesia Treatment Protocol: As Illustrated in the Case of Will

Unless there is an organic basis, amnesia is the result of an unconscious conflict. The amnesia is intended to protect the patient from awareness of unpleasant and self-derogatory motivations. The patient "commits" amnesia to conceal certain conflicts from conscious awareness. Hypnosis is a primary key to unlocking such repressed memories. Because hypnosis is also a threat to breaching the patient's wall of defenses, it will meet with much resistance if presented as a technique rather than part of the ongoing resonate relationship with the patient. Although flexibility of technique and resonance are the keys to the treatment of amnesia, the following is intended to serve as a general guide to the steps in its treatment:

1. Introduce the patient to hypnosis with your choice of a series of hypnosis and hypnosis-like (Kohnstamn phenomenon) experiences as reviewed in Barabasz & Watkins (2005), Chapters 5 and 6, pp. 121–184.
2. Measure the patient's hypnotizability using the Hypnotic Induction Profile, the Stanford Hypnotic Clinical Scale, or the Stanford Hypnotic Susceptibility Scale Form C to determine not only the patient's hypnotizability score (the primary use in research) but more importantly to reveal the specific types of abilities the patient may have with regard to the experience of dissociative hypnotic phenomena as well as any specific triggering of resistances.
3. Hypnotize the patient and go back to nontraumatic events, that is, events before the trauma in question.
4. Begin with tiny experiential details and expand into broader areas (for example, with patient Will, you will recall the initiation of associative responding to "water").

5. Approach the trauma slowly, in great detail, as exemplified by the reliving of the funeral that Will witnessed. Get the person into the scene (e.g., "Watch the funeral; what's happening now?").

6. Suggest an affect present at the time of the trauma. "Your getting to feel and think just as you did then." Use the affect bridge technique (see Chapter 5).

7. Repeat important sentences ("Get rid of this damn cycle." "I wish I could be in his place.").

8. Ask the patient to express orally what he or she is thinking ("Think out loud. What are you thinking?").

9. Build up a "feeling state" by the use of repetition ("There goes Ivan!" as Ivan was lowered into the grave, "There goes Ivan!")

10. Develop a "we-ness" by involving yourself with the patient in what is being relived and what is being felt. This allies the therapist's ego with that of the patient and provides key support ("O.K., let's go get the bike." "Where are we now?").

11. Build up tension with your voice just as you would in a typical abre-action ("What's happening?" "Look out! Look out!").

12. Anticipate and respond to expected behaviors. For example, when Will was silent after reliving the accident, J.G.W. responded as if he was in the hospital and said, "Good morning, Will."

13. Review reconstructed material both in hypnosis and after normal alertness has been reestablished. Repeat it at later sessions. Do not let the material slip back into amnesia. Remember the patient has much practice with the amnesic defensive maneuvers; repetition, once brought to consciousness, essentially prevents the key information from slipping back into repression. Reiterate the reconstructed events.

14. Always interact with your patient at the level of the patient in both vocabulary and thinking, and at the level of his or her various child states when using regression. When involved in the "we-ness" of the resonate relationship, you are strengthening the patient's ego by being with the patient rather than serving as a "teaching" mentor.

As the patient's therapeutic mentor you must live the experience in the closest possible resonance with your patient to be most effective.

Dissociative Identity Disorder (Multiple Personality)

Almost invariably, patients suffering from this disorder report much abuse during childhood: physical, sexual, and/or psychological. Such trauma elicits dissociation, complicating and preventing the necessary working through of the traumatic memories. Dissociative identity disorders include what was formerly termed "multiple personality," dissociative amnesia, acute PTSD,

ASD, and fugue. Dissociation is also seen in consciousness disorders such as depersonalization disorder and dissociative trance disorder. All may result in an array of symptoms that affect both interpersonal as well as intrapsychic adaptability to the environment. The acute response may be an adaptive and useful means of putting aside threat cues so the person can respond adaptively in the moment, but the persistence of this dissociation influences long-term adjustment, which can lead to chronic dissociation (Kluft, 1985a, 1985b, 1985c; D. Spiegel, 1984). As D. Spiegel and Cardeña (1991) pointed out, these disorders can be understood as chronic and severe post-traumatic stress disorder (PTSD).

The severe abuse suffered by the child forces the abused child to learn that expression of anger back at the abusers (frequently parents) only results in more abuse (Chu & Dill, 1990; Chu, Frey, et al., 1999; D. Spiegel, 1986a, 1986b). Accordingly, the patient is more often female than male. She creates imaginary playmates, who serve as receptacles for dissociated anger. This permits the primary personality to maintain a "good girl" or "good boy" role in the hope of receiving better treatment. If early dissociations are effective in adjusting to a punishing home situation, still more may occur as new problems are met by the creation of new alters (personality entities). Most classic DID patients manifest anywhere from 2 to 15 different alters; however, some have been reported as exhibiting many more, perhaps even a hundred. Such larger numbers appeared when the diagnosis was less clearly defined in reports of case studies published a hundred years ago by Prince (1906) and again later, a half century ago, by Thigpen and Cleckley (1957).

The key mechanism in dissociative disorders is the separation of one personality segment from another by a relatively impermeable barrier. There is often a shifting from one state to another. The primary or "executive" personality is generally unaware of what has happened when one of the secondary or "alter" personalities has emerged and takes over the behavior and the patient's thinking. Frequently, the patient may report no memory of what transpired between certain hours or certain days. The primary personality entity is usually not aware, at least before treatment, of the thoughts and actions of the alters. The alters are quite often aware of everything said and done by the primary state. They sometimes will "communicate" with the primary executive personality through dreams or "internal voices."

Dissociative identity disorders can be traced back to reports in the Middle Ages. Then it was typically considered "demon possession." Some of these reports are quite fascinating but beyond the scope of the present text. For the interested reader, we recommend Ellenberger (1970) and E. R. Hilgard (1986).

Historically, dissociative identity disorders, particularly those at the level we would consider to be true multiple personalities, were considered to be "rare." With better understanding, improved diagnostic tools, and recent research, we now know otherwise (Bliss, 1986; Braun, 1984, 1986; Kluft, 1982, 1984, 1985a, 1985b, 1992, 1993, 1999; E. R. Hilgard, 1986; Putnam, 1989; Ross, 1989; D. Spiegel, 1986a, 1986b; J. G. Watkins, 1992, 1984; J. G. Watkins & Johnson, 1982; J. G. Watkins & H. H. Watkins, 1997).

DID cases have suffered greatly from misdiagnosis and mishandling. The average specialist in this area usually gets contacted by patients only after a long record of their having been misdiagnosed with schizophrenia, manic depression (a frequent misdiagnosis), or sociopathology, and having been in and out of many clinics and hospitals. Patients with borderline DID, who have some permeability among the personality entities (in other words, some awareness of their alters), often manage to function well enough to stay out of the hospital for treatment as late as their late 20s to early 30s. To that ill-defined point, even experienced clinicians and counselors would perhaps see them as having *DSM IV-TR* Axis II disorders, most frequently borderline personality disorder. Indeed, the bizarre behaviors manifested by such individuals are more tolerated (even expected) of younger members of our society. As such, desperately needed diagnosis and treatment for these patients, as well as their own recognition of the need to seek therapy, is delayed as the disorder becomes more and more firmly entrenched.

Many clinical reports and research studies have been available for some time. Unfortunately, the most recent comprehensive bibliography of literature in this field, listing over 250 references, was published over 20 years ago (Boor & Coons, 1983). The reader will have the opportunity to be brought up to date with the most recent findings in a special issue of the *International Journal of Clinical and Experimental Hypnosis* under the guest editorship of Richard Kluft (in preparation).

Given that DID patients are unable to recall parts of experience that are critical to bring to consciousness, pre-existing problems will be intensified over time. As H. Spiegel and D. Spiegel (2004) pointed out, there is evidence from experimental studies with hypnosis that a patient's lack of awareness of an increase in arousal intensifies the physiological consequences of arousal. As Kluft (1982) and D. Spiegel (1987) pointed out, hypnosis can be a critical aid in clarifying the diagnosis of DID as well as in facilitating psychotherapy because the induction of hypnosis can elicit dissociative phenomena. H. Spiegel and D. Spiegel pointed out that, although symptom activation is viewed by some as a worrisome side effect of hypnosis, it actually provides the best opportunity to explain to patients the nature of their symptoms as well as a means of accessing and controlling them.

Hypnoanalytic Treatment of a DID Patient

Dissociating in the face of acute trauma can be very adaptive at the time, because dissociating from threat can get one through the situation, but habitual dissociation results in avoidance of working through the trauma later. This can lead to chronic dissociation, which might be more easily understood as a form of chronic and severe post-traumatic stress disorder (Kluft, 1985a, 1985b, 1985c; D. Spiegel, 1984; H. Spiegel & D. Spiegel, 2004). Given that dissociation is a component of hypnosis, its use with DID patients is advocated, and there is research (Cardeña, 2000) as well as numerous clinical reports showing that psychotherapy with hypnosis is superior to psychotherapy alone (Putnam, 1992; D. Spiegel, 1981; van der Hart et al., 1990; Brom, Kleber, & Defares, 1989).

A brief case will be described to illustrate some of the hypnoanalytic treatment procedures that may be used. Jamie, now age 38, clutched a pillow and a small doll when J.G.W. first saw her in the hospital. She looked like a frightened 3-year-old, which in fact she was at the time: "little Jimmy." As J.G.W. gained her confidence, a mature personality emerged that described many instances of being abused as a child. There were also numerous blanking-out periods throughout her life. Gradually, J.G.W. became acquainted with other personalities: "Jill," who was forthright, strong, and friendly; "Megan," an idealized mother state, who pontificated as mothers often do; "Betty," who had good common sense, was jolly, and knew what was going on inside of Jamie; and a hint of a more malevolent personality, "Jeri," who would cut Jamie with knives or broken glass.

A key technique is to attempt to find an ally inside the patient, who can furnish reports of what is happening and the relationship of the various personality alters (entities) to the primary state, to each other, and to the world, who can make therapeutic suggestions, as well as describe the effect of therapeutic maneuvers, which can sometimes backfire.

Perhaps most important of all is to develop a friendly relationship with each of the alters, especially the more destructive ones. An alter that has been angered by a therapist, who perhaps has inadvertently or innocently transmitted a message that he or she might like to eliminate that personality, or more frequently does something that is construed by the alter as reminding that alter what the abuser did to them, can easily sabotage the entire treatment, unless the therapist actively demonstrates a willingness to honor that alter and take whatever the alter feels it must "do to the therapist." J.G.W. failed to do this and recognized making such a mistake in the well-described case in J. G. Watkins and Johnson (1982). Many errors occurred before J.G.W. learned to correct his intervention techniques and turn the malevolent alter into a friendly, cooperating "cotherapist."

After each of the alters had been interviewed in some detail, Betty became J.G.W.'s internal intelligence agent.

B.: I think Jamie is very angry at Jamie's mother, but is afraid to say so.

J.G.W. note: Jimmy was activated by hypnosis by simply asking for her. Her doll and pillow were placed conveniently near, and while she clutched them, I tried to talk to the frightened, intensely angry little 3-year-old.

J.G.W.:   Jimmy, are you scared? You're scared, aren't you?
J. [Eying J.G.W. suspiciously, nodded cautiously]:   Yes.

J.G.W. note: One must be close enough to give support, but not so close as to frighten the alter.

J.G.W.:   You've been hurt, haven't you?
J.:   [Again a nod, this time more defiantly.]

Slowly and hesitatingly, Jimmy began to talk to J.G.W. Gradually, we steered the conversation into the times where she had been been "hurt." First, an incidence of humiliation at home and mental cruelty, then more severe ones of slappings, then beatings, and finally even molestations. Her attempts to inform her mother were met by accusations of lying. In time, a full-fledged abreaction emoted as Jimmy strode about, beating the walls. J.G.W. did not interfere, hoping to exhaust this childish rage, and left the hospital that day feeling progress had been made.

But as so often happens in the treatment of DID patients, one may make two steps forward to find a step or more backwards the very next day. The supervising nurse reported that last night Jamie broke a light bulb and cut herself. Sure enough, here was Jamie, her arm bound up, but it was really Jimmy clutching the doll and the pillow. We had released much anger but not all of it. This, plus the guilt for attacking "Mommy" had provoked the suicidal gesture of an attack on her own self. Here, we see the dangers to a therapist (A. Barabasz, 2003a; J. G. Watkins & H. Watkins, 1984, 1988). Abreactions are required to relieve the anger, but once the anger is dislodged, it can turn back on the patient or others, including the therapist. Such patients can become both suicidal and homicidal, and the protective environment of a supervised hospital setting may be required unless the therapist can be completely confident in the otherwise resonant relationship with the patient. Nonetheless, the risks to the therapist as well as to the patient are real and must be balanced against the therapist's confidence in a positive treatment outcome.

Outpatient treatment can often be hazardous. If the release of dissociated rage becomes too threatening, a procedure developed by Kluft (1988), which is a slow-release or a slow-burn approach, or the split-screen technique (H. Spiegel & D. Spiegel, 2004) is recommended. These techniques permit the escape of the anger more gradually and spread it over a longer period of time (see Chapter 5 on abreactive techniques).

Given that Jamie was hospitalized, and because her eligibility for paid hospitalization was limited, we decided to continue the more violent abreactions but keep her under close supervision to protect her from self-mutilation. Numerous abreactions were initiated about different frightening and abusing episodes in the life of little Jimmy. However, when possible we would induce Jimmy to "share" or "give back" her memories and feelings of these early experiences to Jamie. We have found that when working with DID patients, this is the most effective approach. It was the destructive environment (people, events) that beat upon the child Jamie in the first place. This caused her to "create" a dissociated Jimmy, who could serve as a kind of "garbage can" for anger that could not be expressed without inviting more abuse. That is why it was stored up in Jimmy. Accordingly, it should be released in the reversed order. Jimmy should release it back into the primary personality, Jamie, through their internal boundary. Jamie should then be able to be the one to abreact it out into the external world, hence, "telling off" the mother of her childhood. This procedure requires a close, supportive relationship with a therapist who will "protect" her from retaliation by the angry mother. The mother, of course, is a mother introject, inside which she must not confront the outside mother. Sometimes the anger is displaced directly upon the therapist or a significant other in the patient's life who is benefiting in some pathological way from the patient's disorder and uses their resonance with the patient to motivate the displacement toward the therapist. No doubt, more than one therapist has been murdered as a result of this phenomenon. Recognize that a patient's significant other or even a "friend," for example, may well have a vested interest in keeping the patient sick to meet his or her own selfish needs.

Obviously, one does not encourage the grown patient to confront or attack the parent in reality. The problem is internal now, no longer external. It must be solved in therapy via transference.

So it was with Jimmy-Jamie. Jimmy existed to absorb the mistreatment, dissociate Jamie's anger, and protect her from further abuse. As the rage was released and dissipated, the need for a separate Jimmy no longer existed. She can be "integrated." This has also happened in these cases where there were many traumas and abusing incidents, and more than one "alter" split off. Soon another state (entity) emerged called "Becky." She, too, was loaded with anger, but apparently split off at an older age when Jamie was estimated to be about 9.

Betty, again, became a main source of information as to how well the abreactions had relieved Jimmy's rage, what were the backfire behaviors, the possible dangers (like who was planning suicidal or homicidal actions), and what should be the next therapeutic step. The cooperation of such an internal entity (term "internal self-helper," or ISH, by Allison, 1974) is a valuable resource to the therapist.

Becky reported the existence of another malevolent personality, called "Sue." We use the word "malevolent" to indicate that its present behavior was destructive, but remember that every alter or dissociated state was created to protect the patient. It emerges to improve survival as a better option when childhood suicide or a breakdown into full psychosis might have occurred. Viewed this way, destructive alters can be treated as potential allies. A.F.B. (2003a) viewed this to be a critical factor in the treatment of these patients. These alters come to protect; the problem is that their "protection" has become both ineffective and maladaptive (J. G. Watkins & H. H. Watkins, 1988, 1997). We must get Becky's cooperation.

J.G.W.:   Becky, would you please come out and talk to me?
Becky: What do you want?
J.G.W.:   I want to understand you and help you if I can.
Becky: Jamie is no good. She's bad, and I am going to kill her. [Becky looked most unfriendly.] And besides that, you don't want to help me. You just want to get rid of me like all the others did.

One assumes that when Becky was "out," the patient was viewed with great rejection by her family, because rebellious Becky was not the smiling, acquiescing Jamie. We repeated the same therapeutic strategy: making friends, then inducing release of anger through abreactions, strong-immediate or controlled-flow, just as we had done with Jimmy. It is not at all uncommon that as one begins to release rage and integrate one personality, the battleground will shift to another, all of which makes the treatment of dissociative disorders a most demanding and thankless task. The therapist must be resilient and confident in his or her skills and "love" for their patient.

To add to those problems, the therapist more often than not does not have the cooperation of other medical personnel. Nurses and even many physicians, including some psychiatrists, and psychologists with little knowledge or experience with DID refuse to accept the reality of the DID diagnosis. They haven't seen one, perhaps because DID patients do not reveal their multiplicity to clinicians whom they perceive as unbelieving and lacking in understanding. These patients have a history of abuse and rejection, and they are already in a defensive posture to begin with. Other, often less educated psychologists and medical personnel merely misdiagnose the patient commonly with borderline personality disorder, bipolar disorder, or even schizophrenia. The entire matter was debated at an American Psychiatric Association national convention by Kluft, Frankel, D. Spiegel, and Orne (1988).

The same is especially true in the case of psychiatric nurses. In the case of Jamie, one psychiatrist, whom J.G.W. had worked with earlier, was most understanding and took the necessary medical responsibilities. A few of the nurses were also supportive. However, J.G.W. often had to hear from the patient that "Nurse Ratchet" told her, "You are just putting on an act, being exhibitionistic, and if you'd only straighten up and behave yourself, all would be well."

Behavioral contracts, signed by the patient, not to engage in suicidal or self-destructive behavior are often used in psychiatric hospitals as well as many outpatient settings. Unfortunately, the staff seldom realizes that such a contract when signed by Jamie did not in any way commit Jimmy, Becky, or any of the other personalities to such control. When subsequent suicidal attempts were made, Jamie was then accused of "lying," not keeping her word, and so on. This is just exactly what her mother had done many years before when she reached out for help when being abused.

Just because a primary personality, like Jamie, may be sweet, compliant, and friendly, and look so normal, not hallucinating or manifesting deep depression, mental personnel who have little or no experience with multiples are easily convinced that this is all an act. One can spend enormous amounts of time attempting to educate hospital staff, sometimes as much time as it takes in treating the patient. Resistance to therapy may be as great in the staff as it is in the patient, and one may be simply viewed as pampering the patient.

In the case of Jamie, after 40 hours of hospitalization with frequent abre-actions, self-mutilation (cuttings), new insights, and integrations, she was discharged. Her alters emerged rarely and generally only when elicited by hypnosis. They appeared then more like normal ego states. These personality segments will be discussed in greater detail in the next chapter. Jamie's adjust-ment was now such that she could return home, hold a job for a period of time without quitting, persevere like an adult in a variety of endeavors, and, at last, properly take care of her children as a single parent.

A wide variety of abreactive, projective, and dissociative procedures were employed. Transference reactions were recognized and often interpreted. Resonant support by the therapist was constantly required. We cannot speak of a multiple personality as being "cured," at least not until good adjustment has been confirmed over several years. There is always the possibly of relapse to one level or another or a new dissociation occurring in response to a new environmental stress. This is how the individual has learned to adapt to stresses in the environment; it is the adaptation (or perhaps better thought of as mal-adaptation) that has been practiced over and over again. Psychotropic medication is virtually always contraindicated in the treatment of these cases. Despite these problems and potentials for relapses, DID, previously thought to be untreatable, can be managed to the point of bringing the patient up to the coping ability and adaptability of a normal or at least near-normal individual. Before leaving the hospital, Jamie made a plaque in occupational therapy. It read:

To Dr. Watkins. How do I thank you for bringing me through a time of fear, confusion, and pain? Your kindness, consideration, and help will long be remembered with fondness.

Thank you, Jamie

On the backside it was signed by Jamie, Jimmy, Betty, Megan, Jill, and Becky plus "Sue" and "Brenda," two alters whose roles we have not described here.

Jamie continued to emerge spontaneously. Some alters remained as ego states, and a few seemed to disappear entirely. Time alone can test how stable her longtime future will eventually be.

Integration versus Fusion

Integration is not the same as fusion. We conceptualize integration as meaning making the boundaries between the various alters permeable, thus increasing cooperation and communication, then returning the various subpersonalities to the status of "covert" ego states, which cannot be contacted except through the use of hypnosis. A normal functioning individual is aware of their various ego states; a DID patient (before therapy) is not initially in the situation where there is communication at a conscious level among the entities. We feel it is unnecessary and, in fact, contraindicated to attempt to "fuse" the entities into a unity, because this is not the structure of a normal "personality." A normal personality has ego states. Unless a person is a flat, colorless, one-dimensional individual, his or her behavior at, for example, a party is quite different than it would be giving a lecture or engaging in a hobby of mountain climbing, race driving, skiing, or playing Scrabble.

The normal personality has its "hidden observers" (E. R. Hilgard, 1986, 1992) and is divided into covert segments for the purposes of adaptive differentiation similar to mood states. Alters in DID personalities are much more resistant to treatment if they are threatened with fusion. In our therapy with DID patients, they can (if they wish) continue to exist as normal, adaptive ego states with loss of independence but still retain their identities. In the patient's internal "civil war," the "states" (like perhaps Alabama and Mississippi) have returned to the "union" as normal personality segments but they have not lost their identities within a "federal jurisdiction" of self.

How to Strengthen an Alter

When a personality has been split into numerous weak fragments, separated by relatively impermeable barriers between each state, the state that becomes executive (primary) has very limited energy resources to confront the problems and stresses of life. It needs help. In unity there is strength; in division, weakness. Such a person can temporarily maintain an apparently effective interaction with the outside world via the energy gained from a dependent relationship with a significant other. But as this is in itself maladaptive, it is doomed to catastrophic failure down the road. Helen Watkins developed a technique that can significantly change an alter or an ego state's outlook, especially when it is lonely, depressed, and perhaps suicidal. The procedure may proceed as follows:

Erika, a previously alcoholic alter in a 30-year-old woman who had been "rehabilitated," emerged during a depressed spell. She was discouraged and lonely, felt isolated from other people in the outside, and had virtually no contact or communication with other alters. She had suffered beatings by her significant other plus a steady stream of criticisms from him. Erika worked hard cleaning the house and cooking meals for her family. In fact, she was an excellent cook, who had once prided herself on her meals. It was the beatings that she endured as a result of developing a dependent relationship on him that had driven her into alcoholism and for which she had been hospitalized. However, she had not emerged overtly now for many months. She stated that life was not worth living, and she was ready to "give up," meaning commit suicide.

Erika was J.G.W.'s patient. However, the late Helen Watkins, my wife and colleague, was sitting in during this session to act as cotherapist. Without a formal hypnotic induction, Helen asked Erika to imagine "being in a peaceful, quiet room, just the three of us." Apparently entering hypnosis, through half-closed eyelids Erika nodded that she could see this. Helen then continued as follows:

H.H.W:	Erika is very lonely, she needs help. She works hard taking care of the children, cleaning, and cooking. She is very tired. Is there anybody there who will help out? Will somebody who is willing to help Erika please come into the room? [Some time was spent in urging before Erika finally reported that somebody was entering.]
E.:	It's Alexandra and she is holding out her hand. [Alexandra was also an alter who hadn't been heard from for many months. She was the artistic one and delighted in decorating the home.]
H.H.W:	Alexandra wants to be your friend. Do you know her?
E.:	Yes, I know of her. We have often worked together about the house side by side. But we never spoke to each other.
H.H.W.:	Ask her if she will be your friend.
E.:	She doesn't say anything, but she is still holding her hand out.
H.H.W:	Why do you think she wants to help and be your friend?
E.:	Alexandra is humiliated the same as I am. Her husband makes fun of her art just like he's always finding fault with my cleaning and my cooking. He tracks the house up with mud

	just after I've cleaned and then makes fun of me. Alexandra is so talented and artistic. I am no good and don't have anything to contribute.
H.H.W:	But Erika [Helen objecting], you are an artist too. You cook fine meals, and that's being artistic in your own way. The two of you would make a fine team. Why not reach out and take her hand?
E. [Timidly]:	I am afraid.
H.H.W:	What are you afraid of? She won't hurt you. Besides, Alexandra may be afraid, too. Let her know you want to be friends. Reach out to her.

Erika "reached out" to Alexandra, and the two of them became much closer together. Now, they could be allies in coping with an abusing husband, they could share support and energies. Erika was not so lonely and isolated now, and they had moved toward "integration."

This technique of asking for someone to come in and help can be used in ego-state therapy (see Chapter 10) as well as in the treatment in true DID patients. J.G.W. asked Helen what she would do if nobody came. Helen replied, "It's never happened."

Treating DID Patients (Multiple Personalities)

1. Interview each of the major alters to determine its purpose and function in the whole psychic economy. Determine how it regards itself and how it views the main personality and the other alters. Find out its assets and its liabilities for building a more integrated and functioning person.

2. Formulate a tentative general plan of treatment. Consider what the supports and stress factors are in the patient's environment. Which alters will work with you first? Which ones are probably the most integratable? What dangers to the patient, to the therapist, and to others are likely or possible: suicide, homicide, and so on? Can the individual be treated as an outpatient, or will hospitalization be required? What cooperation will be needed from allied professions including medical, psychological, and social? Are there other therapists available to help in treatment if needed?

3. Erode the rigidity and increase the permeability of the boundaries separating alters from each other and from the primary (main) personality.

4. Increase awareness and communication among the alters.

5. Encourage cooperation among the alters so they can better meet each others' needs.

6. Suggest, both in and out of hypnosis, that alters "share" their symptoms, strengths, memories, and feelings with each other and, most importantly, with the main personality.

7. Make friends with all the alters, especially the more malevolent and destructive ones. Recognize that these personality structures are, or at least have been, essential to the maintenance of the patient's coping, to at least prevent him or her from moving into a full-blown psychosis.

8. Release dissociated fear and rage by abreactions.

9. Insights must be experiential not merely intellectual, hence, affective, perceptual, and motor. Cognitive restructuring alone is ineffective, yet may produce what appears to be a superficial level of functioning, easily misinterpreted by others in the patient's life as curative.

10. Wear out dissociated affect by repeated abreactions. This requires reexperiencing, reexperiencing, and reexperiencing to exhaust the affect.

11. Strengthen the primary personality, but always provide recognition for the patient's alters.

12. Seek integration rather than fusion with each alter and with the primary personality.

Specific Tactics for Implementing DID Treatment Strategies

1. To erode boundary rigidities, name and talk about other alters when communicating with any alter and with the main personality just as you would do in ego state therapy with a non-DID patient. Educate each about the nature and the purpose of the others. Try to get alters as well as the main personality to resonate with the feelings and needs of the others. J.G.W. often speaks of them as "my friends," in the above example telling "Jamie" just how "my friend Jimmy" feels about a recent event. (You'd feel burned up, too, if you had to take everybody else's anger shoved off on you because they didn't want to handle it.)

2. Increase awareness and communication by suggesting that alters talk to one another or communicate their thoughts and feelings to the main personality through internal voices, dreams, written notes, and so on. Suggest to the main personality that he or she can call upon various alters, put questions to them, and ask for their help. ("Jerry, how do you think we should handle the situation?")

3. Encourage cooperation by suggesting that one personality help another. For example, "Dianna, Alex is getting very bored. He thinks nobody pays attention to him anymore. Why don't you take the children on a picnic to the park and let Alex teach Billy [the patient's son] how to play baseball?" Such activities may meet the needs of both Alex and Billy. Alternatively, suggest to an alter that "Georgia" [the primary

personality in this case] "has to go to court tomorrow because of that speeding ticket. You know, she is scared to death. How about you and Jennifer [another alter] giving her some help in court?"

4. Share strength, share symptoms, share memories, and share feelings. "You and Mary have many of the same ideas. Why not share your ideas as to how you can best deal with Father?" or "Make her [the main person]. Take back and share some of the pain she's been giving you over the years. Why should you have to be the one that gets all the anger-garbage? Open up the door between your room and hers, she really needs to be aware of how tough it's been for you."

Speak to the main personality: "Jimmy has been a real heroine. She's taken all the pain from Father's beatings for years. Don't you think it would be fair if you took some of it back and shared a few good feelings with her?"

The patient emerges from hypnosis and reports some depression and "bad feelings." She is not happy about getting them back but she can understand the necessity. Little Jimmy reports feeling better and is, therefore, less likely to commit suicide or some other destructive act.

5. DID patients are often aware of a precursor to the switching of states. It may take the form of a sudden headache, dizzy feeling, having a hard time "keeping it," and so on. These will frequently occur during therapy when one personality entity is being pressed too hard by the therapist to understand or accept some unpleasant interpretation. Soon, after the warning sign, the alter abdicates and there is a shift to another state. Try to be aware of this; it will become second nature with experience.

When patients come to recognize this warning, they can protect themselves from a possible switch to a destructive alter. For example, the patient is under some stress, perhaps during an argument with a significant other. A warning sign appears. She feels dizzy, indicating that the current executive state (primary personality) can no longer accept this stress and is about to abdicate, perhaps to be replaced with a suicidal or even homicidal one. By recognizing this danger, the current executive personality can break off the argument and go for a walk, so she can "calm down." The patient has learned a defensive behavior designed to protect herself and others, at least for that moment. Therapists should point out this precursor to the patient and note that if the stress is being caused by an offending interpretation, back off, unless forced change of state is desired.

6. Establish a policy of fairness and benevolence toward each of the alters but concentrate especially on winning over the bad, malevolent ones. A destructive alter is usually a very frustrated and hurt child state; how does one win over an angry child? At heart it wants acceptance,

understanding, and affection. Keep building up your relationship with this friend. A 3-year-old furious little girl was partly won over to the therapist when she brought the little alter a small teddy bear. After that, she was never angry at the therapist again. The prerequisites for constructive abreaction and building of new, less angry attitudes were laid. Never, never indicate that you are out to "eliminate" a malevolent alter, no matter how much you may feel this would be of benefit to your patient. It won't; no one likes to be killed off, especially malevolent alters. Bear in mind, those alters can completely sabotage treatment, just as a significant other in the patient's life can (J. G. Watkins & H. Watkins, 1984, 1988).

7. Release bound-up fear and anger through abreactions (see Chapter 5). This is the most potent technique of all, especially if it is followed through by true experiential, affective insight. These may range from a few tears through angry exclamations, up to beating on walls and smashing furniture. Once started, the patient must not be released until the rage has exhausted itself. If you or your patient cannot stand the violence, release it over time with the slow-burn approach (see Chapter 8). Alternatively, try the "poison pen therapy technique" (see Chapter 5), pounding or sobbing into pillows at home when alone, and so on. Probably the best procedure is to ask the alter containing the rage to release it into the primary personality, but this should be done through the internal boundary communication that is permeating that internal boundary. Get the personality to take it back, and then do the abreacting. This is essential. This releases it into the reverse order from which it came in the first place. The child was abused. It dissociated into an alter, withdrew itself from perception of abuse, thus anesthetizing the pain, and pushed the pain down into the dissociated alter. The alter must now give it back to the main personality, who then releases it into the outer world via crying, shouting, cursing, pounding, and so on.

We have found this format for the abreaction more effective than simply activating the alter and letting it abreact. However, it is possible to initiate the abreaction in the alter and then ask it to give "that anger and pain" back to the main personality, including the memories of the original events such as the beatings, molestation, or abandonment. The main personality may emerge angry at you as the therapeutic mentor for having to experience the dissociated feelings, but unless you have confronted it with more than it could handle, it will forgive you in time. In one case, reported by J. G. Watkins and Johnson (1982), the patient regressed into a temporary psychotic-like 3-year-old state. But when she returned to "normal" in a few days, she demonstrated a profound, constructive change, almost a recovery.

8. Find an "internal volunteer," someone to come and help a distressed alter or the primary personality.

9. Avoid attempting to fuse personalities. A normal personality is not singular in nature. Instead, seek integration. Integration, as we mean it here, involves returning the various alters to covert ego states (see Chapter 10). They become a part of normal differentiation and adaptation. They exist in the sense that they can be reactivated hypnotically, but they no longer emerge overtly, spontaneously. They report, "We aren't separate persons any longer. We are just parts of 'her.'" Nobody wants to be eliminated, whole people nor alters. When they are threatened with fusion, their resistance to therapy will be greatly increased. Instead, we promise them they will not be eliminated; they can stay and retain their uniqueness if they want to but as "states" within a "federal" self-jurisdiction. The therapist as mentor to the patient's personality reconstruction should endeavour to do whatever it takes to give recognition to the alters.

When one has worked for a long time with a dissociative identity disordered patient, it is usually quite easy to activate an alter merely by asking for it. One need not go through a formal hypnotic induction once this relationship has been established. Bear in mind, though, that the activation of an alter without hypnosis may not be quite the same as making it overt in the hypnotic state. The hypnotic state offers protection to the patient that is not available in the fully alert state of awareness. Whenever J.G.W. did an induction first, it seemed as if there was more progress. Perhaps hypnosis renders the boundaries of the alters more permeable. That means the communication with them will be facilitated, and the moving of their contents from one to another easier. Cornelia Wilbur, in her account of the treatment of Sybil (Schreiber, 1974), reported that although much of the therapy was conducted with traditional psychoanalysis, when she shifted at various times to hypnoanalysis, the work progressed more rapidly.

Recognize that spontaneous abreactions occur but there are signals of their approach that may be visual, auditory, or kinesthetic hallucinations, and even self-mutilating behavioral patterns (Comstock, 1986). Comstock believes that they have three major purposes: (1) to inform concerning past abuse, (2) to educate, such as the victim's recognition she was not at fault during molestation, and (3) to release repressed affect. The therapist must be ready to accept the strong transference that takes place toward the therapist.

Wilbur (1988) called attention to the fact that each alter within the MPD (DID) complex develops its own transferential relationship with the therapist. This means that one alter may be manifesting positive feelings at the same time that another is hostile toward the therapist. Or, hostile behavior may stem from different alters for entirely different reasons, greatly complicating treatment. You need to be familiar with the process of transference and sensitive to the many changes in which it may characterize the therapy of a DID patient. The analysis and interpretation of transference reactions is of equal if not greater significance in the therapy of dissociative disorders as any of the neuroses. Transference reactions will be discussed and elaborated upon in Chapter 11.

Integration

Every DID case has unique characteristics; however, there are certain general stages that the treatment process seems to go through. Initially, the therapist and the various alters need to get acquainted with each other. The alters may reveal themselves spontaneously, or the therapist may activate them: "Is there somebody there whom I have not talked to?" or "Is there somebody who can give me information about why Jan feels so depressed?" These queries can be made either to the conscious executive personality or, more easily, with the use of hypnosis. During this initial stage, which may take many months or sometimes even years, the therapist discovers who the major players are in this internal drama, and the patient's age and the event at which they first appeared. In some ways, what you are doing may seem like taking a social case history, but with different "people." Next, assessment of the attitudes of the respective alters is usually completed, which ones can be counted on for constructive help and which may be destructive. Other information that is desirable includes the likes and dislikes of each and how each regards itself, the primary personality and the other alters, and who is aware of whom. The patterns of likes and hostilities are determined. In this way, the social structure of the patient's condition can be determined.

Recognize also that, as this process takes place, the alters are also simultaneously assessing (sizing up) the therapist and building attitudes of like, dislike, trust, suspicion, hostility, willingness to cooperate, and even affection. All of this is not really treatment but a prerequisite to serious therapeutic intervention. It is in this crucial stage where the therapist can establish relationships that will move towards success or ruin his or her chances of helping the patient, perhaps permanently.

Iatrogenic Alters

As you no doubt know from your experience, bipolar patients can be enormously engaging, yet the phenomenon of multiplicity is far more fascinating. Therapists new to the treatment of DID patients can easily become so involved in "discovering" yet another alter and exploring it that this initial stage goes on interminably, with the patient producing more and more minor personality segments as the therapist reinforces these productions with tremendous enthusiasm: "Oh, so you are not Geraldine. You say you are Marcia. How great to meet you, Marcia. Tell me about yourself." One wonders if many of these cases, in which some therapist gleefully reports, "I had a patient with over 65 different personalities," are not partially iatrogenically created. One should afford every opportunity for important ego states to emerge, but one does not reward simply for the production of every new one. It is our experience that a limited number of alters or perhaps closely bound clusters, perhaps 7 to as many as 15, will account for most of the variance in a patient's behaviors. The resolution of the conflicts among them and "integration" that results either in their independent dissolving, or their close communication and cooperation through highly permeable boundaries as they become more normal, covert ego states, should be more than sufficient in most cases. It is not at all necessary to resolve every minor dissociation to achieve a functioning individual. Once the individual is functioning, these minor dissociations can resolve themselves on their own. All of us have repressions and dissociations, even the most well-analyzed.

During the second stage, "diagnostic evaluation" has, for the moment, become sufficient. Then the real therapy begins. The therapist should by that time have a fairly good map of the condition's "structure" (Emmerson, 2003) and have formulated a general therapeutic strategy. He or she will have established the best communication and relationship possible with each of the alters, including, of course, the most hostile and destructive ones.

Remember, every alter was established as a protective survival measure. Recognize that each one wants to survive, even the most suicidal. One can appeal to the angry suicidal one as follows: "Marianne, you came to protect her back there when father was beating her. That was a fine thing to do, and you deserve a lot of credit for your courage; you also took all of her hurt and anger then, and you shouldn't have to do this alone. I understand your hurt. Will you let me be your friend?"

The patient's defensive structures are threatened in this second stage of treatment. In the eyes of the affected alters, these structures are menaced by the therapist. Like an abandoned old farmhouse that needs to be demolished and then rebuilt, the multiplicity has served a purpose. However, its remaining inhabitants will strongly resist change. The patient knows no other way of coping and fears that giving up these dissociations will reactivate the brutality, pain, and anger originally suffered. When confronted with these recognitions, the patient wants to move on and flee but he or she is in fact fleeing back to the old familiar maladaptive dissociative structures. One can let "Mary" and "Meg" out of the basement hypnotically, but they may come charging upstairs wreaking their newly released violence suicidally or homicidally. This is the most hazardous period of the treatment (J. G. Watkins & H. H. Watkins, 1977). Be prepared for such dangerous acting out. Close relationships, constant communication, and supportive gestures toward aggressive alters: Sometimes periods of hospitalization as the patient releases the fear and bitterness are essential. Alliances with constructive alters and encouraging their potential life-saving interventions may be crucial. Be prepared for the fact that you may find yourself in continuous crisis therapy with the patient, perhaps for as many as several months.

Recognize though, that in time, the dissociated affects will be released. Bit by bit, memories will reappear, as little new insights manifest themselves. The patient less frequently threatens suicide or violence towards others, or less often abuses his or her own children. The time for integrations approaches. We use the plural, "integrations," because it rarely happens that all the alters suddenly disappear into one giant "ah hah" experience. Rather, alters who have much in common begin sharing their thoughts and feelings, and act in concert with one another. The therapist can encourage this with the use of hypnosis: "Why don't you open the door, Jean, so you and your friend Dorothy are free to go back and forth into each other's room?" However, don't try to force them into union by virtue of hypnosis when they are not ready: "When I count up to five you will wake up. Jean and Dorothy will not be separate anymore but will have fused into a single person." If they are too far apart, a new split may take their place, or more likely the patient will simply split from the therapist.

If personalities A and B are very much alike, these are the ones that should be integrated first. A patient of J.G.W.'s had two attorney alters. One did the research on legal cases and the other presented in court. After a while, the need for such a separation no longer existed. They could easily be integrated.

With A and B integrated, one might turn attention to C and F, who have suffered from the same abuser or have even much less in common, but not entirely different agendas for dealing with the problem. If C and F don't spontaneously integrate, the therapist can provide a gentle nudge with the use of hypnosis. But do keep it gentle. Now we have an AB alter, a D alter, and a CF alter. The patient is reducing the number of conflicting states, strengthening those that remain, building internal communication and cooperation, and developing whole-person responsibility for memories, affects, and behaviors that emerge in the "body."

The key "therapeutic motivation" for the therapist should be commitment to the patient. For the patient, it is the increased willingness to take "responsibility for self." Each learns and practices these as the patient slowly moves towards integration, mastery of his or her internal self, adaptation to the outer world, and newfound mental health and well-being.

The stress on the therapist is great, but it is rewarding to reaffirm one's therapeutic self and see the fragmented pieces of a dissociated human being coming together to form an integrated, adaptive person who is usually a very intelligent, talented contributor to society.

Summary

Dissociative disorders represent pathological forms of the normal dissociations that can take place in everyday life. They can be understood as chronic and severe PTSDs. These patients frequently have histories of severe and chronic abuse as children. Hypnosis, in part, is a controlled dissociation, which can be employed to good effect in both diagnosis as well as therapy for these patients.

Dissociated handwriting is a procedure whereby the hand is removed from conscious control and, by writing, can reveal unconscious or preconscious material. A variation is hallucinated dissociated handwriting where, instead of hand movements, the patient sees a dissociated hand writing on a whiteboard and reports what it says. Automatic writing is similar but is done without prior formal induction of hypnosis.

Amnesias are amenable to treatment with hypnosis, but when the symptom is removed simply by direct hypnotherapeutic suggestion, it may not remain eliminated for long. When symptom removal of amnesia is accompanied by or followed up by hypnoanalytic resolution of the underlying unconscious conflicts, recovery without further substitution of other undesirable sequelae is much more likely.

Dissociative identity disorders with independent personality entities are both difficult and time-consuming to treat. They are often accompanied by risks of suicide, homicide, or other violent behaviors toward the patient, the therapist, and others. They require substantial clinical sensitivity and skill in working with them and freedom from a significant other who may be colluding with the patient's psychopathology to meet his or her own needs.

Alters are resistant to attempts to eliminate or fuse them. Accordingly, integration can be more expeditiously accomplished if the boundaries between them are made more permeable, as is the case with ego states existing in a normally functioning individual. There is an exchange of information with such permeability and mutual awareness without eliminating alters. The idea is to recognize that alters may continue to exist as covert entities within an essentially normal personality structure. Examples include the hidden observer as well as ego-state phenomena.

Be particularly cautious about reinforcing the appearance of each new apparent alter. The therapist may iatrogenically stimulate the patient to continue creating more minor dissociations. It is unnecessary for all minor dissociations to be integrated before the patient can be considered ready for release from therapy.

Recovery depends enormously on the "commitment" of the therapist as well as the willingness of the patient to take responsibility for his or her own feelings and behaviors. The presence of pathological significant others in the patient's life can sabotage the patient's progress, sometimes permanently. Abreactions of dissociated rage should be regarded as almost essential in treatment strategy.

10
Ego-State Therapy

To paste a coping skill on the surface of an injured person is to further remove that person emotionally from the "self." The empirical-behavioral tradition, while showing immediate therapeutic results, has done so by ignoring conditions and behaviors which are mediated through subliminal, "unconscious" processes, thus severely limiting the scope of its operational area. Also controversial is the long-term permanence of [apparent] symptomatic improvements achieved through cognitive-behavioral therapies. ... In the past 30 years, a group of hypnotherapists, seeking to develop a more rapid treatment methodology, which would combine the speed and efficiency of the cognitive-behavioral approach, plus the depth of the psychoanalytic tradition, have been developing a therapeutic system known as ego-state therapy (H. H. Watkins, 1976; J. G. Watkins, 2003; J. G. Watkins & H. H. Watkins, 1982, 1986, 1997).

Mathew is in a new relationship with Emma. He sees Emma playing with a child. He feels and believes, "This is the woman for me. I love her and I want to spend the rest of my life with her." Later in the same day she criticizes him about his job as a plumber. He feels defensive and thinks, "What did I ever see in this woman? How can I get out of this relationship?" These responses may sound extreme, but they are not unusual, and it is not unusual for a person to bounce among several ego states in the process of making a major decision (one state may be in favor, one may be against, and another indifferent). In one moment on one day, Mathew may "know" he wants Emma as his partner, and in another moment he may "know" he does not. In this example, Mathew has an ego state that loves and dreams of a family. It is a soft, caring part of him, and when he sees the woman he cares about playing with a child, his "loving/caring" ego state becomes executive. While in this state, Mathew is capable of feeling very positive and interested in Emma. These are honest feelings. It is Mathew who is feeling them. It is Mathew's "loving/caring" part. Later, when Emma criticized his job, another part of Mathew is energized to become executive (comes out). Mathew's "defensive, don't pick on me" ego state becomes executive. This is not a loving, caring part of Mathew, and probably can't even feel love. Its role is to protect, by creating a shell and withdrawing from the attacker. While in this state, Mathew cannot imagine life with Emma. This too is a part of Mathew, just as valid and needed as the other (Emmerson, 2003, p. 2).

The human personality is not a unity, although it is usually experienced as such. Our personalities are separated into various segments. Unique entities serve different purposes. The state that is overt and conscious at a particular time is the executive state. Those states that are not executive may or may not be aware of what is going on at a conscious level. Conflicts among states take up considerable energy, often forcing the individual into withdrawn, defensive postures. A person, such as in the case of Mathew above, will not be "at peace" with him- or herself until the conflicts are resolved (Watkins & Watkins, 1979–80, 1980, 1996).

An ego state is "an organized system of behavior and experience whose elements are bound together by some common principle, and which is separated from other states by a boundary that is *more or less permeable*" (J. G. Watkins & H. H. Watkins, 1997, p. 25). Each is distinguished by a particular role, mood, and mental function, which when conscious (executive) assumes the person's identity. Ego states start as defensive coping mechanisms and, when repeated, develop into compartmentalized sections of the personality (Emmerson, 2003, p. 3). They may also be created by a single incident of trauma such as an auto accident, rape, or even on first day of kindergarten. Ego states maintain their own memories and communicate with other ego states to a greater or lesser degree. Unlike alters in people with dissociative identity disorder (DID; multiple personalities), ego states are a part of normal personalities.

The Evolution of Ego-State Therapy

Pierre Janet (1907) used the term *dissociation* to describe systems of ideas that were split off, thus not in association with other ideas within the personality. But, as discussed in the previous chapter, Janet's focus was on the study of individuals with true multiple personalities (dissociative identity disorder). He also implied that these personality patterns can exist subconsciously in normal functioning individuals even though not overt and available to conscious observation and experience. Janet, therefore, seems to have been the first to describe those covert personality segments with which we will concern ourselves in ego-state theory and therapy.

Often considered to be one of the first psychoanalysts to deviate from pure Freudian doctrine, Carl Jung (1969) also recognized well-established covert structures within the "collective" or "racial" unconscious. These were termed "archetypes." More transient groups of unconscious ideas clustered together were referred to as a "complex." Although the terminology varies from that of Janet as well as our own, both Jung's concepts of a personality "complex" as well as the more structured "archetypes" refer to personality segments that are organized into unconscious patterns.

Paul Federn (1952a) was the first contributor to systematically apply the concept of ego states to provide a psychodynamic understanding of human behaviors. His disciple Eduardo Weiss (1960) translated his papers, published them, and extended many of their implications. Neither Federn nor Weiss ever seemed to fully realize the great significance of ego states in their treatment procedures, nor did they understand that a different theoretical formulation was needed to comprehend its potential as a new sophisticated form of hypno-analysis. This became one of J.G.W.'s greatest contributions to the science and practice of psychotherapy, according to A.F.B.

Although Federn may have been the first to apply the ego-state concept, his theoretical conceptualization and approach was entirely limited to only ego-energized items. J.G.W. (1996b) was the first to recognize this limitation, modify the conceptualization, and develop the theory of ego states with his wife Helen Huth Watkins. This new theory includes ego-energized and object-energized elements. Thus, when they have become organized together in a coherent pattern, the ego state may represent the age of a relationship in the individual's life that may have been developed to cope with a certain situation (J. G. Watkins, 1978b, 2003; J. G. Watkins & H. H. Watkins, 1979, 1981, 1982, 1986, 1997).

Let's say your patient was severely punished as a 5-year-old. Becoming quiet, saying little, and withdrawing passive-aggressively was a way of handling the situation. Such coping patterns seemed to also work in later life. So when in "trouble with an authority figure," the adult now finds the 5-year-old ego state returning no matter how shortsighted, present oriented, and ultimately self-defeating it may be. As Hunter (2004, p. 88) pointed out, those with borderline personality disorder "still cope the way they did when they were 5 years old."

Thus, an ego state includes both ego- and object-energized elements, which we conceptualize as being encompassed within a common principle, a collection of subject and object items that belong together in some way and which are included within a common boundary that is more or less permeable (accessible by the conscious and sometimes, but not always, in subconscious communication with each other).

When one of these states is invested with a substantial quantity of ego energy, it becomes the "self in the here-and-now." We say that it is executive and it experiences the other states, if it is aware of them all, as "he," "she," or "it" because they are primarily invested with object energy. As ego and object energies flow from one state to another, the behaviors and experiences of the individual change, and we may assign the diagnosis of dissociative identity disorder (multiple personality disorder). Defined in this way, ego states subsume what we call "multiple personalities" but also include other clusters of mental functioning, which may or may not reach consciousness and directly change behavior.

The Most Significant Human Experience: Subject-Object

My leg is me. My arm is me. My thought is me, or is it if I am hallucinating? Subject-object, what is within my "self," and what is not, is perhaps the most significant area of human experience.

Perceptions refer to mental images and sensations that are normally elicited by objects outside the body. But a stone in the stomach and infection in the blood are also "objects." An arm is normally considered as "subject," part of me. But if it is paralyzed and devoid of feeling and movement, then it, too, becomes an object. An idea, a concept is normally subject, it is "my" thought. But a hallucination is an idea that is perceived as coming from the outside. The hallucination is not perceived as part of me; therefore, it is perceived as object.

Clearly then, the body cannot be the criterion for distinguishing between object and subject. The entity that does so discriminate is our essence, "the self." That which is perceived as outside "myself," whether it is within the body or not, is "object." That which is experienced as within "my self," hence, part of "the me," is subject. The "self" and not the body is the distinguishing agent, and the difference is judged by our feeling of selfness when we are aware of it.

The Self

The self and what constitutes it has been the subject of numerous theories as well as scientific controversies. Freud (1933) postulated a state of "primary narcissism," an inherent condition in the original child. Later, he viewed the ego as a structure within the mind, which was equated with the self. This was apparent in his topographic conceptualization of the mind when one looks at it as originally written in German. The ego structure was represented as the *selbst*, literally translated into English as the "self." Hartmann (1939/1958) regarded the ego, hence the self, as not only an inherent structure, but partially determined by the impact of the veridical world on the developing infant. Other object-relations analysts, such as Winnicott (1965), saw the self and its feeling of self-existence as coming about as the mother, who acts like a mirror that reflects back to the child his or her own experience and gestures. The child then believes that "when I look, I am seen, so I exist." When the mother resonates to the child's needs, the latter becomes aware of them. This awareness then slowly evolves into this sense of self. It is the "me" inside, sometimes working and serious, sometimes at play, sometimes in pleasure, and sometimes in pain. Mahler (1972) emphasized the maternal role in developing the child's self through a separation-individuation process by which he or she comes to know him- or herself. As the child interacts with mother, the child separates him- or herself to develop a unique identity and sense of selfness. The concept of "resonance" is discussed in considerable detail elsewhere (J. G. Watkins, 1978, Chapter 15).

Hartmann (1939/1958) considered the self as a representation or experiential construct similar to an object representation. Kernberg (1976) extended Hartmann's formulations to reserve the term *self* to "the sum-total of self-representations." By this, he apparently meant that certain experiences, feelings, and images that were endowed with self-feeling interacted with other images and sensations that were felt as "not me," but were also represented within the mind. This interaction was clearly embedded within the ego and constituted the self.

J.G.W. proposed a similar view (1978, Chapter 6) that "existence" occurred only when an object, "a not-me," impacted a subject, "a me." This was in line with Fairbairn's formulation (see Guntrip, 1961) that ego and object are inseparable. An object is not significant (i.e., does not exist to its perceiver) unless it has a bit of the ego in contact with it.

The classical theory developed by Freud in its original form posited that the individual was born with innate drives, sexual and aggressive, and that it was in the satisfaction or frustration of these that personality structure and neurotic conflicts developed. Analysts using this model, "the drive model analysts," operate from this basic assumption. These theorists and psychotherapists are considered members of the relational model school who have increasingly emphasized the role of interpersonal relationships as a basis for shaping all human development.

Kohut (1971, 1977) is one of this group who departed most from "drive theory." In his *Restoration of the Self* (1971), Kohut assigned the classical functions of ego, super-ego, and id to the self. He hypothesized that this entity was developed by the infant's internalization of "self-objects," meaning the significant people in the child's world, usually his or her parents. Through their empathic responses to his or her needs, they provided the experiences necessary for the development of the child's "self." This is an extension of Mahler's concepts, but unlike her, Kohut broke more definitely with the drive theory approach, because he perceived the self as almost entirely a product of interpersonal relations. The self expresses a need for contact with others, not sexual or aggressive drives, as conceptualized to be its basic motivational apparatus.

Because of loyalty to Freud, the founder of psychoanalysis, and their own wish to be identified with the body of classical psychoanalysis, the object-relations theorists kept trying to reconcile their new concepts, derived from clinical experience with classical drive theory (Greenberg & Mitchell, 1983). All of these practitioners were inhibited, at least to some degree, from proposing concepts of personality development that departed too widely from accepted theories. Innovative psychological theories that deviated too radically from Freud's, such as Alfred Adler's (1948), Carl Jung's (1916), and Otto Rank's (1952), had all resulted in the past with their author's being rejected from their membership within classic psychoanalysis. Harper, for example, in his classic book *Psychoanalysis in psychotherapy* (1959), referred to these three major theorists as "first-line deviants" from psychoanalysis. Kohut's views, which were probably the most progressive of the object-relations theorists, were more closely aligned than the other three to the earlier views of Paul Federn, who was a friend and close associate of Sigmund Freud.

The Ego Psychology of Paul Federn

Federn was one of the first to join Freud's group and developed innovative techniques for treating psychosis. As early as 1927, Paul Federn had proposed many of the concepts advocated later by the object-relations theorists. His work was almost completely ignored in the current controversies between drive model and relations model theorists, as he remained all but unreferenced by those credited with the development of object-relations theory. One gets the impression that they never read Federn, and it remained to Eduardo Weiss (who was analyzed by Federn and trained by Freud) to publish an English compilation of Federn's papers. The lack of awareness of Federn's contributions may stem from three primary problems. First, Federn wrote in what almost any upper-level graduate student would view as super-complex, long-winded German sentences. Weiss, who was J.G.W.'s analyst, once said to J.G.W., "Federn is very difficult to understand. That is why I had to write an introduction to his book to explain him." J.G.W. noted, "I had not acquired the courage to say, 'But Dr. Weiss, your writings are also hard to understand.'"

Another reason for the apparent unawareness of Federn's views in even the most read of psychoanalytic circles may be because the concepts proposed 20 years later by the object-relations theorists were being mentioned with the greatest of caution so as not to attack the drive model theory of Freud. They wished to avoid being alienated from acceptance within the classic psychoanalytic movement, as were Adler, Jung, and Rank.

Yet another reason may have been that Federn used alternative terminology to refer to psychoanalytic structures and processes that were then currently in normal usage. Federn himself was not fully aware of the extent to which his view departed from Freud's. At any rate, his theories have not been widely read or understood by the few who attempted their reading. Federn's theories, however, provide a foundation for ego-state therapy, a unified theory that integrates the use of hypnosis to dramatically speed psychoanalytic processes and its extensions.

After more than a quarter-century of development by J.G.W. and Helen Watkins as the primary formulators of the theory and therapy, ego-state therapy is now considered established. The first World Congress of Ego-State Therapy was held March 20 to 23, 2003, in Bad Orb, Germany, with the recognition and sponsorship of both the German and European Hypnosis Societies. Ego-state theory was again a central focus of the European Society of Hypnosis Congress held in Gozo, Malta, September 18 to 23, 2005. A second World Congress was held in Pretoria February 19–March 1, 2006.

Ego-State Theory

As you will recall, Freud based much of his theory on the displacements of a single energy, libido, which originated in the id. In contrast, Fairbairn (see Guntrip, 1961) hypothesized "the attribution to the ego of its own energy rather than energy siphoned off from the id." Hartmann (1955) also referred to "a primary ego energy," which was not derived from instinctual libidinal energy. Later, Freud hypothesized the need for two variants of libido: "narcissistic libido and object libido." Yet this still represented primarily two different allocations of the same energy source rather than two different kinds of energy. Jacobsen (1964) supported an initial state of undifferentiated energy, which then acquires libidinal or aggressive qualities. Kohut (1971), while attempting to appear loyal to Freud's drive theory, proposed that libidinal energy could be divided into two separate and independent "realms," including narcissistic libido and object libido.

All of these psychodynamic object-relations theorists recognized that Freud's single-energy theory, libido, was not adequate to account for the phenomena that they observed in their patients. Their tortured writings show numerous efforts to force these phenomena into a single-energy (libido) mold. Federn had broken with that position much earlier and had clearly formulated a two-energy theory, resolving many of the conflicts in understanding psychodynamic processes and thus providing a rationale for more effective therapeutic interventions (see Federn, 1952a). It also provided a rationale for hypnotherapy and hypnoanalysis, a consequence not envisioned by either Federn or Weiss.

Ego and Object Energy

Federn hypothesized different energies, one which he initially called narcissistic or ego libido and the other object libido. Later, he more frequently referred to them as "ego energy and object energy." He apparently used the term "libido" out of his loyalty to Freud and to gain acceptance from the libido theory advocates. However, the term "libido," as formulated by Freud, meant an instinctual sexual energy emanating from the id. It was also an object energy, because it could be displaced to various objects such as the patient's mother, who then became an object of erotic interest. The term "libido" was further extended by Jung (1966), who regarded it as life energy to differentiate it from that of purely sexual energy. To avoid the confusion, let us follow both Federn's and Weiss's later terminology and use only "ego energy and object energy."

Energy can be defined as an investment of a quantum of energy to activate a process. A motor is "energized" with electricity and then runs. Ego energy is the energy that cathects or activates the ego. It is the energy of the self. In fact, it is the self. Ego energy is what you are; it is the "you" in you. Self is an energy, an organic life energy, not a compilation of feelings, thoughts, behaviors, and so on. Ego energy has but one basic quality, the feeling of selfness, of "me-ness." If an arm is invested or energized with this ego energy, then I experience it as "my" arm. If a thought is invested or activated with ego energy, then I experience it as "my" thought. It has become part of "the me," and therefore, I regard it as within "myself." By calling it "ego energy" and not "ego libido," we will no longer confuse it with the instinctual sexual and object energy.

Federn's second energy was "object energy." It is qualitatively very different, being a nonorganic energy, much like electricity, radiation, and so on. It has but one basic quality. Being an energy it, like ego energy, can activate or make a process go, but any process or body part object energized is not experienced as "me." It is sensed or perceived as an object, hence, outside "my" self. Patients diagnosed with borderline personality disorder (BPD) ascribe only such object energy to other humans in their life space. To them, people serve a purpose, but do not have selfness. When confronted with others' "emotions" ("feelings," as described by one BPD patient), patients diagnosed with BPD can be viewed as children in adult clothing.

Kohut's (1971) early formulations showed no awareness of Federn's contributions. Thus, Kohut's theoretical and technical innovations were proposed within classical Freudian drive theory, with a division of libidinal energy into separate and independent realms: narcissistic libido and object libido. This is explained in greater detail elsewhere by Greenberg and Mitchell (1983, pp. 357–358).

Kohut (1971) and other object-relations theorists did not seem prepared to challenge Freud's drive theory to the point of recognizing that the concept of a single kind of energy called libido had to be eliminated to bring the theoretical structure to fruition in the treatment of patients. Instead, Kohut and the others continued to modify the concept of the manner of cathecting by a single energy, which determined whether a representation became a "true object" or a "self object." It seemed that at some level, Kohut recognized the need for a two-energy approach but could never bring himself to such a conceptualization.

Federn's concept of two different kinds of energy directly challenged Freud's basic views regarding a single, unitary "libido." As such, it has been ignored even to this very day by many psychoanalysts and was dismissed by Kohut (1977) in a single footnote (Barabasz & Watkins, 2005, p. 429) as "hard to integrate with the established body of psychoanalytic theory."

Neither ego energy nor object energy should be equated in any way with consciousness. If my arm has been hypnotically anesthetized, paralyzed that is, and removed from my self-control, its ego energy has been removed (dissociated). The arm is now experienced by me as an "it," an external object and entirely outside of "myself." If the paralysis is hypnotically removed and the "feeling of selfness" restored, that is because we have invested it again with ego energy. From this perspective, hypnosis is clearly the modality of choice for directing the various displacements of ego energies and object energies.

Existence is impact between object and subject, so consciousness in ego-state theory is an economic matter. When the impact of an object-energized element on an ego-energized boundary exceeds a certain magnitude, we become aware, hence, conscious of it. This depends both on how highly energized the object is and how highly energized the ego boundary is. We can become aware of strongly energized objects even if the ego boundary is lightly energized, and the impact of a low-energized object may become conscious if the receiving ego boundary is highly energized. If you stroke my hand lightly, I may not feel anything. If you slap it strongly, I become aware of the touch. As you develop a highly tuned listening ego boundary, hence a sensitive third ear (Reik, 1948), you may become quite aware of an unconscious and symbolic communication from your patient, which the more obtuse practitioner will completely miss.

Introjection and identification depend on the allocation of object or ego energies. When I introject an outside person—perhaps my father—I have erected a mental image, a replica or representation of my father based on my perceptions of him. This introject is an object because at this time, it is invested with object energy. If my father was a critical person, at the time that I introjected him I will feel (perhaps unconsciously) the lash of his criticism, within which I may simply experience as depression. It, a "not-me," is critically and harmfully impacting "the me." There may also be an introject of a partner, or friend. These are always persons who are, or least have been, meaningful at some time in your patient's life. The patient is frequently astounded at the emotions they experience while an introject is executive, yet by such experiencing in the first person, the patient develops a better understanding of that introject and their limitations.

Introjects are not ego states(Watkins & Watkins, 1997). They are not part of the patient's personality, yet they can be treated in much the same way as an ego state is, and perhaps most importantly, they can change to bring greater health to the patient's adaptability and functioning in life (Barabasz, 2003b). Introjects can be scary, abusive and threatening, or kind and helpful. As Emmerson (2004, p. 12) pointed out, when the significant person in the person's life was benevolent, an introject will then also be benevolent. However, an introject that had been internalized as cold and scary may, through ego-state negotiation, become warm and caring. Thus, it is frequently helpful for ego states to be encouraged in therapy to express themselves as introjects. The hypnotized client can express feelings toward the malevolent introject by being encouraged to speak to those interjected emotions and tell them their true feeling: "You only let me hear what he said to me from my ex-boyfriend's opinion. That made me lose it [my temper] and smash things. I couldn't think sanely and think maybe there is another way to understand what he was trying to say. Couldn't think, so you made me say horrible swearing things to one of the most decent, protective, and forgiving guys I'll ever know, What you did to me was wrong!"

No doubt you will have at one time heard the phrase, "If you can't beat 'em, join 'em." Psychodynamically, we call it "identification with the aggressor (Watkins & Watkins, 1978)." For example, let us say you are employing ego-state therapy to treat a patient with borderline personality disorder. You know the disorder was developed in your patient due to abandonment of a significant other, usually a parent, regardless of whether there may or may not have been a good reason for that abandonment (e.g., military service). The child fixates at the age at which the abandonmentoccurred and internalizes the concept that they deserve to be abandoned as they must have been bad or doing wrong. Accordingly, to escape the internal criticism, which as in the case above may have been expressed as depression, I may "identify" with my father. Hence, a common pattern in borderline patients is choosing a series of psychologically or physically abusive, controlling significant others.

What happens here is that I remove the object from this representation and invest it instead with ego energy. I infuse the representation with the feeling of selfness. The introject is no longer a "not-me" object but instead has become part of "the me." I experience it within myself. I am no longer depressed by my father's introjected criticisms, but I am now critical of my own children. The content of the "introject" has not been changed. It has now become an "identofact," a part of "my" self. I have become like my father, and the neighbors say, "He is just like his father." In so identifying with such a significant other, your patient becomes sicker and less able to adapt in any overall sense; thus, maturity and healthy adaptation are precluded. In object-relations terminology, we might note that what had been an "object representation" has now become a "self representation." (At first, the patient sees the serious problems in the individual and then becomes just like that individual.) This same maneuver is possible with hypnotic intervention through hypnotic suggestion. Ego and object energies can be manipulated therapeutically to the benefit of the patient (see Barabasz & Watkins, 2005, p. 49, p. 177, and elsewhere).

Federn did not theorize nearly as much on the development of the self as on its composition and structure. For example, some object-relations theorists use the term "self-object" to mean an undifferentiated representation in the psychotic or the infant who has not learned to distinguish between self and object (G. Blanck & R. Blanck, 1974; Kernberg, 1976).

The object-relations theorists are sometimes difficult to understand because they often confuse introjects and identifications. Kohut (1977), for example, appeared to define the term of what earlier analysts called introjects of significant others, which at first are objects but later are changed into identifications. He believed that such entities are necessary even in mature adults who function adaptively.

In Federn's ego psychology, the term "self-object" is contradictory. A representation of a significant other constructed within the individual will either be activated by object energy, like an introject, as previously discussed, or energized by ego energy, like an identification. The child's "merger" with such "self-objects" may be gradual; a "representation" cannot be both "self" and "object" at the same time, because this is determined by the quality or nature of the activating energy. It cannot be experienced as "me" and as "not me" at the same time.

Hypnosis and Energies

Conceptualizing treatment of your patients on the basis of object-subject energies, hypnosis emerges as the key modality for moving and changing of energies. When one hypnotically suggests to a patient that he or she is now able to move a hysterically paralyzed limb, this may happen because ego energy has now been invested in it, changing it from object to subject, hence, bringing it within the self and back to the patient's voluntary control.

Similarly, by hypnotically moving more object energies into a repressed memory, it becomes strong enough to impact the ego boundary so as to render it conscious. Energies can also move into an object or process whenever we simply pay attention to it.

Federn himself did not employ hypnosis in his treatment, yet he foreshadowed its use in ego-state therapy. Eduardo Weiss, in his introduction to Federn's book (Federn, 1952a, p. 15), wrote, "Ego states of earlier ages do not disappear, but are only repressed. In hypnosis, a former ego state containing the corresponding emotional dispositions, memories, and urges can be reawakened in the individual." This was a rather profound statement for that era.

If a hypnotized participant's hand is made to wag up and down without conscious control, we have simply removed its ego energy. It is anesthetized and apparently not within the control of the amused subject. Its movement is now object energized. The wagging can become voluntary only if it is ego energized. Hypnosis thus becomes a very powerful therapeutic modality for altering ego and object energy changes within our patients.

Psychoses and Ego Energies

Federn's most significant contribution stemming from his two-energy theory was in the understanding of psychotic symptoms and the psychotherapeutic treatment of the psychoses (see Federn, 1952a, Chapters 6–12). Federn characterized a hallucination as a pseudoperception. The schizophrenic individual actually sees, hears, or otherwise senses something that does not really exist in the outer world. To the psychologically ill patient, these perceptions appear to be quite real, as can be well verified by the clinician or counselor who tries to persuade the client otherwise. Yet, the stimuli from these pseudoperceptions arise from within the patient, that is, the patient's own inner cognitions. They represent ideas that are normally experienced as subject, that is, as stemming from one's self. The psychotic, however, experiences them as object and similar to other outside objects that he or she sees, hears, or otherwise senses.

How can thoughts be turned into perceptions? Federn hypothesized that psychotic patients sense the contents of their delusions and hallucinations as real because they originate from repressed mental stimuli that entered consciousness without obtaining ego energy, not because of faulty reality testing (as graduate students are frequently taught and many in our field assume). Federn reasoned that the mental content, that is, the idea, was strong enough, hence, sufficiently energized to become conscious, but its original ego energy had been replaced with object energy. However, when it contacted an ego boundary, even though from the inside, it was sensed by the patient as an alien element, an object, as the perception of an external object, not as "my thought."

Thus, the problem lay in the weakness of the ego boundary. In the psychotic individual, the inability to test reality adequately results from an energy deficiency, a lack of sufficient ego energy to guard the ego boundaries, where the differentiation must be made for normal adaptation to the outside world. Federn's approach was intended to help the patient build more ego energy. Thus, the patient will be able to remedy this deficiency. That, of course, is precisely what we do with relationships, supportive therapy, exercise, and so on. In the implementation of such an approach, Federn often used a nurse, a mother-surrogate, who could provide the nurturing relationship normally received from one's mother (Schwing, 1954).

The mother figure is critically important because her nurturing in developing self-identity and stable object representations, which Federn and Schwing had been emphasizing, has currently begun to receive more attention. The significance of mothers as "transitional objects" in the development of self structures in infants was increasingly recognized in the late 1990s. Baker (1981), Copeland (1986), and Murray-Jobsis (1984) have employed many of these same concepts in treating psychotic patients within the hypnotic modality with remarkable positive and lasting outcomes.

Federn Psychotics: Reality A, Reality B

Now what was happening here is that Federn, and especially his disciple Weiss (1960), stressed the distinction between reality testing and the sensing of reality. We "sense" reality as something outside our self whenever an object-energized item impacts an ego boundary. However, to "test" reality, we need to move our eyes, ears, and body and note that the sensed object moves its relative position accordingly. The schizophrenic individual, for example, fails to take this action, relying instead entirely on his or her weakened ego boundary in a desperate attempt to distinguish real from unreal, thoughts from perceptions. Federn (1952a) reported that there is a felt difference between an impact of an object on the "inside" of the ego's boundary and its "outside," that which interacts with the external world. If this is also true, there would have to be a change in the magnitude of the impact. The psychotic individual then would be able to experience this "reality" of his or her reported experience when it is explained to the patient that there are in actuality two kinds of reality, "reality A" and "reality B." The idea here is to enlist the patient's cooperation rather than risk the patient's antagonism when being confronted with reality as if they were being accused of "lying."

Federn might say to the patient, "When you see me here across the desk, I want you to label that 'reality A.' When you see or hear those people who are persecuting you, I want you to please call that 'reality B.' Now 'reality A' is a kind of experience you can share with others around you because they, too, are aware of 'reality A.' However, 'reality B' is a private reality, which they cannot share. If you talk to them about 'reality B,' they will think you are crazy! Please do this, when you describe to me any experience, tell me, at least for now, whether it is 'reality A' or 'reality B.'"

Testing this remarkable intervention with numerous psychotic patients, Federn concluded that psychotic patients could, indeed, distinguish between reality A and reality B even though both were experienced as real. By teaching these patients to make this discrimination, he was exercising, strengthening, and hence reenergizing their ego boundaries. In time, not only did these patients make this distinction, but by not reinforcing reality B in the strictest behavioral sense here, reality B was de-energized. Reality B was then returned to the world of nocturnal dreams, wherein lie the consciously inactive "hallucinations" of normal people. By reducing the energy in reality B, its impact with self-boundaries became lower than the threshold necessary to become conscious. In Federn's conceptualization, psychotic symptoms were a consequence of the necessity to economize one's deficiency of ego energy. That is, a lack of ego energy meant that too much energy was invested in objects, thus investing object energy in nonrealities.

Psychoanalysis as a treatment modality is contraindicated for psychotic patients, who are already ego energy anemic, because it requires additional energies to uncover and integrate repressed material. However, for the borderline psychotic patient, an uncovering analytic therapy may well precipitate a full-blown psychosis, and there are more than enough examples of this to preclude the necessity of listing references here. This danger can be substantially lessened, however, if the treating therapist, through a close, intensive "therapeutic-self" relationship involving mutual resonance (J. G. Watkins, 2005), gives to the patient a "loan" of ego energy. The total energy available then may be adequate for him or her to tolerate the confrontation with his or her primitive unegotized material and reintegrate (egotize) it into self structure.

By positing a two-energy system, Federn provided a new rationale to explain many psychological processes that cannot be satisfactorily accounted for by Freud's one-energy (libido) system. For example, if a thought of my dead mother crosses my mind and reaches consciousness, but is activated with object energy, I will experience it as a perception of my dead mother. I will "see" her. And if I report this perception as real, others will say I am psychotic and hallucinating.

Years ago, J.G.W. was trying to explain the mechanism of projection to a paranoid patient. As we all know, that is usually a futile task. Much to my surprise, the patient smiled and said, "Well, Doctor, if you are trying to tell me that those men who persecuted me were a product of my own imagination, you don't have to. I arrived at that conclusion myself over the weekend." In utter amazement, I spent some time evaluating him before accepting that somehow, for reasons unknown to me, his delusions and hallucinations had disappeared. The patient's own unconscious hatreds, externalized into a perception of "men out there" who were persecuting him, had been de-energized of object energy and were now energized with ego energy. He experienced them as his thoughts and not his perceptions. The critical point is that a one-energy system would not give us an adequate explanatory rationale even though psychodynamically we are still unaware of just what caused this energy shift.

Psychologists and psychoanalysts frequently confuse subject and object. Thus, an introject is supposed to be an internal object. Yet, analytic writers portray a patient as "introjecting" another person when they describe that individual as acting and talking like the other person. The image of the other, when internalized, is at first invested with object energy. That is why it is an internal object. An introject is like that submarine sandwich you ate one late evening that lies in the stomach ready to resurface at midnight. It is within the self but not part of it, ingested but not digested.

For the individual to act and talk spontaneously like the other, the object energy must be withdrawn and the image ego energized. In object-relations theories, we would simply say that the object representation has changed into a self representation. Then we no longer have an introject; we have an identofact. The internalized has become part of "the me."

For example, a teenage girl "in love" imitates the behavior of her boyfriend, eating what he eats and regressing to earlier behaviors by acting as immaturely as he does. This action is at first an introject, of that same age as the immature boyfriend's behaviors. Eating like him, behaving like him, taking on his views are simply internal representations of the boyfriend, copied but not part of her own self. However, in the course of time, it may become automatic. The behaviors have become egotized, that is, invested with ego energy. It is now part of her own self. Her same-aged but more mature girlfriends watch her behaving like her boyfriend does and are amazed. If he lacks future goal-directed plans, she too loses focus; if he is opinionated, bitter, or selfish, she is too. She has identified with her boyfriend. An identification with a previously introjected other may be minimal or significant, depending on how much of the other's physical attributes or psychological behavior, as in the present example, is taken over.

As J. G. Watkins (1978a) pointed out, an introject is the result of the process of introjection, and a new term is needed to distinguish between the process of identification and the result of that process. Consider our use of the word "identification" when referring to the process, and the term "identofact" to indicate the internal, ego-energized image that has been created by identification. The girl described above has changed the introject, and object representation, of her boyfriend into an identofact, a self representation. This distinction between what is subject (ego-energized) and what is not-self (object-energized) in physical and psychological processes is crucial. The movement from one to the other is fundamental to the practice of ego-state therapy, as well as many other treatment approaches.

Personality Development: Integration and Differentiation

Personality develops through two basic processes, integration and differentiation. By integration, a child learns to put concepts together, such as dog and cat to build more complex units called animals. By differentiation, he or she separates general concepts into more specific meanings, such as discriminating between a cat and a rabbit. Both processes are normal and adaptive.

Normal differentiation permits us to experience one set of behaviors at a party Saturday night and another at the office Monday morning. When this separating or differentiating process becomes excessive and maladaptive, we call it dissociative identity disorder.

When we differentiate two items, both of which are consciously in mind, we can compare them and note their differences. In dissociation, the two items are so separated from one another that comparison is not possible, because only one is within consciousness at any given time. Both differentiation and dissociation involve the psychological separating of two entities, but differentiation is lesser in degree, generally adaptive, and considered to be normal. Dissociation, on the other hand, is considered to be pathological. It may be more immediately adaptive to cope with the stress of a specific situation, but often at the future expense of greater maladaptiveness. These two may be considered as simply resulting from different degrees of the separating process.

Ego States

To understand the nature of ego states, one must consider their origin. Most frequently, they were first created when the individual was quite young. They think concretely like a child. Adult logic, therefore, may not reach them, even though they often talk in an adult voice. It is as if they were frozen in time. Covert ego states, unlike the alters in a true multiple personality (DID) patient, require hypnosis for their activation. But, if they first originated when the patient was a child, then one should think of them like a small girl who is dressed up in her mother's clothes and pretending to be an adult. The ability to think concretely like a child has been lost by the majority of adults, and thus we are at a disadvantage in dealing with child ego states, especially when they are not so clearly differentiated as true multiple-personality-like alters. States that were created during the patient's teens will still think like a teenager, rejecting and suspicious of grown-ups and very defensive of their own (pseudo) independence; they do not want to be told what is right or what they ought to do. This characteristic will be more clearly illustrated in the case excerpts to be presented later. When working therapeutically with child and adolescent states, one should conceptualize to whom one is talking and conduct the interaction accordingly. The clinician or counselor who resonates well (J. G. Watkins, 1978a) will have the greatest probability of success.

Be mindful that a child ego state was developed to adapt to the conditions of days gone by, not today. Its attempts to function today result in maladaptive behaviors (short-sighted present rather than future-oriented actions). As one inquires and secures information about the time and circumstances when an ego state first appeared, one's approach can be modified accordingly, even though one is confronted ostensibly with a full-grown adult. This modification can be done, without embarrassment, by the use of hypnosis. The psychotherapist interacts as one would with a child when the patient is hypnotized.

Bear in mind that an ego state was most likely developed to enhance the individual's ability to adapt and cope with a specific problem or situation in the past. Thus, one ego state may have taken over the overt, executive position when dealing with parents, another on the playground, another when dealing with a significant other, and yet another when participating in a sporting event, and so on.

In the case of dissociative identity disorder, which is manifested by the presence of true multiple personality alters, the specific situation is usually some very severe trauma such as child abuse or traumatic abandonment (Watkins, J. G., 1984). The ego state forms to help in dissociating the pain from the primary alter or to make it easier for the major personality to deal with an abuser (controller) without inviting retaliation. It is to be expected that these specific ego states will be reactivated in the transferences of the present, such as to teachers, employers, supervisors, mentors, colleagues, and of course therapists (J. G. Watkins & H. H. Watkins, 1990).

A common trait is that, once created, ego states are highly motivated to protect and continue their existence. The clinician or counselor who tries to eliminate (kill off) a maladaptive state will find to his or her dismay that the entity probably does not want to disappear, but that one's intervention has now created an internal enemy who resists therapeutic intervention. Part-persons seek to protect their existence, as do whole-persons. This tendency has important implications in the treatment of dissociative identity disordered patients. Perhaps the most important point to remember is that it is much easier to constructively modify the motivations of malevolent and maladaptive ego states, and their behavior, than to attempt to eliminate them.

Persistence in existence is to realize that the original ego state came into being to protect and facilitate the adaptation of the primary person. It remained because it had a certain amount of success. And from what we have learned about behavior modification, we can recognize that it was positively reinforced, first for coming into existence, and then for continuing its presence. It makes no difference whatsoever that now its efforts may be counterproductive to the person. The earlier adaptations, which are now maladaptive, will hold precedence.

First, we must familiarize ourselves as therapists with the differences in the environment of the patient's past and that of the present. We cannot generally induce a state to change into an adaptive stance toward current adult problems when the treating therapist does not understand its earlier struggles. Recognition of these traits is essential in the planning and conduct of effective therapeutic maneuvers such as abreactions and fractionation.

When working with ego states, the internal equilibrium of the patient will change in such a way that a new ego state, or one that has been long dormant, will be energized and make itself known. This state may first manifest itself by slight changes in posture, mannerism, or voice pitch.

Using the explanatory value of Federn's two-energy theory makes it easier to understand. The nature of the past problems helps us to determine the creation and energies of the various states. The adaptational needs of the present must be met with the appropriate dispositions of object and ego energies assisted by an understanding and accepting therapist. Hypnosis is the key modality that facilitates this allocation of subject and object energies. The effective accomplishment of this treatment goal utilizing the many tactics of supportive, behavioral, psychoanalytic, cognitive, Rogersian, and existential therapies constitutes ego-state therapy.

Ego states that are cognitively dissonant from one another or have contradictory goals often develop conflicts with each other. When they are energized and have rigid, impermeable boundaries, multiple personalities (DID) may result. However, many such conflicts appear between ego states only covertly, and these are often manifested by anxiety, depression, or any number of neurotic, maladaptive, and childlike behaviors.

Ego states may be large, encompassing broad areas of behavior and experience, or they may be small, including very specific and limited reactions. They may also overlap. For example, a 6-year-old child ego state and a "reaction to father" ego state both speak the English language. They can range from minor moods to true overt multiple personalities, the difference being the permeability of their separating boundaries.

Ego-State Boundaries: The Differentiation-Dissociation Continuum

Psychological processes do not exist on an either-or basis. Anxiety, depression, immaturity, and so on all lie on a continuum with lesser or greater degrees of intensity. So it is with differentiation-dissociation. On one end of the continuum, the boundaries are so permeable that they are almost nonexistent. The individual's behavior is very much the same from time to time. The difference that does occur is generally adaptive, and we call it normal differentiation. As the ego-state boundaries become increasingly rigid, intrapersonal communication is impeded so that behavior becomes less and less adaptive. When

Ego States

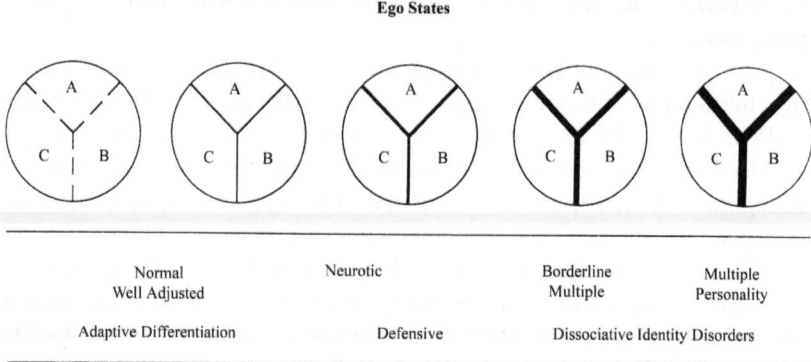

Normal Well Adjusted	Neurotic	Borderline Multiple	Multiple Personality
Adaptive Differentiation	Defensive	Dissociative Identity Disorders	

Figure 10.1 Differentiation-dissociation continuum.

we approach the end of the continuum, the boundaries are very rigid and impermeable, the behavior is maladaptive, and we call it "dissociation." At this extreme end of the continuum, the various ego states no longer interact or communicate with one another, and the individual suffers from a true multiple personality (dissociative identity disorder) if more than one becomes energized enough to assume the overt executive position temporarily.

In between these extremes (see Figure 10.1) lays a body of ego states that may act like covert multiple personalities, but which do not spontaneously become overt. However, they can be activated hypnotically.

As you look at Figure 10.1, note that just to the left of the true DID we have a borderline multiple. The various states are conscious of the existence of each other but refer to the others as "he," "she," or "it," and not as "me." This position on the differentiation-dissociation continuum represents a bordering (almost true) multiple personality and is not to be confused with the diagnosis of borderline personality disorder. The in-between ego states, because of the lesser degree of rigidity in the semipermeable boundaries, retain partial communication, interaction, and sharing of content. In general, they remain covert and do not spontaneously appear overtly, but they can be activated into the executive position by hypnosis. In this region, a conflict between the states may be manifested by headaches, anxiety, withdrawal, plus passive-aggressive and other maladaptive behaviors, such as found in neuroses and in psychophysiologic disorders. It is in this area where ego-state concepts have made the most productive contributions to psychotherapy. We are, therefore, concerned with a general principle of personality formation in which the dispositions of the activating energies and the impermeability of the boundaries separating the organized ego-state patterns have resulted in relatively discreet personality segments that may alternate in assuming the executive position, experienced as "the self" in "the here-and-now." The extreme form of this separating process, as noted above, can result in true dissociative identity disorders.

For some time, true multiples were considered to be extremely rare. However, as recognized in the *Diagnostic statistical manual IV* (APA, 1994) and in the more recent *Text Revised (TR)* edition, many reports of cases meeting full diagnostic criteria are now being presented. The disorder is still uncommon but it can no longer be considered rare. For example, borderline multiple patients are frequently misdiagnosed as having borderline personality disorders (Paulsen, 2007). This is fairly common and particularly prevalent among females and may be due to the higher frequency of abuse of females as children as well as gender-specific maladaptations to abandonment.

Characteristics of Ego States and Dissociative Identity Disorder

Ego states should be regarded as part-persons, except in the case of true multiple personality. They do not normally appear overtly unless hypnotically activated. There is far too much evidence to the contrary to call them simply therapist-created artifacts because they often differ widely from therapist expectations. Some act like complete "persons." Others appear to be very limited personality fragments, perhaps created for a specific defensive purpose. They may have quite differing interests, purposes, and values, even as do the various alters in a true dissociative identity disordered personality. Obviously, then, it is not surprising to find them often in intrapersonal conflict with one another, creating tension, anxiety, psychosomatic symptoms, the desire for flight, and other maladaptive behaviors. As one ego state put it, "I make her eat because if she is overweight, men [who are dangerous] will not be attracted to her." Covert ego-state conflicts may create headaches just like the quarreling of multiple personality alters who struggle to emerge and take over executive control of the body.

Although most ego states are unlikely to be therapist created, it is very important for the counselor or clinician who is working with either a multiple personality or covert ego-state conflict not to create artifacts through suggestion, hypnotic or otherwise. Although ego states will often give themselves names, as do true multiple personalities, we must be careful not to suggest names but let them emerge in classical Rogersian nondirective style. There are still many practitioners today who are hypnotically activating covert ego states and then announcing they have discovered yet another multiple personality. We often find covert ego states among normal students who volunteer for hypnosis studies (Watkins & Watkins, 1988). Even though multiple personalities are usually studied through hypnosis, they should be so diagnosed only when the ego states can become overt spontaneously without the use of hypnosis. We must consider it essential that there be evidence of amnesia in the present. For example, a patient with dissociative identity disorder (a true multiple) may say that he or she was reported to have been at a sporting event yesterday but can't recall being there. In fact, he or she may be quite adamant that everyone else must be mistaken, yet cannot ascertain where he or she was that afternoon. Such lapses of time will be evident in the history of the patient with true dissociative identity disorder but not for the normal person with a variety of ego states.

Consistencies of behavior within a single state and differences in behaviors between states are most clearly observed in true multiple personalities. The "Ken" personality in the "Hillside Strangler" (Watkins & Watkins, 1984) always smoked filter-tipped cigarettes and held them between the first and second fingers, palm toward the face. The "Steve" personality always tore the filters off and held the cigarette between the thumb and the first finger, palm away from the face. Bianchi continued to show this same alteration of behavior during his subsequent incarceration in prison, when he had nothing to gain by claiming a psychiatric defense.

Ego-State Therapy

Ego-state therapy is the utilization of individual, family, and group therapy techniques for the resolution of conflicts between the different ego states that constitute a "family of self" within a single individual (J. G. Watkins & H. H. Watkins, 1997, p. 35). Therapy involves a kind of internal diplomacy that may employ any of the directive, behavioral, cognitive, analytic, Rogersian, or humanistic techniques of treatment but almost always uses hypnosis. These techniques are directed toward the part-persons represented by the ego states and not toward the whole individual. Although it is possible to practice ego-state therapy in the conscious condition (Emmerson, 2006), dealing with ego states with the use of hypnosis is the method of choice for most practitioners(Watkins & Watkins, 1996, 1997). This is because ego states, unlike true, dissociative identity disorder alters, do not usually become overt spontaneously. Most of the time, they require hypnotic activation. Through hypnosis, we can focus on one segment of personality and temporarily ablate or dissociate away other parts. In fact, because hypnosis is itself a form of dissociation, it is not surprising to find that good hypnotic participants often manifest covert ego-state segments in their personalities even though they are not mentally ill. Hypnosis offers access to levels of personality that in classical psychoanalysis require much, much longer periods of time to contact. Because ego-state therapy is an approach involving interpart communication and diplomacy, hypnosis generally becomes essential for practicing it when the states are covert.

At times, an ego state may be exerting an influence as "object" on the primary individual, in which case we might say, "I would like to talk to that part [we don't use the term "ego state" with the patient] of Mary Anne who has been compelling her to overeat (or who knows about her overeating)." A communication back from such a "part" commonly is the result. The content of this part is often at considerable variance with the therapist's expectations, contradicting the notion that these ego states are only artifacts created to please the therapist (a common argument posed by those who incompletely understand ego-state therapy).

Only being part-persons, ego states often think concretely like a child and must be communicated with accordingly. Sometimes ego states appear during sleep or in hypnosis-like dream figures. The same general strategies and tactics used in treating DID patients apply when working with the more covert ego states, except that they must be preceded by a hypnotic induction.

Efficacy Research

Much of the recognition of the efficacy of ego-state therapy has been based on clinical experience rather than controlled research, as evidenced by the acceptance of this approach at the First World Congress on Ego-State Therapy held in Bad Orb, Germany in 2003. Nonetheless, controlled research, although still in its infancy (Frederick, 2005), thus far indicates that ego-state therapy is effective in assisting clients with both psychological and somatic symptoms. Using a time series analysis as the experimental procedure, Emmerson and Farmer (1996) found that women with menstrual migraines were able to experience a significant reduction not only in headaches, but also in depression and anger. This occurred following a 4-week treatment with ego-state therapy. The monthly average number of days with migraine went from 12.2 to only 2.5. Consistent with this decline in headaches was a statistically significant decline in levels of depression and anger. The ego-states text (J. G. Watkins & H. H. Watkins, 1997) reported on 42 clients who had received ego-state therapy for a median of only 11 hours total treatment and those who had received other types of therapy with a median of 145 hours. Twenty-four clients said ego-state therapy met their expectations, while only seven clients said the other therapies met their expectations. Gainer (1993) also reported very positive effects of ego-state therapy. When trauma held by a child ego state was processed, there was complete remission of reflex sympathetic dystrophy (Ginandes, in press; Emmerson & Farmer, 1996).

Amudson, Aladin, and Gill (2003) raised serious questions about the use of efficacy-based research to test the effects of hypnotic interventions. They expressed the concern that to force hypnosis upon such a Procrustean bed might imperil its survival as a therapeutic modality. Their disquiet about the relationship between efficacy studies and clinical practice was echoed by Frederick (2003b), as she noted (p. 1), "Although efficacy studies had been termed the 'gold standard' for clinical care, it is perhaps the better part of wisdom to wonder if all that glitters is truly gold." She went on to point out Gabbard's (2000) unease with efficacy studies where it was noted that "tightly controlled" efficacy studies that are being conducted in academic settings exclude 80 to 90% of the available subjects because of the possible effects of advertising about research upon the experimental population, and the absence of patients. Perhaps the worst offense is the deliberate exclusion of patients with comorbidities from studies to keep the research clean. Real patients in our practices frequently have comorbid disorders. To exclude them in the name of conducting a controlled research study makes the findings from those studies questionable if not entirely useless.

Luborsky, McLelen, Diguer, Woody, and Seligman (1997) were able to demonstrate that identical treatment applications that were both manualized and highly controlled can yield results that vary greatly. There are many reasons why efficacy research using criteria such as that of Chambless and Hollan (1998) may not be the best way to measure the effectiveness of ego-state therapy. As Frederick (2005) pointed out, there are inherent research design problems relating to patient population selection, the issue of comorbidity, and the fact that ego-state therapy is often combined with other forms of psychotherapy. There are, of course, difficulties inherent in making measurements in complex systems. This has been recognized by the National Institutes of Mental Health (Markowitz & Street, 1999), which suggests that more effectiveness as opposed to efficacy research be conducted. Effectiveness studies attempt to research "the process" as opposed to the content and to locate those common, transtheoretical elements that make therapies useful to patients(Watkins & Watkins, 1996, Ch. 12 & 13). As Frederick (2005) pointed out, Oster (2003) in reference to Norcross's examination of available empirical data showed that the therapeutic alliance (resonance, cohesion, empathy, goal consensus, and collaboration) has been demonstrated as effective.

Ego States and Hidden Observers

Little more than a quarter of a century ago, Ernest R. Hilgard (Jack to his friends) was demonstrating hypnotic deafness before a class of students at Stanford University. Before explaining this interesting observation, recall from *Hypnotherapeutic techniques* that to dissociate something, one must first be aware of it at some level. There is now considerable psychophysiological data based on EEG event-related brain potentials (see A. Barabasz, M. Barabasz, Jensen, Calvin, Trevisan, & Warner, 1999; A. Barabasz, 2000) showing that hypnotic deafness produces a statistically significant attenuation of the brain's response to auditory stimuli, rather than an obliteration of the recognition of such stimuli. As foreshowed by Martin Orne's trance logic conceptualization (see Barabasz & Watkins, 2005), you have to hear it or see it before its presence can be negatively hallucinated away. Given that understanding, let us get back to Hilgard's fascinating demonstration. As he was about to invoke hypnotic deafness (which, as with other hypnotic hallucinations, we now know is never complete, see numerous experimentally controlled studies in Barabasz & Watkins), a student in his class asked whether some part of the apparently deaf subject might be aware of what was going on. Hilgard then said, to the hypnotized subject, "Although you are hypnotically deaf, perhaps there is some part of you that is hearing my voice and processing the information.

If there is, I should like the index finger to rise as a sign that this is the case." Much to Hilgard's surprise, the finger lifted! Later, he discovered that individuals similarly reported being aware of pain (but without its sensation) in a hypnotically anesthetized hand, which has been supported with experimental research using actual pain patients (A. Barabasz, M. Barabasz, & Rickard, in preparation). Hilgard ascribed this phenomenon to a cognitive structural system, which he called "the hidden observer." Those few (Christensen, 2005) who still adhere to the socio-cognitive role-play notion of hypnosis frequently misunderstand it.

A.F.B. once had the privilege of taking a workshop from Jack Hilgard in Melbourne, Australia. Demonstrating a more difficult variation of this phenomenon, Hilgard hypnotized Diana Elton, a psychologist participant in the workshop, who was known to have a Stanford Hypnotic Susceptibility Scale Form C score of 11. Passing 11 of the 12 possible items on the scale showed her to be highly hypnotizable. Interestingly, the only item that she could not pass was the item calling for an auditory hallucination. Thus, she was unable to hallucinate voices although she could hallucinate images. Hilgard created a hallucinated Dr. Barabasz in a chair sitting next to the actual Dr. Barabsz in front of the workshop. He asked Dr. Elton to question the two Dr. Barabaszes, knowing that there could only be one real person. Her task was to determine which was the real Dr. Barabasz. The questions went on for over 20 minutes with me answering and with the hallucinated Dr. Barabasz apparently sitting in the other chair dressed exactly as I was, remaining quiet. Hilgard pressed her as to which one of the Barabaszes was real. At first she said, "I can't tell; they both look exactly the same," then in a very different voice she said, "Well, of course that one must be real because he is talking to me and the other one isn't and I know I don't have the ability to produce hypnotic auditory hallucinations." Hilgard had, once again, demonstrated the hidden observer phenomenon rather convincingly. What impressed me greatly was that Dr. Elton's voice had changed to almost that of another person. What I had witnessed, without knowing it at the time, was the hidden observer expressed as one of Dr. Elton's ego states, apparently a very logical and scientific one.

At that time, J.G.W. and H. H. Watkins (1979–80, 1980) were conducting a set of experiments in which they activated hidden observers in former ego-state therapy patients using the same procedures and verbalizations employed by Hilgard in his studies, repeating with both hypnotic deafness and hypnotic analgesia. What emerged were various ego states with which they had dealt in treatment over a year earlier. They hypothesized that hidden observers and ego states are, therefore, the same *class* of phenomena. Hidden observers, ego states, and dissociative identity disordered personalities were then compared in much greater detail in work outside of the scope this book (see J. G. Watkins & H. H. Watkins, 1997).

To conclude our discussion here, let us note the differences between Federn's original conception of ego states and J.G.W.'s view of them as a function in therapy. To Federn, the ego remained a constant. Different contents could pass in and out of it by being ego-energized. The movement was by these contents, which were then organized by the ego into the ego states. When an ego state was de-energized of self energy, it retained its organization and continuous existence as an object representation and, therefore, was perceived as such. An ego state consisted only of self-energized items. In our view, the self consists of pure ego energy, not contents, such as motivations, affects, and ideas. This energy is not the energy of the self, it is the self.

When this ego energy passes into contents, these are then experienced as part of the self; in other words, they are experienced as "me." The movement is on the part of the self energy as it passes into and out of various organized behavior and experience patterns we call ego states. Such a state may contain both object and self representations, which on repression, removed from consciousness, still retain their respective and relative structures. Thus, this ego state, whether self- or object-energized, is the unit to be dealt with in therapy. It takes on the character of the major amount of energy within it, ego or object, and is experienced by the individual as such, "the me" or less frequently as "the it." Looking once again at Figure 10.1, the differentiation-dissociation continuum, it is worth noting that hidden observers and other partially separated personality segments exist as ego states within the middle range.

Ego-State Therapy as an Internal Family: Group Therapy

The ego-state therapy session typically resembles family therapy in that one member speaks, another is asked to respond, and an exchange of communications begins. Sometimes it is necessary to call on specific states to come out and speak. At other times, they will emerge spontaneously so long as the hypnotic state has been adequately established. Sometimes no one will abdicate if pressed too hard, and another will appear. The important point is that you think of it as talking to a multiplicity and not a unity. This is probably contrary to what you have been taught in almost all of your training as a clinician or a counselor. There is a single body in view but you are dealing with a family. What one says to one ego state may well be heard by others who can take offense and oppose one's treatment efforts.

The counselor or clinician operates like a group therapist. Any therapeutic maneuver, such as reflection, ventilation, desensitization, abreaction, free association, interpretation, reinforcement (approval), or clarification, that is part of your armamentarium may be employed. These can be used within the basic theoretical orientation that you have been trained in. However, they are to be applied with the use of hypnosis and to the various personality segments rather than to the entire patient.

Sometimes, the awareness of what has been done with an ego state may be brought to the attention of the conscious person. At other times, efforts will be made to strengthen some of the more constructive ego states. Occasionally, an ego state can be found that may serve as an assistant therapist, consulting with the clinician about strategy, advising of the effects of earlier maneuvers, and helping in planning future steps. We have taught ego states, who at first were destructive, to become behavior modifiers after constructive relationships had been established with them (see H. H. Watkins, 1978, Chapter 22). In one case, "Dark One," previously "the Evil One," provides systematic desensitization therapy to a child ego state to help eliminate a phobia of being on an oxygen mask.

It is our job to try at all times to discover and meet the needs of each ego state. Where they are conflicting, modification, negotiation, and compromise are indicated. Your role as a psychotherapist is frequently that of a communicator and a mediator between the clashing states. For example, "George" (a teenager ego state) was asked, "Would you be willing to do your homework during the week if 'father' [a parental ego state] doesn't bug you about playing on the weekends?"

Remember that ego states, like dissociative identity disorder alters, originated for defensive adaptive purposes during the person's critical developmental years or in response to trauma such as faced by soldiers in the Iraq wars, so they may no longer now be adaptive for the individual. As they were developed when the individual was a child or for immediate survival, defense mechanisms do not serve well for normal functioning adults. It is, therefore, unwise to eliminate "bad" ego states. Rather, one can avoid much resistance if you treat all the ego states with the utmost courtesy and respect, secure their cooperation, try to meet their needs, and play the role of a good friend to each. Attempts to eliminate a state mobilizes much resistance, which can sabotage treatment. Perhaps the role of a therapist in reconciling ego-state conflicts can best be described by presenting segments from a significant treatment session.

The Case of Mikale, Treated by Helen H. Watkins

This patient, who had suffered for 18 months with severe depression and insomnia, was referred to Helen Huth Watkins after she reported hearing "voices in her head." She also suffered from allergies and a recurring rash on her thighs and buttocks, also diagnosed as hives. Her mother apparently was a very strict and controlling individual. Mikale reported being molested by a man in the basement, but when she told her mother, she was not believed. During the first session, three ego states were located: a mother figure, a hurt child, and a "Silent Center," who listens as the above continue to argue. In the second session, she described her rash, and on being hypnotically regressed to the basement scene, she cried, "He's touching me there, and it hurts," referring to her buttocks.

By session three, the rash was gone; however, she now discussed her fear of the wind. At the age of 3, her mother, during a storm, had locked her out of the house for misbehavior. She was rescued by the return of her father. Following the reliving and a full abreaction of this incident, she was given hypnotic suggestions that she would never be afraid of the wind again, and perhaps more importantly, that she was not bad.

In session four, the "mother" ego state emerged and revealed that she had started the allergies for Mikale. "Mother" agreed to work on getting rid of the allergies. The next week, a most important session resulted in a compromise between the three major ego states and subsequently a considerable improvement in the symptoms. The following was taken from a recording from that session, which illustrates interactions typical of ego-state therapy.

H.H.W.: And now I would like to talk to just part of you, and the part that I'd like to talk to again is the part that I talked to the last time. I'd like to talk to Mother, and when Mother is there, just say, "I'm here."—You don't want to talk to me?

M.: I'm here. No, that was Mike or Misha or whoever she is. She wanted to talk but …

H.H.W.: Oh, she wanted to talk, the Little One?

M.: Yes.

H.H.W.: O.K. Maybe I'll talk to her later. I'm glad you told me. Tell me what happened. You told me you were going to work on her allergies, and apparently for several days it was much better, and then she spent some time with her mother and then suddenly the allergies became worse. Tell me how you perceive this.

M.: Well, I did go home, and I did the thinking like I told you I would.

H.H.W.: Um hum.

M.: And I decided maybe you were right. I was being a little overly harsh in my punishment. Umm … and so I started, and it seemed to work. She was feeling better, but when we got there it was like I just lost control, kind of. Strange …

H.H.W.: It isn't like you to lose control, is it?

M.: No. It was like the real mother had more control over what was going on than I did, and she just kind of took over, and I tried to stop it, and I managed to keep it semi-flat level until Saturday, but I couldn't fight anymore.

H.H.W.: And you don't know why, is that it?

M.: I don't understand why. I don't understand how she on the outside could have more effect than I do on the inside. It just don't make any sense, but it wasn't me doing it. I was trying not to do it.

H.H.W.: Um hum. Well, maybe we could find out from other parts in there what's going on, and maybe they had something to do with it. I

	don't know. Do you think that'd be all right if I try to find out for you?
M.:	Yes. I don't understand this, and I'd like to know.
H.H.W.:	Well, why don't you stay where you are? You can stay in the room, and I'm just going to call on someone else, but you can listen in. O.K.?
M.:	O.K.
H.H.W.:	All right. The part that I'd like to talk to is Little Misha, and when she's there just say, "I'm here."
M. [exuberantly]:	I'm here. I'm here.
H.H.W.:	Oh, you're happy to be here.
M.:	You should go faster down those stairs, though, because I wanted to run down the last part ... it's like [Pants].
H.H.W.:	I didn't realize you were there.
M.:	Well, I was.
H.H.W.:	O.K.
M.:	I took 'em slow but I didn't want to.
H.H.W.:	O.K. Well, next time I'll pay attention to you. O.K.?
M.:	O.K.
H.H.W.:	All right. Do you know anything about their allergies, Misha?
M.:	Well, you said something that was really interesting earlier. You said guilt, and that fits.
H.H.W.:	Oh, it does?
M.:	Yeah, because Mommy always told me I was a bad girl and I should feel guilty and I would, but I didn't like it.
H.H.W.:	I see. That doesn't feel good, does it?
M.:	No. It made my tummy hurt.
H.H.W.:	Oh, sure.
M.:	It also fit last night. We had this naughty dream last night. Well, it wasn't real naughty because nothing happened, but it fit. It's really strange.
H.H.W.:	Tell me about it.
M.:	The dream?
H.H.W.:	Yes. Whatever you want to tell me about it.
M.:	Well, it's real strange because, because the big person, the one on the outside, well, she's been having problems with her sex life because something's been holding her back, and she had this dream last night, and she kept kissing her fiancé, and it felt so good, but they kept stopping because she was like afraid to push too far, and that's why because she feels so guilty. She's not supposed to feel like that because Mom doesn't like her to feel like that.
H.H.W.:	Oh.

M.:   It's not right to have those types of feelings.

H.H.W.: Oh, she shouldn't feel sexual. Is that the idea?

M.:   Yeah, because they are naughty feelings.

H.H.W.: Oh, I see.

M.:   And she even calls them naughty feelings, kind of, but I think it's because she feels guilty.

H.H.W.: That's a very good thought on your part.

M.:   I don't know where it came from, but it fits, but don't tell Hardnose over there.

H.H.W.: Who, Mother?

M.:   Yeah. She's grumpy. She'll tell me I'm wrong. She always does.

H.H.W.: Well, I think that sounds like a very ...

M.:   I like the feeling like that.

H.H.W.: Well, sure, that's normal and natural.

M.:   But I'm not supposed to ... but I think that's how come we can't, because we feel guilty.

H.H.W.: You know what, maybe it's O.K. now. Maybe it's O.K. now to feel that way. You know you're kind of growing up yourself. You're having some fine ideas. And maybe your ideas are better that what Mother on the outside used to say. Because you're just acting normally and naturally and healthy like. Maybe it's O.K. to feel those feelings and to let the grown-up part feel those feelings. After all, those are just normal feelings, and she's going to be married pretty soon, and it's no good to have all those guilt feelings about sex when you're married. You're not free to be happy with your sexuality.

M.:   Well, I try, but Hardnose always goes [yuck].

H.H.W.: Ohhh.

M.:   That's Hardnose. I always wonder who did it. But it's Hardnose always.

H.H.W.: Oh, you're talking about Mother.

M.:   Yeah. Whatever her name is. She doesn't have a name, she doesn't like names. She's above names. So I call her Hardnose.

H.H.W.: I see. You have a good time, don't you? Well, tell me what do you know about the allergies?

M.:   Well, I don't know much about them. They itch.

H.H.W.: Well, you don't have anything to do with it, huh?

M.:   Nope. I don't like them.

H.H.W.: Mother inside would ...

M. [Interrupting]: They're kind of disgusting.

H.H.W.: Yeah. She was trying to stop, and then all of a sudden she found out that the Mother on the outside had more influence than she did,

	and she was very surprised, and I thought, well, I'd talk to you and see if you know anything about it.
M.:	It probably has to do with guilt, but I don't know. I would tend to think it would have to go through Hardnose. ... I don't like guilt. I'm the one that makes us do things we end up feeling guilty for.
H.H.W.:	You're the one that's fun, huh?
M.:	Yeah.
H.H.W.:	You like that.
M.:	I feel pretty good, too.
H.H.W.:	That's nice.
M.:	After you rescued me, I feel much better, or after Mike rescued me, I feel much better.
H.H.W.:	Good. Now you're out of that basement. You don't have that rash anymore either, do you?
M.:	We itch, but that's because we got sunburned.
H.H.W.:	Oh, sunburned. That's a good reason to itch.
M.:	We're going over that, too.
H.H.W.:	Well, I'll let you go play and do whatever you want to do, have fun and ...
M.:	Those stairs.
H.H.W.:	Oh, those stairs.
M.:	I want to run down 'em.
H.H.W.:	Yes. I'll have to remember, but not everybody can run as fast as you can. That's the only problem.
M.:	O.K. O.K.
H.H.W.:	O.K. All right. Now go where you need to go or want to go, and I'd like to talk to any part of the personality that knows about the allergies and what happened this weekend.
M.:	I think I did it.
H.H.W.:	Who are you?
M.:	I'm Mike.
H.H.W.:	Oh, you're Mike. Why did you do it?
M.:	Well, I don't know for sure. Misha was having a good time, and she was trying to avoid unpleasantness, which is Misha's purpose, I guess.
H.H.W.:	She's the child, and she wants to have fun.
M.:	Yeah. And Mother was doing things that were, you know, this Mother.
H.H.W.:	The inside Mother or the outside?
M.:	Yeah, the inside Mother.
H.H.W.:	O.K.
M.:	Was doing things that were contradictory to what normally happens. Like, you know. ... She was fighting the outside Mother, and I guess I got to feeling bad, and I let them come back.

H.H.W.: The allergies? Oh, for what purpose? I'm kind of confused.

M.: It was so different, and I was afraid that if things changed they're gonna get worse. At least with them being the same, I know how to deal with that.

H.H.W.: I see. In other words, you could predict. You knew what to do.

M.: Yeah.

H.H.W.: I see. Sometimes you got to take a little risk. There is risk in change, isn't there? You don't know what's going to happen; you got a little scared, huh? Do I have it right, you're 19? Do I have that right? [Nods assent] Well, Mike, you did a nice job with the Little One, and I really appreciate that, but you notice how that change that you promoted and that you helped me with, that change was for the good, and Misha is much more predictable now, much more fun, much more willing to play but no more rash anymore. But that was a change, and you were part of that change.

M.: I'm afraid she's going to do something. Even now I am afraid. I don't want her to do something that's going to hurt us.

H.H.W.: How can you get hurt?

M.: She may do something that somebody on the outside doesn't approve of.

H.H.W.: So? Neither you nor Mother inside need to be so concerned about what other people think. What other people approve of or what they don't approve of. You realize that the main personality is an adult. She's, I guess, what, 22 years old? The main personality. O.K. Well, she's going to get married. She can make decisions for herself. She doesn't have to do what the outside Mother says anymore."

M.: But Misha is so unpredictable and so carefree now, and the other Mother is acting really strange. Normally she's the one who keeps Misha in line, but she's not keeping Misha in line anymore.

H.H.W.: Wonderful.

M.: But, but somebody's got to, don't they?

H.H.W.: Do they? You know you have to have a little trust in the main personality, who's now an adult. She can make judgments for herself on what behavior is appropriate or not appropriate. I haven't seen Misha do anything crazy, inappropriate, wild, dangerous. She's just a delightful kid. I think you need a little more faith.

M.: Could be.

H.H.W.: And she really doesn't need the allergy. That main personality doesn't need that allergy. I'll tell you that, and besides it doesn't stop Misha anyway.

M.: That's true.

H.H.W.: I think you can let go and just trust the process a little more. And, of course, Mother has been changing. She was a little confused.

She tried so hard to get rid of those allergies, and all of a sudden she didn't know what happened. It got worse and she thought it was because of the outside Mother. She didn't understand why but now I think …. I asked her to listen in so she could hear what was going on, so she could find out what was going on. And I appreciate your listening, and do you think maybe you could let go a little? Do you think you could let the process just happen and not worry so much? Just trust the main personality. Really.

M.: I'll try.

H.H.W.: O.K. I would appreciate that. Now you go where you need to go, and you can certainly listen in. You don't have to go away. You can listen in, and I would like to talk to Mother again.

M.: Yes.

H.H.W.: Did you hear what Mike had to say?

M.: It's interesting, very interesting.

H.H.W.: Um hum.

M.: But why would she try to take over my position?

H.H.W.: Very interesting, isn't it?

M.: I don't understand it. Usually she's so noncommittal to anything. You know, she's like Silent Center. It's really strange. I kind of understand why she did it. I understand how she did it, but I don't understand the motivation, I guess.

H.H.W.: I think the motivation is, if I understand it correctly, that you have been kind of, as Misha calls it, hardnosed.

M.: She can be a little insightful, but she's probably closest to correct.

H.H.W.: And you have been controlling, you see, the Little One, so then Mike has not been doing much, as you call the Silent Center, non-committal. So, all of a sudden you changed, and the Little One changed, and she got confused as to what the rules were and what she was supposed to do, and then all of a sudden the allergy went away, and she didn't know what to do. And of course the allergies were based on guilt from starting at age 16, as you told me last time. And so with the guilt there, in a sense, but not there, not a physical manifestation of that guilt, she just didn't know what to do.

M.: Yeah. I can kind of see that.

H.H.W.: She got kind of confused as to what the rules were. In other words, when you feel guilty you're supposed to have an allergy.

M.: And I wasn't creating allergies.

H.H.W.: That's right.

M.: But the guilt was still there, so the allergies had to be there. So she let them in. That makes some sense.

H.H.W.:	O.K. But now that she understands this, and I ask her (I'm sure you heard) to have a little bit more faith in you and the main personality, there's no reason for the allergy. In fact, there's no reason for the guilt. I mean, after all, the main personality is a grown woman, and she can do what she wants in terms of decisions in her life and her wedding, and she doesn't have to feel guilt about what Mother says. That's from the times past when she was young, and she needs to get away from that. And as I told the main personality … I don't know if you heard more or not … did you hear me say she needs to accept the idea that the real Mother will not change?
M.:	Yeah, I heard that.
H.H.W.:	All right. Now acceptance doesn't mean she has to like it, but she needs to face that, that she can't change the world or change Mother, and that's just the way it is. And I thought the behavior of the main personality in terms of dealing with Mother is really quite adult. What do you think?
M.:	Yeah. I think … Yeah, she's starting to catch on.
H.H.W.:	Yeah. She didn't have a tantrum or act like a little kid, and I was wondering if you had anything to do with that?
M.:	Well, it's really strange. It's like Misha and I both kinda met in the middle instead of arguing.
H.H.W.:	Oh, I see.
M.:	And so we kind of decided on a line of action that was neither of us but a combination of the two.
H.H.W.:	That sounds great. I see, and that's why the Silent Center, as you called it before, and she calls herself Mike, didn't have a function, didn't know what to do.
M.:	Well, Misha, I guess, Misha and I aren't used to dealing with her because she's like you said, the Silent Center, and so we're used to fighting, and now we're cooperating. You're right. She doesn't have much of a function.
H.H.W.:	But maybe she needs a function.
M.:	That's what I was thinking, but I don't know what kind of a function, you know.
H.H.W.:	Well, what kind of a function do you think she had before?
M.:	Well, she would take … well, when Misha and I were fighting all the time, we would fight and whoever was the strongest, that was the decision made, and she would kind of implement it.
H.H.W.:	Oh, I see. She would just do it for you.
M.:	Yes.
H.H.W.:	Seems to me she had to do a lot of hard work, and you two didn't take much responsibility for the behavior.

M.:	Ohhh, probably true.
H.H.W.:	Doesn't feel good, does it?
M.:	No.
H.H.W.:	… to admit it. Maybe we ought to ask … why don't you ask Mike to come in where we are, and maybe we could ask her what she'd like to do in the future, what kind of functions she would like to have. Why don't you bring her into our room? Are you there, Mike?
M.:	Um hum.
H.H.W.:	Have you heard what we were saying, what Mother and I were talking about? … We'd like to hear from you, what kind of function would you like to have? I'm sure you heard that Mother and Misha got together in the last few days, since the last time I saw them, and instead of being separated and arguing they kind of got together, and so I guess you weren't needed at that point.
M.:	I guess I've really never been needed and I don't know why I'm here.
H.H.W.:	Umm. Well, you were the arbitrator, I guess, in a sense, or you had to listen to both sides and then, I guess, whoever was the strongest, said Mother, you did that particular behavior. I wonder the function you would like to have now that maybe that's not necessary.
M.:	I felt bad when they went around me.
H.H.W.:	Ohhh.
M.:	I guess I feel that should still be my job now, but now in a positive sense. I wish, you know, instead of them meeting and going out if they would come to me.
H.H.W.:	You'd like to be a partnership, a part of the group.
M.:	Yeah. Yeah.
H.H.W.:	O.K., Mother, why don't you talk to her and say whatever you want to say about the idea of being part of the three of you?
M.:	Well, it's going to take some work … umm, especially with cooperation. But I think we can try. Well, we can try. I don't think, I know we can try. Maybe a little rough on all of us for a while, and maybe some unpleasantness as we're working all of this out, but I'd be willing to try.
H.H.W.:	Mike, what do you think?
M.:	I think it'd be fine.
H.H.W.:	And let's bring Misha in here, too. Misha, I'd like you to come back. I'm not sure if you heard what the other two were saying, but I'd like to hear from you.
M.:	I was listening. I think it'd be great 'cause then I wouldn't have to think anymore.
H.H.W.:	Well, good.
M.:	Then I can play, and she can think.

H.H.W.:   Who's she?

M.:   Mike. Then she could do the thinking.

H.H.W.:   Oh, she can do the thinking.

M.:   'Cause right now I have to think, because I have to take what I'm doing and feeling and kind of convert it into words, so that what's-her-name up there …

H.H.W.:   Mike?

M.:   Mother.

H.H.W.:   Oh, Mother.

M.:   Mother can understand me.

H.H.W.:   Oh, I see.

M.:   But if I funnel it all into Mike, then Mike can do the thinking, and I can do the fun.

H.H.W.:   How about that! Whee!

M.:   I better put the brakes on. I better be careful [tips chair back].

H.H.W. [Laughing]:   I wouldn't worry about that. O.K. Well, now that sounds like a good idea. Mike, did you hear what Misha had to say? She'd like you to have an important function. She'd like to funnel all the thinking into you. Mike, how would you like that?

M.:   I would like that a lot.

H.H.W.:   Great, then you'd have an important function.

M.:   Yeah.

H.H.W.:   O.K. Now, Mother, what about you? … What do you think about that idea that you just heard?

M.:   Well, yeah, Misha's thinking isn't always real logical. She's a little young, but I think it will work. Yeah.

H.H.W.:   Well, Mike is older anyway.

M.:   Yeah. Quite a bit older. Misha's not real old sometimes.

H.H.W.:   She's around 4 or 5. What is she?

M.:   She doesn't stay the same age.

H.H.W.:   Uh huh.

M.:   From 3 to 6.

H.H.W.:   Oh, I see.

M.:   She's …

H.H.W.:   She's up and down. Anyway, she's young.

M.:   Yeah.

H.H.W.:   Well, that sounds like a pretty good compromise. And now maybe with the two of you working on the allergies, I have a feeling you can get rid of them.

M.:   I do, so do I. I'll stop letting them in.

H.H.W.:   Mike's talking huh? You say you're going to stop letting them … who's talking just now?

M.:   That's me. I'm Mike.

H.H.W.:   All right, I know Mother agrees, you agree, so that ought to work out very well and I appreciate the cooperation. O.K. Now I want to talk to the total personality. In a moment I'm going to count up to five, and when I count up to five you will be wide awake, fresh and alert. Coming up now at the count of five. One, two, three, four, five.

H.H.W.:   Now, what do you remember?

M.:   That's weird, they're both talking … all three of them. … Sometimes I wish I could just turn my eyes around and see what's going on.

H.H.W.:   Strange, huh. Well, it sounds like a compromise. That should give you a little peace and get rid those allergies.

M.:   Yeah.

H.H.W.:   O.K.

After 12 sessions (J. G. Watkins, 2005), the depression and insomnia had ceased completely, and the treatment was terminated. Follow-up showed no return of the allergies, and the patient no longer heard "voices" in her head. The boundaries between the ego states became more permeable, and they were more "integrated" with one another. However, when she was serious she spoke in a "Mike-type" voice. A nurturing "Mother" voice appeared when she was taking care of a neighbor child, and a "Misha" voice when engaged in playful activities.

Marathon Ego State Therapy

Freud and other analysts wrestled with the frequency and length of sessions (Freud, 1953b). They finally agreed upon 50-minute hours, three to six times a week. Freud preferred the six times a week. Recently, therapy sessions are generally scheduled on a one-a-week basis, partly because insurance companies will not pay for greater frequency.

Helen Watkins practiced an innovative and very uncommon scheduling of ego state therapy session in weekend marathons. A patient was seen for 2 hours Friday evening, followed by 4 to 6 hours nonstop Saturday, then 3 to 4 hours nonstop Sunday. He or she then flew home on Sunday afternoon. Helen reasoned that progress in treatment conducted 1 to 6 times per week involved a kind of ratcheted effect. During the interval between sessions, the resistances and defenses of the pathology counterattacked so that there was always two steps forward during the session and one step back during the interval before the next session, etc. If no nontreating interval existed between first hour and second hour, third hour, fourth hour, etc., then therapeutic momentum was maintained and progress proceeded most efficiently (Watkins & Watkins, 1997). A analogy might be in the military campaigns of World War I. An attack would gain 2 miles. Then, when the attacking army rested, the opposing side would counterattack and regain 1 mile.

This timing was also most convenient to Helen's patients, largely mental health professionals who traveled to her office in Missoula, Montana, and did not want to be absent longer than necessary from their own practices. The disadvantage was that insurance companies did not want to pay for so many sessions within 3 days. However, her patients came because of her national and international acclaim (J.G. Watkins, 2005), and were willing to pay personally for sessions with her and generally achieve solution of their problems in so short a time (J.G. Watkins, 1995, Ch. 12 and 13).

Summary

Ego-state therapy was derived from the study of multiple personalities and experiments with normal hypnotic subjects within the general theoretical structure of hypnoanalysis. These include J. R. Hilgard's work with "hidden observers." The theories of Paul Federn served as an origin for its conceptual structure. However, we have elaborated on its original formulations and altered them in certain significant areas based on our experimental studies and clinical experiences.

It is essential to recognize that the "separating function" in the formation of personality structure, like almost all psychological processes, exists on a continuum ranging from normal, adaptive differentiations through defensive operations to maladaptive dissociation as exemplified in true multiple personalities (dissociative identity disorder).

Ego-state therapy may use any of the directive, behavioral, cognitive, analytic, or humanistic approaches to treatment. But it applies these to personality segments, that is, part-persons, and not to the entire individual. Generally, it does so with the use of hypnosis because covert ego states do not typically appear spontaneously without having been hypnotically activated.

Our orientation here is essentially eclectic-psychoanalytic; hence, we have termed it hypnoanalytic ego-state therapy. However, a therapist with a different theoretical orientation might prefer to practice a hypnocognitive ego-state therapy, applying his or her interventions to part-persons (ego states) rather than to the entire individual.

Ego-state therapy is a very potent treatment procedure because it focuses on the specific areas of the personality that are most relevant to the presenting problem. This tactical advantage not only is valuable in dealing with the occasional true multiple personality, but it extends to the vast array of neurotic, psychosomatic, and behavioral disorders ranging from simple problems such as stopping smoking and losing weight to severe phobic and anxiety cases. When used with skill, ego-state therapy can provide approaches for handling borderline conditions in ways well beyond the scope of other therapies currently available or, for that matter, in any case where some measure of dissociation, mild or severe, is found.

J.G.W. (2005a) has made a recent modification to ego-state theory based on his observation of simultaneous translation at an international congress and a documentary on the life, emaciation, and destruction of singer and actress Judy Garland. He posited that self existence depended on the amount of ego energy (ego cathexis) with which the self is activated. If inadequately energized, the self will finally be extinguished. It is like a kerosene lamp whose flame is extinguished when there is no more fuel in the tank.

Superior therapists may resonate almost completely with their patients as did Judy Garland with her stage roles, e.g., "Dorothy" in *The Wizard of Oz*, or the simultaneous translator. Each threw their entire self into the objects of their resonance: therapist—patient; Judy—role; translator—translation. This total switch of identity required the expenditure of enormous quantities of ego energy from their own store. But if this store is not replenished by love and other rewards, then the life of each will dwindle and die. Therapists, if you would achieve superior results by totally resonating, then ensure that your love life and other rewards replenish your self energy.

In the documentary, one sees Judy as a frightened, sick, depressed little waif, who is then pushed by greedy promoters to perform. She switches ego states, and the vibrant old Judy is temporarily reactivated within the role. Afterwards, she retreats to the depressed ego state, exhausted, functioning only on drugs until her store of ego energy is exhausted. Then, because there is nothing, no love or satisfactions, left to her (and unlike in the role of Dorothy, she cannot return to the brief happiness of her early childhood), she leaves this world for the heavenly one above—"Over the Rainbow."

11

Hypnotic Transference, Counter-Transference, and the Therapeutic Alliance

"Transference phenomena are part of every therapy, and indeed of everyday life. The well-prepared, intelligent student suffering from examination fear ascribes to the authority figure, his professor, the wish to let him fail regardless of whether the examiner is a mean, overly demanding, or a benign person who would like to see the student pass and become a colleague. The student transfers upon his teachers the Oedipal fantasy he had as a little boy: that his father would not allow him to grow up and become an equal" (Erika Fromm, 1968, p. 77). Between the ages of 3 and 6, nearly every little girl has the normal Oedipal wish that her father take the initiative and have a sexual relationship with her. When a patient has not resolved this Oedipal wish in childhood, it keeps throbbing in her unconscious. Later, she transfers this wish to a father figure, the hypnotherapist. She wishes to be seduced by the hypnotist and unconsciously she may revenge herself on him for *not* having seduced her. She blames the seductive wish on the hypnotist, transferring to him the unfulfilled hope she had with regard to her father (p. 79).

The phenomena of transference is the most powerful psychoanalytic technique (S. Freud, 1938). It is a simple but basic process. Humans tend to perceive present figures in their life and react to them as if they were former significant individuals in their lives, such as a father, mother, sibling, or teacher. The current individual is endowed, unrealistically, with characteristics of the earlier person. Thus, the patient may begin to feel that the therapist is uncaring and manipulative of him or her even though the treating one has been sitting and listening passively to the patient's memories. The transference reaction is a powerful technique, because it involves a "reliving" of the past, not merely a remembering. It occurs also in ego-state therapy (Phillips, 1994; J. G. Watkins & H. H. Watkins, 1990). It may be greatly facilitated when the patient is in a hypnotic state, and because hypnosis is a kind of regression, the regression of transference reactions may be precipitated earlier in the treatment (Erika Fromm, 1968). Therapists often are somewhat "seduced" by the patient into behaving like the parent of the past. They, too, are influenced by transference reactions. When the therapist unconsciously views the patient as perhaps a younger bother figure, and then talks to or behaves toward the patient like he or she would toward that brother, then the therapist is experiencing counter-transference (J. G. Watkins & H. H. Watkins, 1990, 1997, pp. 97–98).

The Nature of Transference

Transference is a phenomenon that occurs with all people. In the analytic and hypnoanalytic situation, its understandings and interpretation provide the basis for therapeutic change. It refers to the process by which an individual experiences feelings and attitudes in relation to a present-day person or situation that was originally acquired much earlier toward another (J. G. Watkins, 1963).

Quite commonly, a patient will see in the therapist traits that he or she originally perceived in a parent as a child. Thus, if a daughter had been rejected by her father, she may have the feeling that her therapist is rejecting her when in reality he has done nothing of the kind. She "transfers" onto him the image of her father and attributes to him her father's characteristics. She feels emotions toward her therapist similar to those she once felt for her father and which she now retains unconsciously. In fact, she may demonize him and accuse him of precisely that: "You don't really care anything about me. You would like me to go away and not bother you." The patient's thoughts and accusations are a "psychotic-like" distortion of anything the therapist may have done or said.

In the psychoanalytic situation, where the analyst has been sitting quietly and patiently behind a couch on which the patient reclines, he or she is in a position to point out to the patient that his or her view of him is in contradiction with his or her true behavior. The analyst "interprets" the patient transference reaction, which forces him or her to confront the discrepancy between his or her perceptions of him and the analyst's actual behaviors. Because the therapist has not behaved in ways to justify the patient's feelings, they must be reexamined and the true source determined. In this way, the patient acquires "insight" and comes to realize that perhaps his or her feelings that the therapist (and perhaps all men) has rejected him or her are not justified. He or she takes a significant step forward toward maturity: perceiving, feeling, and behaving realistically toward the real world. To this point in his or her life, fears of rejection have led him or her to unrealistically comply with whimsical as well as irrational demands that have been placed on him or her, often by a series of significant others.

The term *transference* has often been used erroneously to mean all feelings that a patient has toward the therapist. The clinician or counselor may say, "She has a positive transference toward me," when the feeling does not stem from some early childhood learning experience but from good impressions about normal interactions with each other. Fenichel (1941) attempted to bring such reactions under the umbrella of transference by terming it "rational transference," which is also often referred to as "mature transference." This aspect of interaction might better be thought of as the "therapeutic alliance" (Phillips & Frederick, 1995; Frederick & McNeal, 1999). Transference should be reserved for those feelings and attitudes (positive or negative) that come from experiential patterns learned from early significant figures in the patient's life.

Let us consider how transference was originally acquired before we go on to our investigation of transference in hypnoanalysis. As a child develops, he experiences different feelings in relation to its perception of the world and the important people in it. If a mother is rejecting, administering too much scolding and discipline, then the child might develop a constant fear toward her. This fear may be reinitiated when the child contacts a person later in life who reminds him of his mother. The child may have been ambivalent toward his mother, but on one hand, he loved her and needed her, and on the other hand, there was fear of criticisms and punishments. Because of his need for her, he may marry a woman who somehow reminds him of her. As an old song put it, "I want a girl, just like the girl who married dear old Dad." The cue that brings back this reminder may be a personality trait that both the mother and the wife possess. Or it could simply be that one or more physical features of his wife, such as hair color, size, posture, and face, are similar to his mother's. This constitutes the source of the attraction that draws him to her. The young mind interprets this as "love." Correspondingly, the brain (via subcortical structures [amygdala] stimulates a strong physical attraction.

We must remember that the image of the mother, which is preserved in the unconscious of the individual, is not that of the old lady of the present but of the young woman who gave birth to him and governed his early years. This may well have been a woman whose age would not be greatly at variance with that of his "love." However, after marriage or partner commitment where they are living together, the interaction becomes closer. He begins to feel, rightly or wrongly, that she also has the critical traits that characterized his mother and which he did not want to recognize during the physical attraction phase of their relationship. He develops fear toward her and anxiety in the relationship. This may result in many different symptoms, such as sexual impotence, anger flare-ups, psychosomatic reactions, and so on. Because she reminds him of his mother, on one hand, he chooses her and needs her. On the other hand, also because she reminds him of his mother, he gets the feeling that she is critical, rejects him, and punishes him, whether or not she actually does so in reality. It is in such transference situations that Freud's classical Oedipus complex may be revealed. The foregoing is, obviously, a very elemental explanation of transference, which is well known to all analytically oriented practitioners, but is presented here so that we can agree on the basic phenomenon before extending it and showing its uses in hypnoanalytic treatment.

There is another way by which we can explain transference. Our perceptions of the real world and our understanding of it stem essentially from two sources: the stimuli coming in from that world and the distortions and interpretations that we place on those stimuli that arise from our own memories, feelings, and attitudes, hence, from an amalgamation of both outer and inner stimuli. The resulting "experience" is like a photograph of the outer world but colored and changed by our own early encounters, wishes, hopes, fears, and motivations. Furthermore, from all such experiences, we form inner replications in the form of images and memories. As discussed in Chapter 10, when these inner images are replications of significant people, they are called "introjects" or "object representations." In other words, we "introject" a parent and form an internal replica, an object representation, of that parent, which then acquires a kind of life of its own. If the parent has been a nagging, criticizing parent, we may go through life feeling constantly depressed because this inner introject (self-object, ego state) continues a barrage of unconscious criticism, which is consciously experienced as lowered self-esteem.

It is important to recognize that we not only introject a significant person, we also introject "the drama" around such a person. This drama may continue to be enacted in later life. Thus, if one introject or object representation stems from our original perceptions of mother and another from perceptions of father, and if mother and father were constantly arguing, we may repeat this confrontation unconsciously in our own head and wonder why we suffer from frequent headaches. Then, if a new person in our life reminds us of mother or father, the conflict between these two object representations may be reactivated, and we begin to suffer from transference headaches when we are around that person. We are doing it to ourselves; the person isn't doing anything to stimulate that.

Therefore, transference may occur whenever one's perception of something or someone in the real world is contaminated with a memory of something or person from the past. Perception and reaction to the real world is most likely distorted with inner "memory-perceptions" for all people, even the most completely analyzed individuals. However, the aim of psychoanalytic therapy is to greatly reduce the influence on a patient's behavior and experience from distorted or contaminated unconscious memories or inner feelings originating from the past and to increase the correctness of perception of the real external world as it actually is.

The goal of analysis is to increase realistic perception and behavior, and the goal of all therapy is to improve adjustment and the happiness of the patient. There is an implicit assumption among psychoanalysts that these goals are the same, hence, that well-analyzed persons will be more happy, successful, and symptom free because they now experience and behave more appropriately toward the real world. This assumption may not always be true. There is no reason that a happy, optimistic, giving person, who radiates goodwill to others and continuously enjoys life, should undertake analysis and submit to change simply because psychoanalytic theories say that he or she is living in a "fool's paradise" based on repression.

Consider also the case of people who are in love; when a couple are young, it is likely to be a transference love. Because of their affection, they may overlook flaws in each other and enjoy a happy life together. The problem does not arise from an adjustment based on repression or other defenses; it only becomes overt when that adjustment breaks down because of the great disparity with external reality.

In (chapter 15, on dental hypnosis), we suggested a technique for helping patients to relieve some of the strangeness in the feel of new dental fixtures Barabasz & Watkins, (2005). The memory "of how the original teeth felt" is hypnotically reactivated and tied to the stimuli received from running the tongue over the new cap. The reality perception of the new teeth is distorted or contaminated with a past memory of what one's original teeth felt like. This is transference hypnotically activated and manipulated in the service of that patient to alter an unpleasant sensation in present reality. If successful, the patient becomes adjusted to the newly acquired prosthetic device and is happier and better adjusted.

The examples above are presented to point out that human happiness and reality orientation are not necessarily identical. Still, in most cases, the long-term well-being of an individual is more likely to be enhanced if transferences are analyzed and resolved than if they are reinforced and maintained, such as might happen when a person "in love" identifies with his or her significant other. Accordingly, hypnoanalytic therapy will be devoted primarily to the same goals as psychoanalytic treatment: the uncovering of unconscious processes, the resolution of unrealistic transferences, and the promoting of maturity and reality behavior.

The human personality is a dynamic system of equilibrium with both input and output. We have mentioned input in terms of the internalization or introjection of outside people and situations, as well as the building of replicas of these within the self. The other side of this equilibrium is output. The personality externalizes or splits off from itself these same replications through a process termed "projection," a form of transference. In its extreme form, projection is at the basis of paranoid reactions. The individual, unable to face his or her own hatred, "projects" this out onto another and accuses the other of hating him or her. Freud (1953a) explained this mechanism in a paranoid individual as transforming latent homosexual feelings toward another male, "I love you," first into its opposite through "reaction formation." This feeling then becomes an "I hate you," which, not being acceptable, is reversed and projected onto the other as "You hate me" before it can come to consciousness. Freud felt this accounted for the patient's delusions of persecution.

Transference may be considered as a special form of this projection. The internalized replica, perhaps of the patient's mother, is projected out onto the person of his wife. He, figuratively, has dressed the perception of his wife with his mother's attributes. He looks at his wife, but unconsciously sees his mother and reacts toward her as he once did toward his mother, be it with affection, fear, or hatred. This mechanism may also be recognized and interpreted in dreams. Hypnosis gives us much flexibility in deciphering, altering, and manipulating images. It also allows us to intervene in their internalization or externalization.

Transference and Hypnosis

The relationship between transference and the hypnotic modality has been the subject of both serious study and conjecture for a long time. As you will recall from Barabasz & Watkins, (2005) (Chapter 3, Theorizing about Hypnosis), many of the theories of hypnosis emphasize interpersonal suggestion, regression, and dissociation. Yet, each of these are essential components of transference. Hypnotic suggestions given by one individual, the therapist, to another, the patient (or research participant), are generally based on the established patterns of feeling and behavior toward each other acquired in their respective childhoods. Regression means a return to earlier patterns of feeling, thinking, and reacting, which is precisely what is involved in transference. And dissociation is invariably a part of transference, because to manifest it, an individual must dissociate to some degree his or her perception of the present to accept one acquired in the past.

Erika Fromm (1977, 1992) viewed hypnosis as an adaptive regression in the service of the ego. She saw the hypnotic state as one that causes an ego-modulated relaxation of defensive barriers, allowing a return to earlier, less realistic primary-process thinking. She emphasized that this is also temporary and limited to the time of relatively deep hypnotic trance, one that Schilder and Kauders (1926) noted is controlled by the subject and consciously reversible. Erika Fromm viewed regression in the service of the ego as healthy. She pointed out that letting go of one's usual controls and going backward a step on the developmental ladder to enable forward steps is indeed the definition of "regression in the service of the ego," or as Hartmann (1939/1958) also termed it, "adaptive regression." Brenman and Gill (1947) preferred to emphasize the relationship aspect of hypnosis. J.G.W. (1954, 1963) first considered hypnosis itself as a special form of transference behavior and then later held that its induction, deepening, and termination reflected transference and countertransference needs within the two participants, both the hypnotist and the participant.

The late Ronald Shor (1979) proposed that hypnosis consisted of three essential factors: role-playing (although not taken to the extreme as discussed by Sarbin, 2005), trance, and "archaic involvement," by which he meant transference. A. Smith (1984) examined the hypnotic relationship from an object-relations point of view, whereas Murray-Jobsis (1988) proposed an integration of adaptive regression, dissociation, and transference to form a more comprehensive theory of hypnosis. Many contributors to the field emphasized that hypnosis is founded on the parent/child transference relationship, but Meares (1976) disagreed. Based on his theory of hypnosis of "atavistic regression," he pointed out that this regression is to a primitive mode of behavior, not to the parent/child relationship. This position has been supported by experimentally controlled research (A. Barabasz & Christensen, 2006). Obviously, parent-child transferences can and sometimes do arise during hypnosis, but they are not basic to the hypnotic modality itself.

Brenman and Gill (1947) made a clear distinction between "the changing transference manifestations which take place during the course of the therapy and the relatively constant transference relationship, which we assume to underlie the hypnotic state." In fact, they held that the hypnotic state should be termed a hypnotic "relationship," a view with which many hypnosis researchers would not agree because research studies often require an effort to minimize or control the relationship factor. In this respect, Brenman and Gill believed that hypnosis takes place because it is the gratification of unconscious fantasies or wishes in the subject. Later, they (1959) extended this position to maintain that hypnosis must be viewed as a two-way (transference-counter-transference) relationship in which the overt behavior of one is the covert fantasy of the other. In other words, if the subject is overtly passive and acquiescent, the therapist then behaves in a dominant manner. Simultaneously, the dominant behavior of therapists may be a reaction formation against their own passive-dependent needs, which are then gratified by resonance with the patients. Likewise, the patient is resonating with the aggressive, dominating therapist and satisfying his or her covert desires for omnipotence.

Brenman and Gill (1959) presented even more significant data concerning the interactions between transference and the depth of the hypnotic state/relationship. The ability of the patient to enter into a hypnotic state, and how deeply, varies with alterations in the transference-counter-transference situation. When resistant to hypnosis alterations, interpretations of the negative transference are often followed by more rapid inductions and regressions into deeper hypnotic states. Gill and Brenman noted that they did not normally interpret the basic transference that underlies the hypnotic contract between a given therapist-patient unit but did so for changes of transference manifestations that arise as they normally do in traditional psychoanalysis. They preferred to leave the underlying constant transference situation alone. Now if this is based on "fear," or if it is interfering with the hypnotic induction or the therapy, then it warrants interpretation.

Brief hypnotic states often appear during traditional analysis when transference changes occur. As discussed in Barabasz & Watkins, (2005), these are examples of spontaneous hypnosis (J. G. Watkins, 1963). The patient becomes momentarily glassy-eyed and manifests other trance behaviors. This happens when there is a change in the impulse/defense balance. Transference then becomes an equal precursor for induction with "attacks on the sensory-motor level," such as eye fixation, postural sway, hand levitation, and so on. H. Spiegel and D. Spiegel (2004) noted that dissociative disordered patients may have serious losses of function, exhibit psychotic symptoms, and be quite manipulative but that the underlying conflicts are usually of a positive libidinal nature. The therapist can still establish rapport relatively easily with them, and they tend to be trusting in therapy, as A.F.B. observed at Sunnyside Psychiatric Hospital in Christchurch, New Zealand, with a series of 12 such patients. All of them complied with the hypnotic protocol. In contrast, patients with genuine borderline disorders are frequently hostile and paranoid. As Kernberg (1975) pointed out, this becomes a major work in any psychotherapy of patients with borderline disorders. Such patients, when functioning at that level, tend to not allow themselves to experience the sensory motor changes characteristic of the trance state due to their underlying hostility and suspicions.

Those of us who have worked for some time with a patient may find that lengthy, formal inductions are no longer necessary. A simple request, such as, "Please go into hypnosis," is sufficient (Spiegel, 2008). Occasionally, A.F.B. established this as a posthypnotic suggestion such as, "When I talk to you like this, and you hear my voice like this, and you are ready to go into hypnosis, if it's O.K. to let yourself go down into hypnosis, indicate that to me by raising a finger." This technique is used with full awareness of the patient and reviewed consciously after its implantation in the hypnotic state. J.G.W. would simply say, "It's been a long time since I conversed with 'Meg.' Would you please come out, Meg, and talk to me?" Reportedly, the patient would respond with the requested dissociation, although some coaxing might be required if Meg was angry with J.G.W. at the time. The close transference relationship made unnecessary the use of formal induction procedures. Here, as pointed out by Nash (2005), the initial suggestion constitutes the hypnotic induction.

The examples above highlight the dissociative aspect of hypnosis (E. R. Hilgard, 1986). Herbert Spiegel (see H. Spiegel & D. Spiegel, 2004, pp. 24–25) noted that some highly hypnotizable subjects actively seek situations in which they feel they can place themselves under someone else's control. This may happen unconsciously in spite of conscious protest. Dr. Herbert Spiegel provided an example with his study of hypnosis exploring 16 of 20 patients on a particular hospital ward. He noted that during his absence from the ward, there was apparently much discussion about what went on in the examining room (the hypnotic sessions with Spiegel). A patient suddenly appeared and said, "Sir, you could not hypnotize me even if you wanted to." Spiegel noticed that as he was saying this, his right eye fixed on a penciled dot used for the trance induction, and then closed. Dr. Spiegel challenged him: "Then why can't you open your right eye?" The patient struggled to open his right eye but was unable to do so. Simultaneously and in a defiant tone, he maintained his eye was open (the eye was actually closed). The patient was actually begging for the signal to enter trance just as the other men on the ward had described it. Spiegel simply said, "All right, now both your eyes will close." The patient's eyes did close and he went into a deep trance state. The point is that it is not unusual for people with significant hypnotizability to enter trance states spontaneously as long as the hypnotherapist does not interfere with the process (Barabasz, 2005, 2006). In A.F.B.'s research (A. Barabasz & M. Barabasz, 2006) on tailored versus manualized hypnotic inductions for irritable bowel syndrome (IBS) patients, we often found that interference could be constituted by insisting on the long, drawn-out, manualized induction that was part of the standard protocols, which are the norm for IBS (Palson, 2006). The scripted inductions lend themselves nicely to research protocols, but for some patients they interfered substantially with their entry into hypnosis. Brief tailored inductions became the preferred mode for these difficult patients and facilitated positive treatment outcomes. The point is that underlying transference-counter-transference relationships can be so developed that sensory-motor level changes can be automatically triggered, thus in some cases contraindicating the use of long drawn-out hypnotic induction procedures (A. Barabasz & Christensen, 2006).

Erika Fromm (1968) described a number of transference manifestations that occur in hypnosis, such as Oedipal and sibling transference. She recommended that in hypnotherapy, the transference be "utilized" and not necessarily "analyzed," and gave the example of a patient who competed with her by reporting that self-hypnosis was deeper than that induced by the therapist. Instead of analyzing this transference reaction, Fromm simply suggested that the patient use her self-hypnosis to unearth more material for hypnoanalysis. This particular paper is very readable and one that we highly recommend for advanced graduate students or readers who may be beginning their work in hypnocounseling or hypnoanalysis (see also Watkins & Watkins, 1990).

Hypnosis is a modality by which the therapist and the patient can regulate the amount of closeness or distance between them (Gill & Brenman, 1959). They noted the resistance encountered when an attempt was made to analyze and interpret the "meaning" of hypnosis to the patient. Both consciously and unconsciously, patients generally show that they want this area left alone. Therefore, it is best to accept this and work with its transference meaning than to remove it by interpretation. Confronting the patient with the interpretation might, at least temporarily, render the patient unhypnotizable.

Another example of how to utilize transference is as follows: A 28-year-old patient reported to J.G.W. that he was very much afraid of his father, but when accused of being like his father, he would feel "strong" and his speech would not be blocked. In hypnosis, he was asked to imagine a stage with a man and a boy on it. He was told to "fuse" with the boy and identify with him. The patient then manifested much fear. When asked to describe the theater, he blocked and was unable to talk well. It was then suggested that he remove himself from the boy and approach the man, fusing with him. The patient's blocking ceased and his speech cleared. In this example, we have changed an object representation hypnotically: the boy to a self representation (me) and then reversed them again by making "the boy" the object and "the man" self.

After some exploration to determine what negative traits might be acquired by identifying with his father, the fusing was fixed posthypnotically by hypnotic suggestion. The patient emerged from hypnosis with no apparent speech blocking. The clearing of speech was not permanent following this first session. However, after a number of repeats, the blocking apparently disappeared. In this case, the transference was not interpreted but simply utilized in a subject-object hypno-suggestive approach to treatment. In object-relations theory terminology, this father object representation had been turned into a self representation—an introject had been turned into an identofact.

As in psychoanalysis, the successful resolution of a transference reaction can be the significant turning point in hypnotherapy. This will often concern a block in the treatment related to the specific emotions (love or fear) that are evoked in the patient by the hypnotic relationship. Lazar and Dempster (1984) described a case in which a woman who had been sexually abused by her father reported an "overwhelming sexual desire" toward her male therapist. He correctly recognized this as a transference related to her father. Her first reaction was indignation, and she regarded it as a rejection. However, she soon came to see that the sexuality was a way of continuing contact with her "therapeutic father," because she had "given" sex to her original father to reduce his abuse. Following this, she began to feel that the therapist truly "loved" her in a way she had not previously experienced (without sexual contact), and the treatment progressed to an effective conclusion.

A.F.B. treated a somewhat similar case. Now in her mid-30s, this attractive patient had spent her life drifting from one job and one relationship to another despite her high grades in attaining a bachelor's degree in her early 20s. Her one marriage ended in her husband's tragic accidental death, which was then followed by a series of highly controlling "boyfriends." As a child, she learned to give oral sex to her father while showering together, which continued to her latency years when she finally confronted him. Guilt-ridden and embarrassed, he left the home, providing the abandonment necessary for a precipitation of the patient's borderline personality disorder. A.F.B. worked with this patient for 56 hours in 6- to 9-hour days over a period of several weeks. This patient was not only very beautiful but also exceptionally seductive as was noted in the records of many previous psychotherapists. She expressed considerable sexual desire for me and, very much as in the case above, was, at first, indignant at its rejection. Therapy progressed with a series of abreactions to her father, where I allied with her to make her ego strong enough to resist his insistence of her oral sexual favors as a youngster and the releasing of anger related to the abandonment, which she transferred toward me for many hours/days in therapy before it was exhausted and resolved. In a follow-up session several months later, the patient confided in me that I had been her 19th therapist and that I was the only one that she "couldn't get to hit on her." It was this level of transference, respect, and alliance with the patient that may well have contributed to the successful outcome. And as in the Lazar and Dempster case above (1984), she too recognized she felt that the therapist truly "loved" her in a way she had not previously experienced and discovered that a supportive relationship could be maintained without sexual favors.

When blocks to progress occur, the therapist will be wise to consider carefully the transference and counter-transference situation and resolve them through proper interpretation. This is especially true when a previously hypnotizable patient suddenly becomes resistant to hypnosis. Not only does the patient manifest transference reactions, but the therapist also is subject to distortions of perception and behavior, which stem from his or her own childhood experiences with others. This is counter-transference.

Counter-Transference

Analysts are human, too. Feelings and attitudes can be stimulated in them by interactions in the therapeutic relationship. Many of these are quite normal. When challenged, we may become competitive. When approached seductively, we may develop erotic feelings. These are often termed "counter-transference" because they are developed as "counter" to those initiated by the patient or, as we have been discussing earlier, the reactions of an object to the patient's subject. Even though therapists commonly refer to counter-transferences as any feeling state initiated in them by the patient, let us reserve this term and strictly speak of it only for those therapist feelings and behaviors in which the patient's actions have served as stimuli to activate a reexperiencing in the therapist of patterns he or she learned toward early significant others.

There are clues by which the therapist might recognize his or her own counter-transference (Stein, 1970). These include alterations in the usual fees, signs of familiarity, overlooking failures to take prescribed medications, allowing telephone abuses (allowing this particular patient and only this particular patient to contact the therapist at almost any time), neglecting to take a full history, and repeated discussions regarding this particular patient with colleagues (Freud, 1924; J. G. Watkins, 1992 pp. 284).

The manner of the therapist (aggressive, seductive, etc.) may often represent clues to counter-transference (Gruenewald, 1971). Erika Fromm (1968) noted that such reactions are to be considered counterproductive therapeutically, and that unless they are understood and resolved, the therapist will be unlikely to help the patient. This view seems more than a bit extreme because all people are subject to counter-transferences, most of which are analyzed and resolved. By such a yardstick, most therapists could not help people. In some cases, the natural counter-transferences of the therapist may actually be helpful to the patient by fitting in with the patient's needs even though based on distortions of the therapist's perceptions of the patient. Perhaps instead we should take the position that counter-transferences *may* interfere with therapy and should optimally be understood, analyzed, and resolved. However, helping humans do not have to be perfect.

Counter-transference can not only impair therapists' reactions to their patients, but also may be equally a distorting factor in the interactions of researchers with their subjects. This possibility seems completely ignored by those conducting research in hypnosis and psychotherapy in general and is, to the best of our knowledge, never controlled for in the design of studies in hypnosis or, for that matter, other experiments.

In Chapter 3, The Psychodynamics of Hypnotic Induction, we have already given considerable attention to the effect of transference in initiating a hypnotic state. Our emphasis here will be the consideration and use of that process in dealing therapeutically with patients who are working within a hypnoanalytic relationship. In psychoanalysis, the purpose of having the patient recline in a passive condition and concentrate on his or her internal processes is to encourage a regression in which transferences may become manifest (Menninger & Holzman, 1973). In hypnoanalysis, we establish the regression more directly by the induction of the hypnotic state. This brings the patient more rapidly into contact with childhood behaviors and experiences and saves considerable therapy time.

As the patient sinks deeper and deeper into a hypnotic trance state, reality perception fades, and regressive material becomes more and more evident. However, this does not give us permission to immediately interpret the transference. Conducting analysis in the hypnotic state does not mean that resistances are removed. It does not mean that the hypnoanalyst needs less skill or less sensitivity than the psychoanalyst. Quite the contrary. Even though the hypnotic modality has given him or her access to regressive processes far more rapidly than otherwise, it does not indicate in any way that resistance disappears and that we can immediately interpret the transference and achieve genuine insight. Luckily, if a newcomer to this form of therapy mishandles the situation and interprets directly while the patient is in the hypnotic state, more often than not, we will find that upon emerging from hypnosis the patient has "forgotten" what was said, re-repressed, or merely recalls an "intellectual" interpretation. The patient does not at that time fully recall the "experience."

It is like confronting an alcoholic with his or her intoxicated behavior later when sober. He or she will either not remember it, remember it vaguely, misconstrue what happened, or perhaps simply deny it ("That wasn't me, I was drunk and not responsible for my behavior then." "I didn't mean any of those things, it was just because I was drunk or I had too much to drink."). What we must do is recognize that the experience had not been "egotized," recognized as part and parcel of the person's self. As one patient once said to A.F.B., "My husband would always say to me something like, 'I didn't mean those things, it was just because I was drinking.' It took me years to realize that it was his true self that came out while he was drinking and not the other way around." Unfortunately for this poor woman, she had believed him for years, had had children with him, suffered through a difficult divorce, and was finding it difficult to find a new partner to meet her needs at a mature level.

We can give the transference interpretation ("You're acting as if I was your father") in hypnosis and find that it is not well remembered subsequently or not re-experienced and integrated. Or we can interpret it after the patient has emerged from hypnosis. Then the transference interpretation cannot be compared with the conscious reality perception because the interpretation is no longer tied to the experience that the patient had in hypnosis. The experience of the transference, the reality perception, and the interpretation should be tied together, hence, experienced simultaneously.

This objection is one frequently used by classical analysts as an argument against the use of hypnosis, and it is not without some merit. However, all is not lost. The experiencing of the transference in hypnosis may be considered as a forerunner or precursor of it in the conscious state later, even as the experiencing of the transference in psychoanalysis may come first of all in dreams and only later in the relaxed semihypnotic/light hypnotic state, which is normal on the psychoanalytic couch. The next time the experience is reactivated hypnotically, it will be closer to "the surface." Like a dress rehearsal in a play, the elements are approaching "the real thing." This is the leverage that the flexibility of the hypnotic modality offers to the analyst. He or she not only can elicit repressed and dissociated material, not only can vivify this into affective experiencing, but can, to some extent, control the state of the patient's ego for its reception, acceptance, and integration. The therapist can have the remembering and experience occur in deeper to lighter stages of hypnosis and thus approach the fully conscious, egotized state. "Working through" may still be required, but it can be done in far less time when using such hypnotic interventions.

In classical psychoanalysis, the tendency is to attempt to get the patient to focus transference on the analyst. This has considerable advantage because the crucial experiences (compare fantasy from the past with the reality behavior of the present) are immediately available and being experienced within the analytic hour. Because the analyst has always acted in an objective and neutral way, the behaviors and attitudes imputed to him or her transferentially by the patient are more easily demonstrated as false.

There is also a restricting effect by this great concentration of inducing the transferences to manifest him- or herself on the person of the analyst, and this is a significant limitation. Transference is operative in almost all relationships, and it often takes a long time before these are projected on to the analyst. That is one of the reasons why psychoanalysis is so time-consuming and expensive and, therefore, limited in its availability to the wider population.

The hypnotic modality, in addition to stimulating such reactions earlier, makes possible greater attention to the analysis of transferences that occur outside the analytic hour because of its ability to alter both object and self representations. The great impact of transference interpretations occurs because of the disparity between an externally perceived reality and an inner experienced fantasy-reality. There is no reason why the individual analyst who makes the interpretation must also be the person on whom the transferences are targeted. Freud discovered transference when, as an outsider, he observed its projection onto Breuer by a hysterical patient!

The important point is that to be believed, one whom the patient trusts must give an interpretation. Although the analyst's objectivity helps build trust, a person who is actively our friend and supporter may be able to make suggestions and interpretations to us with enhanced credibility whether or not they are accurate. Interpretations concerning transferences that are being manifested toward other relationships *outside* the analysis that are made by analysts who have real, positive rapport with their patients may be more effective than those voiced by a completely "neutral" analyst. Consistent with the intensive weekend therapeutic approaches pioneered by John and Helen Watkins, A.F.B. has found that working intensively with patients in 5- to 9-hour days, sometimes even 7 days a week (including contact outside the therapy office during that time), greatly enhances the speed and progress of therapy by developing rapport and the therapeutic alliance on several levels. This is not to be construed as creating a dualism in the relationship and must be acknowledged as part of the therapeutic process in some states (the state of Washington being just one example) in the legalistic disclosure forms that patients are required to sign at the beginning of therapy.

The clinician or counselor not being party to outside transferences can utilize these continuous, underlying positive levels of rapport that can become indigenous to his or her credibility regarding these transferential manifestations. It was precisely the aspect of contact outside of the therapeutic office with the case A.F.B. noted earlier that was a critical aspect in her therapeutic progress. As Arnold Lazarus (1994) showed, "Those anxious conformists who go entirely by the book, and who live in constant fear of malpractice suits, are unlikely to prove significantly helpful to a broad array of clients and that the worst professional/ethical violation is to permit current risk-management principles to take precedence over humane interventions."

Today, the positive relationship aspects of good therapists are being increasingly emphasized by object-relations theorists (Greenberg & Mitchell, 1983) and others over the "objective" manner, which sometimes is perceived by the patient as cold and rejecting. This is especially true in the treatment of psychotic and borderline patients. The comparative values of an objective, neutral analytic attitude with a more warm, Rogersian supportive approach is worthy of controlled research.

The first impressions a patient gets of his or her analyst are both real and "transferred." This is because the analyst is relatively unknown to the patient then. As the two work together, more material emerges and the patient "works through" transference manifestations. However, he or she is also gathering more real perceptions, and his or her therapist is becoming better known as well. Simultaneously, as therapy progresses, there is less and less new material to be transferred. Even though the therapist is behaving non-directively and minimizing his or her "real" presence, as advised in classical psychoanalysis, the analyst cannot escape becoming more and more real to the patient.

As the psychoanalysis or hypnoanalysis progresses, this is not necessarily bad. Personal comments and self-disclosures about him- or herself by the therapist will not have the distracting effect they would have had earlier in the relationship. They now permit the patient to gradually make the therapist into a "real" person. Obviously, to the patient suffering from borderline personality disorder, the therapist is an object similar to everyone else in his or her life. When the termination of a successful treatment arrives, there is no further need of the patient to use the therapist as a transference target, and he or she should become a real object.

In the earlier days of psychoanalysis, a "rite" of great significance to both parties celebrated this change from analyst to friend (J. G. Watkins, 1978, pp. 73–74). The analyst invited the analysand to dinner. This signified the transition in their relationship from analyst/client to friend/friend in which both become reality objects for each other. Again, this should not be construed by ethicians as a dual relationship; it is, indeed, part and parcel of successful therapy. Because this usually occurred with analysands who were undertaking a "training analysis," it meant that the two were now colleagues. This delightful and meaningful event is all too rarely practiced today, partly because we view treatment far too much as "taking analysis," not as completing an analysis. It is never finished, because analysis is not a discreet undertaking but a continuing growth process carried on in self-analysis by the "patient" who is no longer in face-to-face contact with his or her hypnoanalyst.

Transference in Hypnoanalysis

Transference can be worked with, managed, or interpreted. In working with a transference, usually a positive one, we may recognize its transferential nature but choose to keep and utilize its motivation to achieve symptomatic and behavioral changes. As long as the transference remains positive, the patient (for love of the therapist) tries to please and works hard at the treatment. As emphasized at various points in Barabasz & Watkins, there is nothing wrong with symptomatic change if the patient is improved thereby, and if the underlying conflict needs are not so strong as to render the improvement only temporary. Sometimes for good psychodynamic reasons, constructive symptomatic improvement becomes permanent and analysis is unnecessary and economically contraindicated.

A situation that can threaten both the therapist and the treatment occurs if the positive transference becomes sexualized. Such a situation requires special attention. There are a number of warning signs that can alert the clinician or counselor to this problem (Soskis, 1986). They include finding the patient unusually attractive or appearing in the therapist's sexual fantasies or dreams. Other alerting signs are a patient with a past history of sexual relationships with clinicians or teachers, one who emphasizes the erotic aspects of the hypnotic relationship in discussions, or one who acts in sexually provocative ways. This problem was discussed by Freud (1924) at considerable length in his "Observations on transference love." He warned the young analyst against being entangled in it.

The analyst risks being caught up in a dilemma. If he or she rejects the patient's overtures, the patient may turn against the therapist and discontinue therapy or even bring a lawsuit or make allegations that he or she was seduced by the therapist. Alternatively, if he or she succumbs to the temptation and acts out the situation, then the possibility of ever interpreting this transference to disentangle the patient from an early erotic transference on a parent is forever lost. As Pope, Sonne, and Holroyd (1993) have shown, acting out sexual activity with a patient is now not only unethical and illegal in most states, but it also does not have positive effects on the patient's treatment outcome. When resistance arises in the therapy, the patient will seek a repeat of a sexual affair, the treatment will fail, and the lives of both the therapist and patient eventually become miserable.

Sexual activity with one's patient only became viewed as unethical by the American Psychological Association during the last 20 years of the 20th century. State laws governing the practices of psychologists and medical practitioners rapidly followed suit. Interestingly, by the time A.F.B. became a member of the State Board of Psychology Examiners for the state of Washington and eventually chair of that board, complaints regarding such activities had all but vanished. Public information on one rather interesting case that occurred before my tenure on the board provides a grim reminder to the therapist who might consider becoming so involved. A complaint was raised with the board by a psychologist about a former colleague regarding his engagement in sex with one of his patients. The patient refused to testify against the psychologist and they eventually married. It may be that a borderline patient seduced the psychologist, but the story does not end there. Seven years after the marriage, they were divorced. Given that the state had no statute of limitations on complaints of such a nature, she then filed a complaint with the board against her now-divorced husband. Apparently, he then lost his license to practice. Both the American Psychological Association and many states indicate that sexual relations with patients are considered unethical/illegal for a period of 2 years or longer after termination of a therapeutic relationship.

It is essential to keep the transference positive and not to analyze its source. Then its sexual aspects can be minimized by interpretations like this: "You are indeed a very attractive person. But you have come to me to help you with your problem [illness]. An affair might be very pleasant temporarily, but it would completely spoil our efforts to help you in therapy. Lovers are easier to come by than good therapists. I respect you and care too much about your welfare to ruin it in this way. Let us keep our relationship on this level of high regard and respect for one another." Interpretations of such a nature are usually sufficient to retain the positive transference and not let it denigrate into a treatment-destroying sexual affair. If the therapist's erotic counter-transference toward the patient is too strong for him (and it usually is a male) to accept a stabilization of the relationship at a "respecting, caring" level, then the patient should be referred to another clinician or counselor.

Warning of this hazard when treating a dissociative identity disorder, Wilbur (1988) stated that one alter may be very seductive toward the therapist. Another may also have erotic transference toward the therapist, and another may also have an erotic transference but manifest it by denial and a hostile defense. Interpretations that resolve the transference when dealing with one alter may still leave a sexual transference masquerading in another. A transference situation becomes extremely complex when treating dissociative identity disordered patients with many alters (J. G. Watkins, 1963; J. G. Watkins & H. H. Watkins, 1990).

When simply managing the transference, the therapist is aware of the changes in its manifestations and adjusts the therapeutic interventions for maximum impact. No attempt, whatsoever, is made to resolve them by interpreting their origins. More than half a century ago, Alexander and French (1946) described many cases of psychoanalytic therapy where the transference was simply managed or at least given minimal interpretation. They did not use hypnosis but did achieve significant symptomatic improvements with comparatively few sessions for that era. It is when transference interpretations are employed to counter resistance and reveal underlying conflicts that we can truly speak of the therapy as being "analytic." Let us now consider techniques for implementing this within the hypnotic modality.

The Interpretation of Transference in Hypnoanalysis

A dissociated patient, having experienced both the pain and subsequent relief in previous abreactions, reacted to a new induction procedure with considerable resistance:

Patient: I don't think I can be hypnotized today.
J.G.W.:   You act as if you are afraid of me.
Patient: Yes, I seem to be very afraid of you right now.

Given these reactions, the patient was permitted to enter hypnosis in her own way (nondirectively). Soon she was again reliving scenes where her father had molested her, and J.G.W recognized that like her father, he had given her pain. Transference interpretations both in hypnosis and afterward brought relief from the fear and a renewal of the positive transference.

As foreshadowed in Chapter 7, Realities, Dreams, and Fantasies, dreams often reflect the current state of the transference between the therapist and the patient. This phenomenon has been well documented by psychoanalysts too numerous to mention. Often, the analysis of a dream through the use of hypnosis can permit a transference interpretation that removes a block and significantly moves the treatment forward (M. V. Kline, 1967). In hypnoanalysis, the patient who reports a dream that probably stems from transference can be hypnotized and its meaning more easily derived than would be possible in the conscious state. However, the hypnoanalyst often discovers that the resistance in a negative transference dream may be manifested by greater difficulty in hypnotizing the patient at that specific time. The resistance to the induction is, itself, evidence that the dream represents a negative transference manifestation. The resistance will require interpretative removal before the content of the dream can be activated and analyzed.

Psychoanalytically oriented clinicians and counselors will find that the principles they learned for interpreting transference manifestations apply equally well in hypnoanalytic therapy. The hypnotic state does not result in any basic changes but has the advantage of providing greater flexibility and numerous options. For example, interpretation of negative transference is commonly followed by a change to the positive and visa versa. Interpretations generally require a subsequent "working through," hence, repetition and elaboration. Interpretations are most effective when given at the time that the transferred affect is strong. A new dimension for control of the amount of ego participation is added by the use of hypnosis. You can protect your patient and at the same time facilitate the speed as well as the quality of therapeutic progress.

Most traditional analysts fail to recognize that, almost invariably, hypnosis is spontaneously involved in the traditional psychoanalytic situation. The patient, reclining on the couch, is instructed to concentrate on his or her inner productions and to report them without alteration or censorship. Both relaxation and attention to inner processes, especially fantasies, are in themselves induction techniques. It is, therefore, not surprising that many psychoanalytic patients do their "couch work" in what those of us educated in the field of hypnosis would recognize as a light hypnotic state, which is controlled by the patient's own internal and transference processes active at the time.

Just as the traditional analyst does, the hypnoanalyst recognizes the presence and potentialities of transference. He or she interacts with the patient in ways to control this factor so as to optimize the balance between the uncovering of repressions and the ego integration (egotization) of material so elicited.

It is, of course, customary during psychoanalysis to be patient and wait until the transference feelings are quite strong and the ego is conscious and highly alert. Thus, Fenichel (1945) noted, "The fact that the pathogenic conflicts, revived in the transference, are now expressed in their full emotional context makes the transference interpretation so much more effective."

For the best ego integration, this is true. However, the hypnoanalyst accepts this fact that the relaxed patient on the analytic couch is probably lightly and sometimes more deeply hypnotized through spontaneous self-induction (Barabasz & Watkins, 2005, pp. 76, 78, 226, 413; H. Spiegel & D. Spiegel, 2004, pp. 4–6). Accordingly, what appears overtly to be a genuine re-experiencing "reliving" of conflicts "in their full emotional context" may be less than psychoanalytic theory would predict. The ego is not fully conscious and alert, but only partially so because of the hypnotic state the patient is engaged in. This may be one of the reasons that the psychoanalyst frequently has to make his or her transference interpretations more than once and why they often require more substantial subsequent working through. As you will recall from Barabasz & Watkins (2005) and earlier discussions in this book, patients can experience amnesia or partial amnesia for hypnotic experiences.

One of the advantages of the hypnoanalytic approach, therefore, is that it provides a working methodology for controlling and observing the depths of hypnosis from light, to medium, to deep, to profound. This is an enormous advantage for the therapist in that hypnoanalysis allows us to optimize a level of ego participation, which in the traditional psychoanalytic treatment is left uncontrolled and unnoticed by the analyst. The argument might be waged that the patient might be better left to setting his or her own hypnotic, thus ego participating, level for uncovering repressed material and its integration.

However, patients left entirely to themselves seldom analyze anything nor work through or become free of their conflicts without professional assistance. In fact, left to their own, patients lead a life of seeking out relationships and do nothing but confirm and exacerbate their own pathologies. For example, an abandoned or abused patient is likely to lead a life of resonating with significant others who are also controllers and/or abusers. As a child, one can only blame him- or herself for somehow being bad and, thus, deserving the abandonment. Without professional assistance and a working through of the underlying conflicts, the self-defeating, maladjusted behavior will be repeated again and again throughout the patient's life. The patient never learns to become an adaptive, mature, giving, and truly happy individual.

If interpretations are given when the patient is deeply hypnotized, they will probably require much repetition and working through in subsequent, lighter states. If the interpretation is made when the transference manifestations are near consciousness, hence, in the lighter states of hypnosis, less repetition will be required to meet the analytic criteria of genuine insight. In general, the hypnotic interpretation will have some effect on moving the patient forward; however, occasionally the premature hypnotic interpretation may well alert defensive processes. The patient will then resist hypnosis and interpretations must be against these blocks (the defensive transference) before a return to activating and interpreting the original conflict transference can be made. Managing this transference resistance is quite important and, in fact, was termed "the core of analysis" by Fenichel (1945).

Hypnoanalysis with Psychotic and Borderline Patients

According to classical psychoanalytic theory, psychotic individuals cannot be analyzed because of their inability to establish a stable transference onto the analyst. Cognitive behaviorists using hypnosis followed suit with the notion that "the presence of a severe psychosis is a prime contra-indication to hyp-noanalysis" (Korger & Fezler, 1976). However, work by hypnoanalysts over the past quarter-century have shown otherwise (Baker, 1981, 1983c; Cope-land, 1986; Scagnelli, 1974, 1976; Zeig, 1974). Apparently, despite the difficulty psychotic patients have with contact with reality, there are some psychotic patients who respond to hypnosis even though unstable and vacillating between externalizing and internalizing their representations; psychotic and also borderline patients can and do establish transferences.

Interestingly, Gordon (1973) reported significantly higher hypnotizability in a group of 32 schizophrenic patients compared to age-matched nonpsychi-atrically diagnosed patients in a general medical and surgical inpatient service, using the Stanford Hypnotic Susceptibility Scale Form A. The scale was modi-fied to delete any reference to the term "hypnosis." If the word "hypnosis" was so important to the induction and establishment of hypnotic responsiveness, as held by the sociocognitivists (Braffman & Kirsch, 1999), why would a popula-tion known to be resistant to hypnosis show a higher responsiveness when the word was deleted? Obviously, there are worries about precipitating delusions, but nonetheless the hypnotizability scores were above the general patient popu-lation. Pettinati, Kogan, and Evans (1990) measured the hypnotizability of 113 psychiatric inpatients and 58 healthy control subjects; they found significantly lower hypnotizability on the Hypnotic Induction Profile (HIP) but not on the Stanford Hypnotic Susceptibility Scale. H. Spiegel and D. Spiegel (2004) noted that this may have to do with the Stanford Scale's greater emphasis on behav-ioral observation and compliance in contrast to the HIP's emphases on cogni-tive flow and subjective reports of patient perception regarding response.

Literature reviews of this area, although thorough, are all now quite dated (Baker, 1983; Scagnelli-Jobsis, 1982; Pettinati, 1982; Lavoie & Sabourin, 1980). Baker reported that psychotic patients have now been found to be as hypno-tizable as any other patient population and that apparently the same tech-niques that are employed with other conditions can be applied to them. The research continues and so does the controversy about the hypnotizability of this population (D. Spiegel, 1983; H. Spiegel & D. Spiegel, 2004; Scagnelli-Jobsis, 1983). However, many therapists are now reporting success using hypnosis with psychotic patients as well as borderline personalities.

Baker (1981) asserted that hypnosis can be one of the better modalities for stabilizing transference onto the analyst. Furthermore, Biddle (1967) found the hand levitation induction effective with psychotic patients (Barabasz & Watkins, 2005, pp. 136–143, for details on how to use this technique). A. Barabasz' verbal-nonverbal induction for resistant subjects incorporating a hand levitation variation based on the Kohnstamn affect has also been found to be a bridge to hypnotic responding with this population (Barabasz & Watkins, pp. 159–162). Beahrs (1986) described in detail the dramatic disappearance of psychotic symptoms in a severely schizophrenic patient after a brief treatment by hypnosis. H. Spiegel and D. Spiegel (2004), based on their discussion of the work of Copeland (1986), might conceptualize such a "recovery" as the use of hypnosis or hypnotizability testing in discovering dissociative "mimics" of schizophrenia and serious mood disorders. Copeland discussed several patients who were seemingly psychotic but who were easily hypnotized and subsequently recovered quite quickly. They viewed those patients who were not hypnotizable and whom had worse outcomes as being more consistent with the course of severe affective or thought disorder. Nonetheless, these reports suggest that we need to take a good second look at treating psychosis hypnotically.

This chapter has been essentially about transference and its manifestations in psychoanalytic therapy. However, because the problems of treating psychotic and borderline patients depend so much on the ability to establish, elicit, and work with transferences, this seems an appropriate point to consider these conditions.

Psychotic and borderline patients did not generally establish stable object relationships early in life. Thus, there is great difficulty in the application of classical psychoanalytic methods with this population. They cannot usually start treatment by introjecting the analyst and forming an object representation of him or her. Baker (1981) used hypnosis in the early stages of therapy to help the patient establish such an object, a therapeutic object, with which he or she can interact. This may be considered as a "transitional object" (Winnicott, 1965). Because the psychotic or borderline patient did not establish object representations because the objects (parents) in his or her early environment were not accepting and nurturing, he or she cannot distinguish an object from subject, external reality from self.

Additionally, if we have been through an experience ourselves, it is easier to resonate and understand another in a similar situation. A very excellent psychotherapist with psychotic patients known by J.G.W. has herself been through a psychotic episode. This enables her to understand deeply many communications of her patients, which most clinicians and counselors would miss. However, therapists generally have not had this experience personally.

Some have, but only when sleeping and dreaming, a time when we do exist in a temporally "psychotic" internal world (see Chapter 7). The boundaries between the "me" and external reality are at that time laid aside, and we cannot differentiate between self and object representations. Like the psychotic or borderline patient who has not established ego boundaries, we too may have difficulty in the middle of a dream pulling ourselves out unless there is some transitional object embedded in reality to provide the needed stimulus for recathecting our ego boundaries, such as an alarm clock or the voice of another person. These are specifically noted because most therapists think of transitional objects as being things such as a child's teddy bear or doll.

Try an experiment on yourself if you are accustomed to sleeping soundly throughout the night. Determine that you will awaken at 3:00 a.m. without an alarm clock. Often you will fail and continue to sleep until your accustomed time for arising. Even if you are successful, you may find yourself struggling desperately to pull yourself out of a dream and re-establish contact with an external world in which the touch of the bedsheets provides only a very weak transitional object. Perhaps in such an experience, you can appreciate the difficulty facing the psychotic or the borderline patient who is trying to regain contact with external reality.

Borderline and psychotic patients are frequently in conflict between wishing to merge with a loved object, the therapist, and fear of being engulfed and destroyed by that very object. Copeland (1986) used hypnosis to regulate the amount of "distance" between therapist and patient so as to optimize motivations for the patient to establish an object relationship with him or her. This takes advantage of the focusing ability of hypnosis. The loss of reality contact-distractibility of the psychotic patient is temporarily held in abeyance via the hypnotic modality.

Psychosis, in a sense, is like an individual turned inside out. In neurosis, the id is repressed and the ego contacts the outside world. In psychosis, it is the reverse. The id is released to interact with the outside world, hence, the hallucinations and primitive behavior. Alternatively, it is the ego that is repressed and that needs to be contacted.

Bowers (1961) conceptualized schizophrenia as a defense. In treating schizophrenic patients, she used hypnosis to contact the "little me" or "inner self" of the patient. She believed that the schizophrenic individual uses auto-hypnosis to ward off outer reality and to maintain inner reality, which is less threatening. Perhaps the "schizophrenics" she treated were in fact examples of dissociative "mimics" of schizophrenia identified by Copeland (1986), as discussed earlier by H. Spiegel and D. Spiegel (2004). Nonetheless, object-relations theorists would maintain that the patient needs a "transitional object" to make contact with the outer world (reality). How can we make use of these observations and conceptualizations in treating these patient populations with hypnoanalysis?

One way we can help this type of patient is by becoming for him or her a transitional object that gives a sense of some external, anchoring reality that can later be extended to significant others in his or her world. In this respect Bowers used herself as such an anchoring object, reaching out to contact the "little me" of the patient (1961). However, she warned that sometimes the schizophrenic patient would "merge" with the therapist in a symbiotic relationship, which, if reinforced, might continue indefinitely. In such a case, the patient fails to establish a self/nonself boundary that is achieved by most children in relation to their mothers during the separation-individuation developmental process and which is normally completed by the age of 24 months (Mahler, 1972). Bowers warned that this was one of the greatest hazards in treating schizophrenic patients.

Sometimes a real relationship with a live person in several contexts (as employed by J.G.W., Helen Watkins, and A.F.B.) may seem too threatening to such a patient. Then, a teddy bear or inanimate object may be less fearsome, enabling him or her to establish some contact with external reality and start the process of differentiating self from nonself. Teddy bears or even ragged fragments from the child's security blanket should not be taken away from young children until their "objectivity" has been extended to include other people and things. The behavior modification technique of withdrawing such objects from children for "misbehavior" is one reason why A.F.B. began to move away from an early emphasis on behaviorally conceptualized therapeutic procedures.

Perhaps a brief case study will make this point remarkably clear to even the most casual observer. A middle-aged professional woman was so detached from the world that she existed only in a schizoid fog. She was successful in her occupation but she never had a sense of reality. She lived in a kind of dream world. Hypnosis, because of its ability to provide focus for a patient, seemed especially indicated in her case. Accordingly, hypnosis was used to mobilize her self energies (ego cathexes) and focus them all on her fingertips, a small area of her physical ego boundary. J.G.W. then gave her a pencil. In a flood of tears, she exclaimed, "For the first time in 30 years I'm feeling something real." For her, the differentiation between "the me" and the "not-me" was started. She had experienced an external object, if only a pencil.

This was the beginning of an extended treatment that J.G.W. referred to at the time as "existential hypnoanalysis" (1967a, 1967b). The aim was to establish "meaning" to self and to the external reality as they impacted one another. First, she impacted a pencil, next the therapist, then other people in the world. Finally, a normal, albeit neurotic, transference could be established, permitting therapy to continue along more traditional analytic lines. Existential hypnoanalysis will be discussed in the next and final chapter of the present volume.

A.F.B. was working with a mid-20s, intellectually brilliant, schizophrenic male who was in a similar dream world. In the session, the patient was expounding esoterically and with great bitterness about unfairness in the world. He became more and more withdrawn as the bitterness overwhelmed his facial expression. Any attempt at a standard hypnotic induction would have been futile. I tossed him an orange that was sitting on my desk. Reflexively, he caught it (not a great feat, as we were less than 4 feet apart). I said loudly to him, "Hold it, feel it, squeeze it, squash it, peel it, squeeze it harder. What does it feel like?" "Sticky, gooey," he said. "Yes, it's real sticky, gooey," I said. "Smell it now, taste it!" His facial expression began to change and began to normalize. At that point, I took the risk of him losing contact with reality again by saying, "It's O.K. to let your eyes close now, it's O.K., it's O.K. to let your eyes close now, you're focused on the here-and-now, you can still feel the orange, you can still taste the orange in your mouth." It was in this manner, following J.G.W.'s techniques, that A.F.B. helped the patient develop his ego cathexes. This patient was unlikely to be one of those dissociative types mimicking schizophrenia in that he did respond, to some extent, to antipsychotic medication. A treatment by medication alone was insufficient to provide a basis for him to hold a job for any period of time. Laborious work in therapy using hypnosis and mobilizing ego cathexes provided a basis for him to hold his first job for more than a year, which was my last follow-up on that patient. As in J.G.W.'s case above, the orange, which facilitated the hypnotic induction, became the basis for initial impact. This experience with an external object, which was then extended to other people in his world, made it possible for him to maintain sufficient reality-based perceptions so that he could maintain a job position for a reasonable period of time.

Federn (1952a) distinguished between an "estrangement" and "depersonalization." Estrangement means the inability to sense the external as real. Today, we would call it a deficiency in forming object representations. By depersonalization, Federn referred to the inability to experience one's own self, the inadequate energizing of self representations. In his theoretical conceptions, estrangement meant the lack of object cathexis vested into perceptions. Individuals feel "depersonalized" when they cannot cathect self representation with ego cathexis because of the weakness or lack of self energies. However, the two are interactively related. For us to have the impact of reality, an object representation must be innervated by a certain quantity of object cathexis in contact with a minimally energized ego representation (J. G. Watkins, 1978). Unless object plus ego energies add up to a certain quantum, the "experience" does not take place or does so only at an unconscious level. Unless the magnitude of light from an object plus the degree of sensitivity of the retina exceed a certain threshold, vision cannot take place. Hypnosis with hypnotic suggestion can be used to focus object and ego energies on different physical or mental points of contact.

Elgan Baker suggested several hypnotic techniques for building self and object representations. First, the patient was asked to visualize an image of self accompanied by a pleasant feeling. Second, the patient was instructed to open his or her eyes and see the therapist, then close them again and return to the image of self. Next, the patient was helped to visualize an image of therapist, a step that borderline patients often find difficult. The hypnotized patient was then asked to alternate between the images of self and of the therapist. Next, the two would be pictured together, letting the patient set the distance between them. And finally, fantasies would be developed involving the patient and the therapist in parallel activity and in interaction. As ego functioning stabilized, the process was extended to include other significant objects and to integrating positive and negative images. In this way, the therapist was first established as a transitional object, followed by a strengthening of the patient's ability to form other object relations.

Christensen (personal communication to A.F.B., July 2007) recommends the adjunctive use of EMDR to obtain and enhance a positive cognition of the therapist or to assist the processing/resolution of transference issues the patient has toward the therapist.

Much of Federn's treatment of psychotics was in collaboration with Gertrude Schwing (1954), a motherly nurse who provided the "holding environment" that Winnicott (1965) described as being an essential feature in helping psychotic individuals to establish a stable object representation. Federn also believed that the analyst-patient transference should be kept positive and interpreted only when it became negative. There seems to be no reason why Federn's techniques could not be applied far more effectively using hypnosis.

In using hypnosis with psychotic patients, it should be remembered that the activation, or only the memory enhancement, of psychotic dreams or other regressions will likely reprecipitate the psychotic episode associated with them. Accordingly, the "analytic" methods of free association and dream interpretation are quite clearly contraindicated. Interpretations should center on blocks to ego control and the development of defenses, not at all on remembering and releasing primitive id-related drives. The psychotic patient's ego has already been overwhelmed by such. It needs integration and building-up, not tearing down. In fact, because psychotic and borderline conditions represent developmental failures, Dan Brown and Erika Fromm (1987) have suggested that the therapy should be "hypno-integrative" rather than hypnoanalytic. Fromm reported a patient who, using hypnotic visualization, conceptualized himself floating inside a protective bubble, which protected him from merging with the therapist and could establish the safest and most acceptable distance from outside people. In the early stages of treatment with this patient, the bubble would break up easily, but as the patient's boundaries became more stabilized, it would burst only under intense emotional interactions (a precaution to note if treatment becomes too abreactive).

Scagnelli (1974, 1976, 1977, 1980) developed effective procedures for using hypnosis in the treatment of psychotic and borderline patients. She recommended autohypnosis because patients are less fearful when they are not forced into a one-to-one close relationship with the therapist and they are more in control of their own therapy. Apparently, most of her patients used hypnosis for ego strengthening and the formation of self or object representations and not for uncovering (although a few borderline patients did do uncovering). She also recommended autohypnosis for the therapist, a state in which she reported being able to better concentrate and be more sensitive to her patients' needs. Scagnelli/(Jobsis) is most empathic in coexperiencing with her patients. This is similar to "resonance," a term that will be discussed more in the next chapter. Most recently, Ginandes (in press) has been working to expand the ego strengthening concept by using hypnosis to help foster "healthy narcissism."

J.G.W. had a dissociated patient enter a psychotic state following several days of severe abreactions (J. G. Watkins & Johnson, 1982). She regressed to the age of 3, carrying her teddy bear around the ward. However, after contacts with her mother and continued perseverance by the therapist, she returned to normalcy and showed great improvement in her dissociations. The point is to be persistent. Don't give up. The regression into a suicidal, psychotic, or child state may be the most potent possible request for help and "love" that the patient can make. The therapist who doesn't run, and who meets the challenge, will often be rewarded by the patient taking a big step forward.

The Safe-Room Technique

Helen Watkins used a "safe-room technique" to help the patient restore boundaries and save energy when stress (external or internal) becomes too severe. The therapist may then proceed similar to the following: Hypnotize the patient and ask him or her to go down a long staircase with you. At the bottom, ask the patient to walk along a hallway and visualize a door on one side: "A door to a room of your own choosing in which you will feel safe and comfortable. Look at the door and tell me what it looks like. Have you ever seen this door before?" (Such a question is designed to elicit possible past associations.) She then continued, "Would you like to enter this room alone, or would you like me to come with you? Either way is fine." The answer reveals the patient's dependency needs. The patient can close the door in this place and be "safe" while he or she rests and restores self-integrity and energy.

Inspired by Helen Watkins' approach, A.F.B. uses a substantial elaboration of this technique for patients who are unwilling or unable to explore in depth the problems at hand due to the nature of a limited relationship (short-term therapy). I use a long descending escalator induction such as one might find outdoors at the San Diego Zoo, where one is able to experience various smells of flowers, trees, and earth, then an entrance into a hall with several doors; the patients have a choice of a door, which leads to a hallway that again has several doors. All the time, the patients are carrying a backpack full of stones, which represent their problems. Each of the stones has a label on it, giving the nature of the problem, but some stones are unlabeled and these represent conflicts or problems that the patients have not come into contact with yet but that they may know, at some level, are affecting their ability to lead a more adaptive life. Eventually, patients pick a door in the hallway and are asked to describe the door in detail: What sort of handle is it, where is the handle, what does the door look like, does it have panels, etc. Then patients are asked to enter the room and close the door and lock it. The patients are then told, "This is a safe room that you can always enter anytime you want to. No one can come into the room after you." In the room, they are asked to "unload the backpack and pour the stones on the floor; some are large, some are small, and others are only pebbles. Spend some time arranging the stones in piles of big problems, medium problems, and even little pesky ones." The patients are then allowed some time for calm contemplation.

The above segment of images only proceeds after an ideomotor finger-raise signal is observed to verify that the images had been experienced. Progression is then made to the point of asking the patients to put the now-empty backpack on and to indicate when they are ready to leave the room. When they have done so, they are asked once again to check to make sure they haven't left some pebbles in the backpack. They are told that some people are pebble gatherers, that even when things can be experienced successfully they tend to pick up pebbles or sometimes even stones that will stand in their way. They are asked once again "to look in the backpack and make sure it's truly empty." The patients are reassured that "these stones will be in the room," and that they "can come back and examine them at anytime." Some patients choose to have colored stones to represent different things and thus facilitate interpretation. Red stones often represent sexual problems or sometimes menstrual problems, brown retentive problems, and so on.

None of this is explored at that time; patients are simply left to leave the room with the now-empty backpack on, slowly brought back down the hall, and out of hypnosis. If the relationship is severely limited at that particular point,they are reassured that I will never ask them about those stones. It is up to them to bring that up. Reassurance is given that I will always be ready to listen and to help the stones talk to each other and work their problems out. Patients are reassured that they can always go back to the room to work with the stones and rearrange them in ways that may work better. Recognizing that "the stones" might also represent part-persons of the patients, it is important that the patients are clear that we are not trying to eliminate the stones, although we have pointed out that they do represent problems. Each person is alerted from hypnosis by walking back down the hall and then through ascension via the escalator. "The day is now sunny and bright and you are feeling just fine, feeling just fine without the burden of the heavy, heavy backpack full of stones. They are working together in your safe room and you will know when to go back and see how they are doing."

One patient Helen Watkins worked with (1978) was pursued by a malevolent ego state called the "Evil One." At times, he would emerge as a full-fledged auditory hallucination. He kept trying to follow the patient into the safe room, shouting and yelling. Helen said she would hold onto the Evil One while the patient went into the safe room and closed the door. The patient did so. The hallucination of the Evil One temporarily ceased and the therapist's role as the patient's protector was further strengthened.

Hypnosis and transference are regressive processes. Normally, we think of regression as taking one back to more primitive and childlike behaviors. It is a bit strange to report the reverse. The hypnotic regression took one patient back to an earlier time and in this case a much better adjusted existence.

Clarence was a paranoid schizophrenic in his mid-30s. He had been hospitalized for 8 years with chronic psychosis, plagued by hallucinations of the "Its," a malevolent gang who constantly persecuted him and whose machinations he continually talked about. After J.G.W. (2002) worked with him hypnotically for 6 months, and after having established a good therapeutic relationship, J.G.W. regressed him back to a time before he had become psychotic and hospitalized. The initiation of the hypnotic state was difficult, but with persistence, it was achieved and the patient regressed back to the age of 19. At that point, when he emerged from hypnosis it would be 1942 instead of 1951 (World War II ended in 1945).

To J.G.W.'s astonishment, he came out of hypnosis and showed not the slightest sign of psychosis. Gone were all of his delusions, his hallucinations, and his concrete verbalizations. Instead, the patient appeared perfectly normal. Hardly believing it, J.G.W. invited Clarence to join him and a colleague for lunch. My friend knew nothing about Clarence. During lunch he, a very experienced psychologist, and Clarence conversed normally, exchanging childhood reminiscences and their impressions of certain communities. At no time did my colleague suspect he was talking to a patient with chronic paranoid schizophrenia. In fact, Clarence's manner was so completely normal that the only time a puzzled expression appeared on my friend's face was when Clarence mentioned that he was expecting to receive his draft notice soon (World War II having been over for 6 years then).

Later that day, J.G.W. rehypnotized Clarence and removed the posthypnotic suggestion. He immediately reverted to his usual psychotic ideation. J.W.G.'s colleague, when asked about the lunch, assured him he had no idea he was talking to a chronic paranoid patient who was hospitalized with schizophrenia. A few days later, J.G.W. again tried to rehypnotize Clarence. The patient was extremely resistant and after that was no longer willing or able to enter a state of hypnosis. Apparently, the paranoid structure had a life of its own and would not accept permanent elimination. Bowers (1961) observed that "the schizophrenic who is hypnotized successfully by a therapist who he is not ready to trust completely" may be "consequently most difficult to hypnotize the second time." Perhaps living in his earlier life of reality was too frightening unconsciously to Clarence, and in suggesting doing so, even for an hour or two with the protection of hypnosis, J.G.W. had stretched the credibility of his relationship with the patient too far.

Unfortunately, just a few weeks later, J.G.W. was transferred to another veteran's hospital facility and never saw Clarence again. However, 3 years later, on revisiting the hospital he was observing a group of patients some distance away being taken to the gym for exercise. From the middle of the group, a hand waved in J.G.W.'s direction and Clarence was shouting, "Hey Doc, we got the 'Its' on the run."

J.G.W. has often wondered what would have happened to Clarence if he had not removed his posthypnotic suggestion. How long could the regression to "normalcy" have been maintained in the face of the world of reality and the absence of a continuous hypnotic relationship with his therapist? Apparently, he could act the role of a normal individual, but the world would not have allowed him to live in 1942. As soon as that point came up, and he had been informed that "now" was really 1951, his regression probably would have been broken; his paranoid condition would have returned. Nonetheless, the possibilities here for treating psychotics with hypnosis are intriguing and clearly warrant further study.

Summary

Transference, a common phenomenon, occurs when an individual reacts to a present-day person (frequently his or her therapist or mentor) as if he or she was a significant person in the individual's past. The interpretation of this transference is a powerful technique in analytic therapies. When the therapist perceives the patient similarly, hence, experiencing feelings that stem from early relationships in his or her own past, this is called "counter-transference." The elimination of transferences and the developing of reality perceptions is a basic goal in both psychoanalysis and hypnoanalysis. Hypnosis makes it possible to activate transference reactions far sooner in therapy than traditional analysis would allow. They can be utilized, manipulated, or interpreted. Hypnotizability and resistance represent changes in transferences. The timing and skill with which transferences are interpreted are highly significant in both psychoanalytic and hypnoanalytic therapies.

The common position in the past has been that psychotic individuals could not be analyzed because they are unable to establish stable object relationships and, hence, transferences on the analyst. Hypnosis makes it possible, at least in some cases, to build the therapist into a "transitional object" for the patient. In this way, the patient learns to establish stable object and self representations so therapy can progress. These approaches have brought even schizophrenia within the possibilities of treatment through hypnosis.

12
Existential Hypnoanalysis and the Therapeutic Self

Symptoms are ways of creating the illusion that time does not pass, that it is not moving at all or that it can be stopped at will, an unconscious means of managing existential anxiety.

Yalom, 1980

There seems to be a close relationship between an individual's implicit sense of the passage of time and his or her psychopathological state. Many defenses—isolation, displacement, avoidance, denial, and projection, for example—can be seen as attempts to avoid the movement of time; to act as though time were really like a clock and one could start over, be young again, and avoid the significance of the moment. These defenses deprive a situation of its novelty, making it seem familiar even when it is not entirely familiar. Growth occurs as individuals learn to seize each moment and make the most of it rather than expending psychological energy in denying the importance of time and its fleeting quality (H. Spiegel & D. Spiegel, 2004, p. 195).

There may be an essential interplay between the unconscious presumption that time does not move on and the perpetuation of psychological symptoms. The very preservation of the symptom carries with it an implication of indifference about the passage of time. The rigidity of a dysfunctional pattern of keeping other people at a distance, for example, presupposes that other people will always be available to be fended off. The transference in therapy can blossom only if the transference object, the therapist (or mentor), is still available for projection (H. Spiegel & D. Spiegel, 2004, p. 197).

Severely disturbed patients are trapped in an expanded present. They are selfish beings where references to the future, if any, fail to incorporate immediate plans to make wishes for happiness come true. As clients responds to therapy, becoming more adaptive, happier, successful, and symptom-free, and interacting more appropriately with the real world as a giving person, they evidence intermediate and long-term plans for the future. Their temporal orientation becomes future oriented and the behaviors to make that positive future possible are in place (A. Barabasz, 1974a, 1974b).

Bored Patients

En route, I proceeded across Mercer Island and the Lake Washington floating bridge. As usual, morning traffic was bumper to bumper. Some passengers dozed, some read the morning *Post Intelligencer*, others listened to the radio. My fellow commuters were various. Some appeared sad, worried, grim, bored, or passive, but not many appeared happy about going to work. As on many past occasions, I thought how fortunate I was to be a pilot with everyday work that was not only a challenge but a joy. How fortunate not to be confined to mundane tasks, repetitious procedures, and boring environments. But most significant was the challenge of the job ... (Johnston, 1991).

The new patient slumped into the easy chair. "What seems to be the trouble?" inquired the therapist.

"Well, nothing I guess," replied the patient slowly.

"Then why are you here?

"You know, Doc, I really don't know. I have everything, a good wife, children, an excellent income, big house, two cars paid for, a cabin at the lake, job security, and nothing to worry about, and I am really happy. It's just—well, it's just that I don't seem to get much of a kick out of life. I build things in the shop. My wife and I play tennis at the club. No sexual frustrations. The kids are in college. We're thinking about a round-the-world sailing cruise next year, but there is something missing."

The wheels inside the therapist's head started spinning. Low-level depression? Mid-life crisis? Borderline? Maybe an obsessive-compulsive personality? Silently, the therapist reviewed the many diagnostic categories found in the *Diagnostic and statistical manual*. None of them seem to fit. Why would an apparently happy and successful person come to a psychotherapist merely because he wasn't getting a "kick" out of life (J. G. Watkins, 1967a) ?

The usual suggestions passed through the therapist's mind: medical checkup, diet checkup, exercise program, more "together" activities, join an organization, meet new people, change work, get a hobby, start a garden, become involved in community activities, and so on. None of these seemed to fit either. Why?

Psychotherapists are being increasingly confronted with patients who don't show the classic anxieties, conversional symptoms, or psychosomatic disorders for which treatment strategies have been primarily developed. True, more low-level depressions are being uncovered, while schizoid and borderline characters are diagnosed with greater frequency, but increasing numbers of people are manifesting a kind of ennui with life, individuals who according to present societal standards "have it made." They don't demonstrate clearcut symptoms, such that they can be regarded as "sick." Somehow, they are a product of a general cultural malaise in a society that has everything, a society in which most of life's frustrations can be gratified, where there is a pill for almost every symptom, but a lack of challenge. One can get away with building credit card debt and living in an expanded present of gratifications for years without having the perseverance to create the wealth required to earn them. Our forefathers struggled against a hostile nature, a harsh environment, all sorts of diseases, sometimes starvation, and sometimes unfriendly natives to wrest a continent from the wilderness. They were often defeated, but they were never bored!

Today, we are confronted with a cultural deficiency. We have "things," yet increasingly, people who have more and more that they have done little to earn are bitter and envious of those who have what they do not. We lack "souls." With the greatest number of conveniences, labor-saving devices, activities, and luxuries of any society that ever existed, we have the most number of "bored" people. As therapists, analysts, or human engineers, we have many skills for enhancing perceptions, improving motivations, integrating dissociations, and developing our patients' self-understanding through hypnosis, hypnotic suggestion, interpretation, plus other numerous devices. We are strengthened by our knowledge of unconscious processes and our facilitative techniques of clinical hypnosis and hypnocounseling. But can we do something about improving the "quality of life"? We have the psychological "tweezers" for removing a fly from the soup. Can we also enhance the taste of the soup? Must we only "eliminate the negative," or can we also, as suggested in the song of old, "accentuate the positive," and add to the zest for living?

For many people, there is lack of "meaning" in their life's activities (Frankl, 1963). They interact with others, have affairs, listen to T.V. evangelists, donate to causes, and sometimes, just sometimes, see therapists. There is no dearth of stimulation. They have developed object representations, and they also have self representations, but somehow the two don't significantly contact each other.

Humans have always wrestled with the problem of existence. Existential philosophers, like Kierkegaard (1954), Heidegger (1949), Marcel (1948), Buber (1970), and Tillich (1952), have addressed this area. We can also refer to the classical debate between Locke (1823/1963), who felt that reality existed in external objects, in "matter," Berkeley (1929), who noted that external reality would not exist unless there was the self of a perceiver, hence, mind, and Hume (1963), a skeptic, who used three arguments to "prove" that neither mind nor matter existed. This brought philosophy to a nihilism that required the rescue of Kant (1934), who questioned the validity of a "pure" reason that destroys its own self.

The question of what is real, what exists, and what has "meaning" became the focus of the mid-20th-century group of therapists who developed a school of psychological treatment that became known as "humanistic." That conceptualization contrasted with the behavioral and psychoanalytic approaches.

Emphasis is put on the role of the "self"(J. G. Watkins, 2001a, 2001b, 2001c, 2004) and human adjustment and the ability of the patients to heal themselves with minimal intervention and control by the therapist. Humanistic-existential approaches to treatment were proposed by Bugental (1967), Satir (1967), Burton (1972), Shostrom (1967), and Jourard (1971). These writers emphasized the encouragement of "authenticity" in the therapist and spontaneity in the patient. Born of that era was the idea to call the patient "a client" to de-emphasize the concept of "illness." They drew inspiration from the writings of John Dewey (1916) who, railing against the widespread authoritarianism in schools, advocated a liberal democratic approach to education, which stressed more permissiveness and freedom for students to develop their own interests. The mood was toward less parent-control, less teacher-control, and less therapist-control. Human behavior was to be improved by the development of inner self-resources rather than by the control of outer stimuli, as advocated by the behaviorists of the time. Some psychoanalysts, such as Perls (1969), Erich Fromm (1973), and Erikson (1964), began turning more attention toward the development rather than the analysis of inner processes. The pendulum was moving from a focus on "interpersonal" relationships toward one on " intrapersonal" relationships.

Attempting to provide some integration between the two positions, May (1958) proposed three areas of existence: "*umwelt*," the external or "around-world" (the physical environment); "*mitwelt*," the world of interpersonal relationships, hence, the "with-world"; and "*eigenwelt*," the "own-world" of self. When we use hypnotic suggestion directed at a patient's external behavior, we are intervening in the patient's *umwelt*. When we interpret his or her transference in a hypnoanalytic relationship, we are dealing with his or her *mitwelt*. And when we are developing self-object representations to establish ego boundaries, we are refashioning the patient's *eigenwelt*. Each is a kind of reality that can have some meaning to the patient in the different spheres of his or her existence.

Existential hypnoanalysis (J. G. Watkins, 1967a) is not really a new therapeutic technique that should have a devoted group of disciples ("I am an existential hypnoanalyst"). It is a perspective and a therapeutic goal where the object of our interventions is not merely the symptom, but rather an approach that aims in enhancing "meaning-in-living" for our bored patients. When Elgan Baker (1983a), Donna Copeland (1986), and Joan Murray-Jobsis (1984) hypnotically helped their psychotic patients establish stable ego boundaries so that self-object representations could meaningfully contact one another, they were practicing existential hypnoanalysis. Back when Federn (1952a) taught his schizophrenic patients to distinguish between reality A and reality B, he too was practicing existential analysis, although he didn't label it as such.

Once J.G.W. tried to interest therapists (who were practicing then a strictly (J. G. Watkins, 1967b) behavioral point of view) in an approach that treated "meaning" as a behavior, a behavior that could be enhanced if its discovery was "reinforced" with therapist praise (the classic "approval" counseling lead) as well as by a natural reinforcement that insightful discoveries always receive.

This was an attempt to integrate two very different therapeutic languages. But a paper written on this approach appealed to neither humanistic editors nor behavioral editors and was never published.

Carl Rogers (1961) called our attention to the inherent strengths in the human self, which, when not invaded by directiveness on the part of the therapist, could, through its own resources, make important steps toward new insights and integration. However, the stereotypes of hypnosis as necessarily being a directive approach tended to alienate Rogersian nondirective/client-centered practitioners. J.G.W. suggested to a devoted disciple of Rogers that he try practicing nondirective therapy using hypnosis. In astonishment, he replied, "Why, they are the exact opposite. In hypnosis you suggest and direct. We never do that in client-centered therapy." Obviously, this poor fellow was unaware of the approaches of Milton Erickson. It was decades before publication of the text titled *Hypnocounseling: An eclectic bridge between Milton Erickson and Carl Rogers* (Gunnison, 2004), and the American Psychological Association Division on Counseling Psychology began meetings of special interest groups on "hypnosis in counseling."

Once induced, hypnosis is simply an altered state within an intensive relationship setting, and there is nothing, nothing at all, inherent in hypnosis that requires us to be suggestive and directive. The ease with which hypnotic suggestions can be made operative in hypnosis is seductive to the practitioner whose counter-transference needs for controlling others gain encouragement. However, the principles and approaches practiced by nondirective, client-centered, person-centered therapies can be equally applied using hypnosis if only these therapists were trained in hypnosis. But even decades ago, there were exceptions: Volney Faw, a professor at Lewis and Clark College, practiced Rogersian nondirective therapy with hypnotized clients and reported great success (personal communication to J.G.W.). He utilized the techniques of reflection of feeling ("You feel that your father is hostile toward you"), and clarification counseling leads ("As I understand it, you are telling me that you can't really trust him"), which were advocated by Rogers (1951), throughout the use of hypnosis. His experiences with this approach were sadly not available in published form for general distribution. It was from this contribution of this group of philosophers and therapists, as well as the theories of Paul Federn plus his own experience with patients, that we have attempted to apply hypnosis in the implementation of a more humanistic approach to treatment termed "the therapeutic self" (A. Barabasz & J. Watkins, 2005).

The Therapeutic Self

Psychotherapy may be studied as a science but it is practiced as an art. In spite of the titles of our two texts, *Hypnotherapeutic techniques* and *Advanced hypnotherapy: Hypnodynamic techniques,* the techniques are not as important as the "self" of the clinician or counselor who practices them. J.G.W. notes that two equally trained young resident physicians were rotated on a medical ward at a large hospital. Whenever Dr. Y was assigned to the ward, morale was excellent and healing took place, be it on the gastroenterology, cardiac, or gastro-intestinal wards. However, after 3 months, morale dropped when Dr. X replaced him on these same wards. Urinary infections proved more stubborn, complaints of anginal pain were more frequent, and ulcers flared. These two young doctors had both graduated from the University of Oregon Medical School, had equal training, and were ranked comparably among their class-mates. Yet Dr. Y had something that Dr. X lacked: a "therapeutic self."

Resonance

Can we tell who has it and who does not? What constitutes the therapeu-tic self? How can it be developed in young healing-arts practitioners-to-be? Again, the theories of Federn (1952a) have a contribution to make here. The issue is that of resonance. Resonance is that inner experience within therapists during which they co-feel, co-enjoy, co-suffer, and co-understand a patient, though in microform. It is a relationship, but not an object relationship. Such therapists can "morph" into an embodiment of the patient, yet without the psychopathology. It is a "subject" or self relationship, one in which they com-mit themselves as full-fledged allies with their patients. When resonating, therapists replicate within themselves, as close as possible, a facsimile of the other's experiential world, yet it seems an effortless transformation on the part of the therapist, considering the limitations of communication—verbal, postural, and so on—that identify with that replica. When patients are sad, their therapists are also sad. When the patients are successful, the therapists participate in the resulting joy. When treating another, therapists are involved in a kind of "with-ness." At the moment, the therapist is able to experience the patient's world, almost exactly like the patient does. Resonance, therefore, is a temporary identification established, effortlessly in the good resonator, for the purposes of better understanding the internal motivations, feelings, and attitudes of a patient. Resonance describes from an inner, experiential point of view a kind of "modeling" from the point of view of the social learning theorists (Bandura & Walters, 1963).

"Accurate empathy" is the term used by Carl Rogers (1961). This seems about as close as we can get to "resonance." But although Rogers defined it as where "the counselor is perceiving the hates, and hopes, and fears of the client through emersion in the empathic process," he then delimited the scope of empathy by adding to it, "without himself experiencing those hates, hopes, fears." Unfortunately, Rogers conceived empathy as an "intellectual under-standing process," but not as a fully "co-experiencing process" like we mean by our use of the term "resonance." Resonance assumes that we cannot fully understand a process merely by observing it from the outside, as an object. Some understanding is certainly acquired in this way. But a more complete comprehension requires participation by the therapist (if only in microform), not merely an outside observing.

Resonance is a relationship. It should be clearly distinguished from transference. In transference, we impact our object representations by clothing them with the "psychological garments" of our parents and other early, significant figures. We will respond to them as if they were such. In resonance, we coexist with the internalization of the patient as if it is our own self, not as an object. The image of them is now included within our own ego boundaries, as part of our self, and is sensed in the same way as we experience our own self.

Resonance can be differentiated into "affective resonance," and "cognitive resonance." Resonance as a whole can be objectively rated by individuals listening to recordings of therapy sessions, as we do when we train people to be psychotherapists. In fact, an objective scoring system for evaluating these phenomena has even been developed and subjected to a certain amount of experimental validation (J. Watkins, 1978b).

The initial validation study for this scale employed a world-renowned group of therapists including Albert Ellis, Carl Rogers, John Cameron, Franz Alexander, and John Watkins. Groups of raters, using this scale, scored therapists' responses as resonant (R), objective (O), and simply facilitative (F). The percentages in each category were determined based on sessions conducted by this group of therapists that were both published and audiotape recorded. However, lest it be assumed that the "best therapists" are those who manifest the greatest amount of resonance, another equally important consideration must be taken into account.

If therapists immerses themselves 100% into their patients' feelings and understandings, they will not be able to help the patients achieve more objectivity in life. There will now be a *folie à deux*, and the two will be sick together. Such a folie à deux is commonly observed in young relationships where, more often than not, females might adopt the most maladaptive personality characteristics of the male. Extreme cases occasionally make the news, such as the murderer Charles Manson, whose girlfriends became accomplices to his murderous acts. During the trials, parents and friends of these young women, who knew them as they grew up, were astonished at how such once nice, open, energetic people could turn into murderers. The point of greatest concern for therapists is to remember that they can understand patients through both resonance and objectivity, which is, of course, precisely what Charles Manson's young women friends lacked.

These two perspectives provide different understandings of the patient from different perspectives: the internal and the external. If only an "objective" approach is taken, the therapist will not understand the patient's world as does the patient. Hence, understanding will be incomplete. However, if he or she lacks objectivity, then there will be no adequate comprehension of the ways in which the patient's perspective differs from external reality and from the expectations of society. The therapist cannot, therefore, hope to move the patient from his or her neurosis to the reality of an experiential maturity. The therapist must be like a bridge, a therapeutic bridge, with one foot in the patient's experiential world, including his or her pathology, and the other foot in the world of objective reality. A *balance* between resonance and objectivity is optimal. There must not be an overemphasis on either one.

In the scientific tradition of adhering to objectivity in the design and execution of experimental research, the majority of cognitive and cognitive-behavioral as well as psychoanalytic therapists are trained to be objective when doing therapy. The practitioners are urged to avoid contaminating the outcome with "counter-transference needs." Such a position increases the problem, however, of initiating in the patient the feeling that he or she is only a "thing," an object of interest, but not a "person," who evokes "caring" feelings in the therapist. Because patients are accustomed to being treated as "things" by doctors, especially those who are not their family physicians, they may accept this "object relationship." However, something important is lost therapeutically. As Tillich (1960) most eloquently stated it:

> The other person cannot be controlled like a natural object. Every human being is an absolute limit, an unpierceable wall of resistance against any attempts to make him into an object. He who breaks this resistance by external forces destroys his own humanity; he never can become a mature person.

This interdependence of person and person in the process of becoming human is a judgment against a psychotherapeutic method in which the patient is a mere object for the analyst as subject. The inevitable reaction then is that the patient tries in return to make the analyst into an object for him- or herself as subject. This kind of acting and reacting has a depersonalizing effect on both the analyst and the patient (J. G. Watkins, 1967a).

Just as transference may beget counter-transference and resonance beget counter- resonance (J. G. Watkins, 2005), so does complete "objectivity" beget complete "counter-objectivity." Should the doctor fail to cure, the patient will have no hesitancy in suing. It may well be that more doctors have been sued for their failure to resonate than because of genuine malpractice. Patients may forgive a "caring" doctor, but they deeply resent being treated as objects, as things (J. G. Watkins, 2001a).

An equally regrettable trap happens to the therapist who is an overresonator. In supervising psychology trainees in prison settings, J.G.W. (at Montana State Prison and A.F.B. (at Paparua Prison in New Zealand) would often hear their strong feelings of indignation at the "mistreatment" of the inmates by the prison guards. The poor inmate had been abused by his parents (possibly true), had been "railroaded" into jail by an overly vindictive prosecuting attorney (less likely true), and had been sentenced by a judge who wouldn't even listen to him (least likely true). Our trainees had learned to resonate well, but their own counter-transferences toward their own rejecting parent figures had been stimulated in their resonance with the inmates.

J.G.W. found it necessary to commend these psychology trainees on their ability to resonate but to also say to them, "Whoa! Sit back and look at your inmate client from a different point of view; he is in prison for aggressive acts inflicted on others. Suppose it was your own sister or brother who had been their victims. Would you still feel the same way?" The trainee therapists had to learn to balance their resonating with an at least equal objectivity. Otherwise, they could never help their inmate clients rehabilitate and find places back in society. They had learned half the secret of the therapeutic self. Perhaps because of the emphasis on "objectivity" in the research training that they had received, they had overly reacted against it in the therapeutic side of their training. However, the ability to resonate is extremely important and is not generally studied in the preparation of young counselors, psychologists, and psychiatrists. But why is resonance so effective in therapy?

Resonance is effective in therapy because we are all more prone to fight for our own causes than those of others. When we resonate, we also "cosuffer" the discomforts of the patient and, hence, are more impelled to find solutions that will reduce such anxiety in our own self as well as in the patient. The attorney who resonates with his or her client adopts the position of the client as his or her own and is thus more highly motivated to prepare a strong case. The therapist is more effective when he or she serves as an attorney for the *defense* of the patients, protecting them against their pathology, than if the therapist only strived to be 100% "objective."

Sociopaths seem incapable of resonating with others. They can victimize people and feel neither anxiety nor remorse, except perhaps concern for the possibility of being caught. Other people are simply objects that they manipulate for their own pleasure. Perhaps one of the difficulties in treating sociopaths is because of the inability of most therapists to resonate with such characters.

When listening to the communications of the patient, the therapist is building an increasingly accurate image. The therapist introjects a replica of the other and forms an object representation. The therapist senses the characteristics of this object and achieves some understanding of it. However, a therapist who resonates may identify with this image. The treating one turns it into an "iden-tofact," and it becomes a self representation (J. G. Watkins, 2001a, 2001b, 2001c). The therapist can then cofeel and counderstand the way the patient does. This is additional data not derived from the therapist's original sensing of the object representation and perhaps not derivable if contacted only as an object.

As therapists moves back and forth from resonance to objectivity, they gain greater appreciation of their patients (J. G. Watkins, 2003). The therapist's intervention becomes more knowledgeable and effective. Perhaps from objective observation, the therapist recognizes the that patient has repressed a murderous rage toward a sister. But from his or her resonance, the therapist realizes that the patient is not ready to accept such an interpretation. It would be too devastating because he, himself, would hurt too much if "we" confronted this problem at this time. The ability to resonate and to balance it with objectivity gives the analyst a greater therapeutic sensitivity—an internal "third ear" (Reik, 1948).

Federn's theory of ego and object energy (discussed in Chapter 10) contributes a rationale to the understanding of resonance. The image of the therapist is first introjected as an object by investing it with object energy at the time it is internalized. The sensing of the "object" gives the analyst first knowledge concerning it. Then this object representation is changed into a self representation by removing the object energy and investing it with self energy, "ego energy." The therapist now experiences the patient as part of his or her own self. The therapist gathers understanding from it from within to add to the knowledge received from its sensing as object.

In making an interpretation, hypnotic suggestion, or other intervention, the analyst tests it on self representation to determine whether it is desirable, appropriate, and acceptable before transmitting it to the patient. If his or her resonance has been correct, then the intervention will also be correct and optimal. The therapist and the patient will move, bit by bit, toward a resolution of the problem.

Unfortunately, we can never resonate completely. We have our own personal agenda based on our training and life experiences, which may interfere. Resonance will then be only partial. We may have "self-tested" an interpretation and transmitted it to our client, only to find that we were off-base. Our internal evaluation was faulty. We screwed up. However, if resonance is still functioning, we may notice our mistake and make appropriate correction before damage has been done (see J. G. Watkins, 2005).

The more other people are like us, the easier it is to resonate with them. Middle-class therapists resonate better with middle-class patients than with those coming from other socioeconomic levels, cultures, or races, or who possess quite different value systems. To resonate with a female patient, the male therapist should be experiencing outrage when she is revealing a rape or other sexual abuse. If, instead, he is having sexual feelings toward her, he is treating her as an object. Male therapists who are afraid of their own feminine components (Jung's anima), and the fear that it will "take them over," such that they will become gay, may not be able to resonant with their female patients. It does not mean they cannot treat such patients, but their understanding will, of necessity, come from their objective sensing and thus be more limited.

There is another benefit that enhances the effectives of the therapist who can resonate. Resonance begets counter-resonance. If I deeply understand my patient and correctly transmit this understanding to him or her, then the patient will feel understood. My interpretations will have greater credibility and weight; their timing will be better, and they will be much more effective. The patient senses that a new constructive force has entered his or her world (J. G. Watkins, 2001b). The patient is encouraged. "We" can do what "I" could never do alone. The motivations for recovery are strengthened and renewed. The patient accepts more eagerly the therapist's "loan" of self energy. This is why many studies show that the quality of the therapeutic relationship is so much more important than mere techniques.

The therapist who is willing to commit his or her own self to a resonant, as well as objective, relationship in the interests of greater therapeutic effectiveness should recognize that it does not come easily. The therapist must be willing to resonate, not only with the patient's assets, but also with liabilities. The resonating therapist accepts into his or her own self-structure the pathology of the patient, even though in microform. So temporarily, while the patient is getting well, the therapist is getting "sick." If the therapist undertakes too many therapeutic commitments and resonates too deeply with them, the therapist will be destroyed psychologically.

A young resident physician once said to J.G.W. "I'm no damn good as a doctor; all my patients are dying." This conscientious practitioner had been assigned to manage the terminal tumor ward, a purgatory to which all the elderly patients with inoperable cancer were assigned. In the guise of "getting experience," this young doctor was being systematically destroyed. If he resonated with his patients, he would go down with them; if he didn't, they would be treated as objects and, like so many rejected people, die alone. The solution for such a dilemma is not easy. Perhaps if one can view life as a quality rather than a quantity, then the treating one can be sustained by the recognition that credit is deserved for being a good therapist for every minute of pain-free and meaningful existence that can be offered one's patients. Their therapy then becomes a growth experience for the doctor, not a debilitating trauma. As the patient recovers, the ego-loan, which the doctor has invested into the self representation of the individual, is increasingly paid back. Through resonance, the therapist now coenjoys the therapeutic gains with the patient and grows in strength and maturity as a therapist and as a person. When the therapist overresonates with too many extremely sick individuals, and their ego-economy is on a deficit track, then sooner or later the therapist must either reduce his or her therapeutic commitments, lessen their effectiveness, or face "burnout." The self-economy of a therapeutic self, like that of his or her patients, requires care and nourishment. Vacations, the love and caring of others, plus the rewards of therapeutic success must keep the therapist's ego-energy income greater than its outgo; otherwise, they will become personal bankrupts. Therapists and analysts need to be very aware of their current energy "balance sheets." Don't try to be a lifesaver if you are already exhausted from swimming.

Resonance has another effect. The more people get to know one another, the more they resonate with each other, the better their relationship, and vice versa. When President Reagan and then-president Gorbachev were meeting in Moscow, can trace the development of their relationship from the early days of name-calling to that historic Moscow meeting when they evidenced on several occasions publicly that they had grown to understand one another much better, communicate, and have a genuine friendly relationship. As the two heads of state learned to resonate within one another, tension began to melt and the future chances of world peace began to brighten. A decade later when George W. Bush was reelected, exit poll interviews were telling. Factory workers who had lost their jobs during the first four years of his administration would make statements about voting for him because "he's a regular guy, he's just like me."

What we see today might be likened to the psychotherapy of a neurotic, almost psychotic world which if left unchecked would have made nuclear and mutual destruction almost inevitable. The meetings that Reagan and Gorbachev had together point out the importance of a balance between resonance and understanding of each other's needs and objectivity in which each championed the position of his own country and "did not sacrifice its own assets" to the disadvantage of his own people. The balance between "with-ness" (resonance) and the realities of national security (objectivity) demonstrated the best chance for "treating," at the foreign policy level, the major "dissociation" in our world community at that time. A purely objective interchange would in all likelihood never have brought about the remarkable transformation that occurred in the years that followed.

There is a certain mental health maintenance necessary as the therapist or analyst practices resonance. If one internalizes a replica of the patient in order to understand him or her, one must temporarily introject the patient's pathology as well as the patient's assets. Otherwise, one's resonant understanding will be incomplete. Yet, to do this means ingesting that which has been neurotic, immature, pathogenic, and maladaptive in the patient's experience and behavior. If it were not so, the patient would not be seeking treatment. To do this will require energy on the part of the therapist because inevitably much of this material will be cognitively dissonant with the therapist's own concepts, values, and behaviors. Resonance and therapy, therefore, is energy-demanding. The therapist may suffer anxiety or other symptoms if he or she resonates too strongly, or if his or her resonance is not mitigated by objectivity and ego strengths (J. G. Watkins, 2004). The therapist must now experience within his or her own self something of what it feels to suffer from a phobia or an obsessive thought, being unable to control compulsive behavior, and so on.

We could go on but it should be obvious by now that if some part of one's self, perhaps almost one half, is to enter into a coexperience with the patient's pathology, an internalized reality that has been borrowed from the patient even though temporarily so, then the therapist is in for difficult times.

As the therapist reconciles these cognitively dissonant elements within, the patient, who is coresonating, will receive and integrate the new meanings within. Doctor and patient "heal" together. The therapist experiences these dissonances and maladaptations in microform, permitting his or her own self to serve as a kind of laboratory experiment wherein the patient's problems are temporarily those of the therapist and where they are both searching for solutions. Furthermore, as the therapist increases his or her resonance of the patient, the patient will resonate more with the therapist's objectivity. There is a quid pro quo, a kind of temporary exchange of egos as the patient increasingly incorporates the values, the coping abilities, and the ego strengths of the therapist. Of course, those of the therapist should be more mature, more adjusted, more realistic, more in tune with the environmental demands of the culture as a whole than those of the patient. If that were not the case, the two should change places!

Assuming that the therapist's self is, as can be reasonably expected, more mature and well-adjusted, the patient by counter-resonating with the therapist is erecting within him- or herself a constructive replica of the treating one. Accordingly, the patient is introjecting a mature and healing object representation. (Just as the therapist is giving, the patient becomes adaptively giving, rather than immature and selfish.) This element can serve as a focus for integrative forces and as a defense against regression to immature modes of thought and immature modes of behavior. In fact, this therapist-introject may in time replace destructive object representations built around the much-earlier internalization of rejecting or abusing parent figures. The patient now has within him- or herself an object that will "truly" love him or her, one who can do so unselfishly, one which can issue reassurance and constructive suggestions unconsciously to the patient.

This establishing of an inner therapist object representation can be the beginning of a more benevolent cycle of intrapersonal process, which will replace patients' previous malevolent ones. If patients invest this introject with ego energy, identify with it, and change it into a self representation, their attitudes and behaviors will undergo constructive change. As they have been treated by the therapist, so also will they now begin to treat others. As patients interact with others constructively, patients then are more likely to be rewarded by their actions. It is a matter of a new "being." Therapy takes place, not so much because of the impact of therapist's techniques on the patient, but because of the impact of the doctor's "self."

Theoretically, if the clinician's or counselor's resonance and objectivity were both perfect, every interpretation would be correct. There could never be a false intervention. Through cofeeling and counderstanding, the therapist would understand correctly the current position of the patient and exactly what needs to be said and done. Through the therapist's objectivity, he or she would administer those in terms of the reality of society, the future orientation needed to cope with that reality, and the environment in which the patient exists. Through his or her continuous and correct resonance, the therapist would know just what could be accepted and integrated by the patient. The therapist would not time the interpretation wrongly nor present the patient with more than the patient was currently prepared to handle.

Unfortunately, counselors and clinicians are not perfect, neither in their resonating abilities nor in their objectivity. Good therapists will be closer to this ideal than poor ones. But each of us, through resonance, can probably grasp a faction of what is being experienced by the patient, and each of us is subject to the misperceptions, biases, counter-transferences, and all the other distortions that accrue to humans. We will make mistakes because psychotherapy is not an exact science; it is an art based on the best scientific study of which we are capable.

Psychoanalytic theorists have been emphasizing the importance of establishing good object relationships, hence, interacting realistically with others. But this is not enough! Two people may have clear inner images of the other, but if their relationship is purely an "objective" one, then they will treat each other as only objects. The optimal interaction would be the establishing of a self-object relationship in which each individual balances his or her objectivity with resonance for the other through the formation of constructive subject-object relationships. Parents and children would build better families, teachers and pupils would optimize their education, labor and management would reach better settlements, and international disagreements could be resolved without war.

But what does hypnosis have to do with all of this? We have defined hypnosis as used in the clinical or counseling setting as an altered state of consciousness within an intensive interpersonal relationship. When we are "conscious," we are aware of only part of the communications that may be emitted by a patient. Therefore, both our objectivity and our resonance will lack all the necessary data to fully understand the patient. If we are lucky in being talented and gifted with the therapeutic third ear (Reik, 1948), then we will be more sensitive therapists than those who are not so fortunate. Hypnosis does not substitute for a good third ear, but it can mitigate the deficiency somewhat by eliciting and bringing to our own consciousness data that the patient had previously not presented overtly. Probably, a good third ear plus hypnosis would be better yet. But the many hypnoanalytic techniques for discovering covert processes in patients are simply an extension of both our third ear and the original two. Thus, they permit us to sense aspects of our patient that had previously not been brought to our attention and to transmit interventions to the same deeper levels of the patient's personality.

From the other side of the equation, hypnosis, by being an intensive interpersonal relationship, facilitates resonance. The release of affect in abreactions plus the alliance with the patient necessary for their safe execution demands that the therapist resonate. He or she who neglects to do so, who plows ahead in the release of violent affects without sensing the patient's ability to handle them, risks destructive, suicidal, homicidal, or psychotic episodes. What is a luxury in ordinary conscious psychotherapy becomes a necessity during intensive hypnoanalytic therapy. In hypnosis, we may be traveling both deeper and more rapidly. Dare we be unwilling to coexperience the significant journey with our patient?

Fortunately, there is something about the hypnotic relationship that actively promotes resonance and counter-resonance. "With-ness" is more easily achieved. We are impelled to throw our own self into the interaction and are rewarded by the patient's doing likewise. In hypnosis, patients may manifest increased sensitivity to the cues emitted by the hypnotherapist. Perhaps that is why skeptics and those who research hypnosis with "subjects" frequently do not report observing the phenomena, which experienced hypnotherapists find in their patients. Objectivity alone cannot hope to elicit all that objectivity and resonance together can. Furthermore, research subjects who are regarded as experimental "objects" will not reveal the potentialities in their covert processes to hypnotists who do not resonate. Yet, resonance itself increases enormously the difficulties and scientific control of experiments. Although we might wish otherwise, "experimental selves" do not make the very best therapists, even as "therapeutic selves" do not necessarily do the best experimental research. Human knowledge advances when approached from both perspectives and from their communication with one another.

Perhaps we should briefly discuss the selection and training of "therapeutic selves." Is this an inherent trait or can it be developed? As in musical talent, there are some individuals who seem to be born with it. They exert constructive impact on others even though they have received no graduate training in the healing arts. Others with MD's and PhD's may ply their treatment crafts, yet lack highly developed therapeutic selves. Graduate training does not guarantee therapeutic success, although it makes it much more probable. Success and happiness in life require three key ingredients: talent, luck, and perseverance. In this regard, one does best for others when one does well for oneself. The best therapists must not only have intelligence and the motivation to enter graduate school and complete it, but they also must have the talent to resonate.

The interaction of person on person is generally more therapeutic than otherwise, and especially so if the treating one is not burdened with excessive immature or neurotic motivations. Talented therapists probably begin with natural abilities that, when enhanced by graduate study with a caring knowledgeable mentor, render them sufficiently free of neurotic motivations, more mature, and much more effective.

Learning to become a "doctor" in the sense of a healing person can certainly be enhanced if the student has role models: supervisors, mentors, training analysts, more experienced colleagues, and so on. Not all of these are constructive.

We have seen resident doctors who were chewed out by their clinical professors and have wondered how the future "treaters of men and women" could be developed from models who were "beaters of men and women." If we are to have therapeutic selves in the healing arts, then our medical and dental schools, graduate departments of psychology, and schools of nursing and social work need to be peopled with faculty members who have done more than merely memorized knowledge and therapeutic techniques, be they medical, psychological, or hypnoanalytic. Clinical faculty should be chosen for their impact on the lives of others, not merely for their scientific expertise, for therapeutic selves beget and develop therapeutic-self structure in others.

Finally, if those of us who hold society's mandate to heal would live up to our full potential, then the development of better therapeutic selves along with more scientific and objective knowledge should be our constant life goal. And if the ability to interact with others through a balance of resonance and objectivity can be transmitted broadly, then perhaps we will see a world that through its therapeutic selves can heal its pathologies of injustice, hatred, crime, and war (J. G. Watkins, 1978a).

Summary

Many patients currently confront their therapist with a lack of meaning in life rather than the classical neurotic symptoms. They appear to be products of a culture that emphasizes "things" instead of people and meaningful adaptive relationships. The "meaning" of life has been much considered by many philosophers throughout the years. More recently, the humanistic branch of psychotherapists has been the one to focus on this problem.

Psychotherapeutic interventions have been focused toward the patient's "*Umwelt*," or reactions to the exterior world; his or her "*Mitwelt*," or interpersonal relations; and his or her "*Eigenwelt*," or intrapersonal experience within his or her own self.

The "therapeutic self" is a concept formulated by observing the differential impact of various doctors (who are equally well trained) on their patients. The patients of those who possessed a therapeutic self responded much more favorably to treatment even though all were equally skilled in technical knowledge and therapeutic techniques.

Resonance is the ability to coexperience, cosuffer, and coenjoy with another person. It involves temporarily internalizing the other, forming first an objective representation, and then by investing it with "ego energy," changing it into a self representation. It is a partial identification that may be affective, cognitive, or both.

When there is a balance of resonance and objectivity, therapeutic interventions are maximized, because the therapist or analyst is viewing the patient from two different perspectives simultaneously: as others view the patient, and as he or she perceives and experiences him- or herself.

Underresonance leaves the therapist without the sensitive inside understanding of his or her patient. Overresonance can result in a *folie à deux*, with the two simply being sick together. Also, because resonance takes energy, too much will personally exhaust the therapist unless he or she can renew his or her own store of ego energies from other sources. The therapist must then reduce his or her therapeutic commitments, lessen their intensity, or face burnout. Income must balance outgo in his or her own ego economy.

The hypnotic relationship encourages resonance in the therapist and hence counter-resonance in the patient. The doctor better understands the needs of the patient and can time his or her interventions, and the patient is better able to accept such interventions.

Not only is the "therapeutic self" of the doctor optimized by a proper balance between resonance and objectivity, but such a balance within parents and teachers can greatly improve their interactions with children. Finally, the same balance could assist diplomats and world leaders in achieving better international relations by helping them to understand the needs of the other without compromising the interests of their own country. If more "therapeutic selves" could be developed in such individuals, international conflicts and wars could better be avoided.

The techniques of psychotherapy and analysis, including both hypnotic and nonhypnotic modalities, are our scientific heritage of knowledge as healers. But the full use of these for the betterment of our patients, our students, our children, and other people in our world rests on a balance between our objectivity and our ability to resonate with others. Of such are "therapeutic selves."

References

Adler, A. (1963). *The practice and theory of individual psychology.* Totowa, NJ: Littlefield, Adams.

Adler, G. (1948). *Studies in analytical psychology.* London: Routledge & Kegan Paul.

Alexander, F., & French, T. M. (1946). *Psychoanalytic therapy.* New York: Ronald Press.

Alliance of Psychoanalytic Organizations (2006). *Psychodynamic Diagnostic Manual* (PDM). Silver Spring, MD.

Allison, R. B. (1974). A new treatment approach for multiple personalities. *American Journal of Clinical Hypnosis 17,* 15–32.

American Psychiatric Association. (1994). *Diagnostic and statistical manual of mental disorders* (4th ed.). Washington, DC.

American Psychiatric Association. (2000). *Diagnostic and statistical manual of mental disorders* (4th ed., text revision). Washington, DC.

Amundson, J. K., Aladin, A., & Gill, E. (2003). Efficacy vs. effectiveness research in psychotherapy: Implications for clinical hypnosis. *American Journal of Clinical Hypnosis 46* (1), 11–31.

As, A. (1962). The recovery of forgotten language knowledge through hypnotic age regression. *American Journal of Clinical Hypnosis 5,* 21–29.

Aston–Jones, G., Rajkowski, R., & Cohen, J. (1999). Role of locus coeruleus in attention and behavioral flexibility. *Biological Psychiatry 46,* 1309–1320.

Baker, E. L. (1981). A hypnotherapeutic approach to enhance object relatedness in psychotic patients. *International Journal of Clinical and Experimental Hypnosis 29,* 136–147.

Baker, E. L. (1983a). Resistance in hypnotherapy of primitive states: Its meaning and management. *International Journal of Clinical and Experimental Hypnosis 31,* 2, 82–89.

Baker, E. L. (1983b). The use of hypnotic dreaming in the treatment of the borderline patient: Some thoughts on resistance and transitional phenomena. *International Journal of Clinical and Experimental Hypnosis 31,* 1, 19–27.

Baker, E. L. (1983c). The use of hypnotic techniques with psychotics. *American Journal of Clinical Hypnosis 25,* 283–288.

Bandura, A., & Walters, R. (1963). *Social learning and personality development.* New York: Holt, Rinehart and Winston.

Banyai, E. I., & Hilgard, E. R. (1976). A comparison of active-alert hypnotic induction with traditional relaxation induction. *Journal of Abnormal Psychology 85,* 218–224.

Barabasz, A. (1970a). Galvanic skin response and test anxiety among Negroes and Caucasians. *Child Study Journal 1,* 33–36.

Barabasz, A. (1970b). Temporal orientation and academic achievement in college. *Journal of Social Psychology 82,* 265–267.

Barabasz, A. (1970c). Time estimation in delinquents and non-delinquents. *Journal of General Psychology 82,* 265–267.

Barabasz, A. (1974a). Enhancement of temporal orientation through exposure to audio tape recorded counseling models. *Adolescence 9*, 107–112.

Barabasz, A. (1974b). Enlarging temporal orientation: A test of alternative counseling approaches. *Journal of Social Psychology 93*, 67–64.

Barabasz, A. (1974c). Quantifying hierarchy stimuli in systematic desensitization via GSR: A preliminary investigation. *Child Study Journal 4*, 201–211.

Barabasz, A. (1977). *New techniques in behavior therapy and hypnosis*. South Orange, NJ: Power Publishers.

Barabasz, A. (1979). Isolation, EEG alpha and hypnotizability in Antarctica. In G. Burrows (Ed.), *Hypnosis 1979*, pp. 3–18. Amsterdam: Elsevier/North Holland Biomedica Press.

Barabasz, A. (1980a). EEG alpha, skin conductance and hypnotizability in Antarctica. *International Journal of Clinical and Experimental Hypnosis 28*, 63–74.

Barabasz, A. (1980b). Effects of hypnosis and perceptual deprivation on vigilance in a simulated radar target detection task. *Perceptual and Motor Skills 50*, 19–24.

Barabasz, A. (1980c). Enhancement of hypnotic susceptibility following perceptual deprivation: Pain tolerance, electrodermal and EEG correlates. In M. Pajntar, E. Roskar, and M. Lavric (Eds.), *Hypnosis in psychotherapy and psychosomatic medicine*, pp. 13–18. Ljubljana, Yugoslavia: University Press (Univerzitetna tiskarna).

Barabasz, A. (1980d). Imaginative involvement and hypnotizability in Antarctica. *Proceedings 10th Annual Congress of the Australian Society for Clinical and Experimental Hypnosis*. Hobart, Tasmania, September.

Barabasz, A. (1982). Restricted environmental stimulation and the enhancement of hypnotizability: Pain, EEG alpha, skin conductance and temperature responses. *International Journal of Clinical and Experimental Hypnosis 30* (2), 147–166.

Barabasz, A. (1984a). Antarctic isolation and imaginative involvement: Preliminary findings. *International Journal of Clinical and Experimental Hypnosis 32*, 296–300.

Barabasz, A. (1984b). Hypnosis in the treatment of HPV. Paper presented at Massachusetts General Hospital, Boston, April 7.

Barabasz, A. (1994). Schnell neuronale Aktivierung. Reduzierte Stimulation und psychophysiologische Aufziechnungen bei der Behandlung eines phobischen Piloten. *Experimentelle und Klinische Hypnose 10*, 167–176.

Barabasz, A. (2000). EEG markers of alert hypnosis: The inducttion makes a difference. *Sleep and Hypnosis 2* (4), 164–169.

Barabasz, A. (2003a). Hypnosis for real induction can make the difference. Presidential address from 111th annual convention of the American Psychological Association, Toronto, August 7–10.

Barabasz, A. (2003b). The reality of trance. Keynote address presented at the annual conference of the Australian Society of Hypnosis, Gold Coast, Australia, September 10–16.

Barabasz, A. (2005/2006). Whither spontaneous hypnosis: A critical issue for practitioners and researchers. *American Journal of Clinical Hypnosis, 48*, 2–3, 91–98.

Barabasz, A. (in preparation). Dream interpretation using "specific radiality": An extension of Watkins' technique.

Barabasz, A., & Barabasz, M. (1989). Effects of restricted environmental stimulation: Enhancement of hypnotizability for experimental and chronic pain control. *International Journal of Clinical and Experimental Hypnosis 37* (3), 217–231.

Barabasz, A., & Barabasz, M. (1992). Research design considerations. In Ericka Fromm & M. Nash (Eds.), *Contemporary hypnosis research*, pp. 173–200. New York: Guilford Press.

Barabasz, A., & Barabasz, M. (Eds.). (1993). *Clinical and experimental restricted environmental stimulation: New developments and perspective.* New York: Springer-Verlag.

Barabasz, A., & Barabasz, M. (1994a). EEG responses to a reading comprehension task during active alert hypnosis and waking states. Paper presented at the 45th annual scientific meeting of the Society for Clinical and Experimental Hypnosis, San Francisco, October.

Barabasz, A., & Barabasz, M. (1994b). Effects of focused attention on EEG topography during a reading task. Symposium: Behavioral Medicine, Psychophysiology and Hypnosis, presented at the 102nd annual convention of the American Psychological Association (APA Division 30), Los Angeles, August 12–16.

Barabasz, A., & Barabasz, M. (1996). Neurotherapy and alert hypnosis in the treatment of attention deficit hyperactivity disorder. In S. Lynn, I. Kirsch, & J. Rhue (Eds.), *Clinical Hypnosis Casebook*, pp. 271–292. Washington, DC: American Psychological Association.

Barabasz, A., & Barabasz, M. (2006). Effects of tailored and manualized hypnotic inductions for complicated irritable bowel syndrome patients. *International Journal of Clinical and Experimental Hypnosis 54,* 100–112.

Barabasz, A., Barabasz, M., Jensen, S., Calvin, S., Trevisan, M., & Warner, D. (1999). Cortical event–related potentials show the structure of hypnotic suggestions is crucial. *International Journal of Clinical and Experimental Hypnosis 47* (1), 5–22.

Barabasz, A., Barabasz, M., Lin–Roark, I., Roark, J., Sanchez, O., & Christensen, C. (2003). Age regression produced focal point dependence: Experience makes a difference. Presented at 54th annual scientific program, Society for Clinical and Experimental Hypnosis, Chicago, November 12–16.

Barabasz, A., Barabasz, M., & Rickard, J. (in preparation). Hypnosis relieves phantom limb pain.

Barabasz, A., & Christensen, C. (2006). Age regression: Tailored vs. scripted inductions. *American Journal of Clinical Hypnosis 48,* 4, 251–261.

Barabasz, A. & Christensen, C. (2007). The transitional object as an affect bridge to facilitate age regression. Paper presented at the Annual Convention of the American Psychological Association, San Francisco, August.

Barabasz, A., Crawford, H., & Barabasz, M. (1993). EEG topographic map differences in attention deficit disordered and normal children: Moderating effects from focused active alert instructions during reading, math, and listening tasks. Paper presented at the 33rd annual meeting of the Society for Psychophysiological Research, Rottach-Egern, Germany, October.

Barabasz, A., & Dodd, J. M. (1978). Focal point location and inversion perception among New Zealand Maori and Pakeha children at two age levels. *Journal of Psychology 99,* 19–22.

Barabasz, A., & Gregson, R. A. M. (1979). Antarctic wintering–over, suggestion and transient olfactory stimulation: EEG evoked potential and electrodermal responses. *Biological Psychology 9,* 285–295.

Barabasz, A., Gregson, R. A. M., & Mullin, C. S. (1984). Questionable chronometry: Does Antarctic isolation produce cognitive slowing? *New Zealand Journal of Psychology 13*, 71–78.

Barabasz, A., & Lonsdale, C. (1983). Effects of hypnosis on P300 olfactory evoked potential amplitudes. *Journal of Abnormal Psychology 92*, 520–525.

Barabasz, A., & Watkins, J. G. (2005). *Hypnotherapeutic techniques*. New York: Brunner–Routledge.

Barabasz, M. (1996). Hypnosis, hypnotizability, and eating disorders. Presented at the 47th annual workshop and scientific program of the Society for Clinical and Experimental Hypnosis, Tampa.

Barabasz, M., Barabasz, A., & Mullin, C. S. (1983). Effects of brief Antarctic isolation on absorption and hypnotic susceptibility: Preliminary results and recommendations. *International Journal of Clinical and Experimental Hypnosis, 31*, 235–238.

Barber, T. X. (1962). Toward a theory of hypnotic behavior: The "hypnotically induced dream." *Journal of Nervous and Mental Disease 135*, 206–221.

Barber, T. X. (1965). The effects of "hypnosis" on learning and recall: A methodological critique. *Journal of Clinical Psychology 21*, 19–25.

Barnier, A. (2002). Posthypnotic amnesia for autobiographical episodes: A laboratory model for functional amnesia? *Psychological Science 13* (3): 232–237.

Barrett, D. L. (1979). The hypnotic dream: Its relation to nocturnal dreams and waking fantasies. *Journal of Abnormal Psychology 88*, 5, 584–591.

Barrett, D. L. (1988a). Dreams of death. *OMEGA: The Journal of Death and Dying 19*, 95–102.

Barrett, D. L. (1988b). Trance–related pseudocyesis in a male. *International Journal of Clinical and Experimental Hypnosis 36*, 256 261.

Barrett, D. L. (1991a). An empirical study of the relationship of lucidity and flying dreams. *Dreaming: The Journal of the Association for the Study of Dreams 1* (2), 129–133.

Barrett, D. L. (1991b). Through a glass darkly: The dead appear in dreams. *OMEGA: The Journal of Death and Dying 24*, 97–108.

Barrett, D. L. (1992a). Fantasizers and dissociaters: An empirically based schema of two types of deep trance subjects. *Psychological Reports 71*, 1011–1014.

Barrett, D. L. (1992b). Just how lucid are lucid dreams: An empirical study of their cognitive characteristics. *Dreaming: The Journal of the Association for the Study of Dreams 2*, 221–228.

Barrett, D. L. (1993a). The "committee of sleep." *Dreaming: The Journal of the Association for the Study of Dreams, 3* (2), 1–7.

Barrett, D. L. (1993b). The "committee of sleep": A study of dream incubation for problem solving. *Dreaming: The Journal of the Association for the Study of Dreams, 3*, 115–123.

Barrett, D. L. (1994). Dreams in dissociative disorders. *Dreaming: The Journal of the Association for the Study of Dreams, 4* (3), 165–177.

Barrett, D. L. (1995a). The dream character as a prototype for the multiple personality "alter." *Dissociation 8*, 61–68.

Barrett, D. L. (1995b). Using hypnosis to work with dreams. *Self & Society 23*, 4, 25–30.

Barrett, D. L. (Ed.). (1996). *Trauma and dreams*. Cambridge, MA: Harvard University Press.

Barrett, D. L. (1998). *The pregnant man: And other cases from a hypnoanalyst's couch*. New York: New York Times Books/Random House.

Barrett, D. L. (2001). *The committee of sleep*. New York: Random House.

Barrett, D. L. (2002). The "royal road" becomes a shrewd short cut: The use of dreams in focused treatment. *Journal of Cognitive Psychotherapy 16*, 1–1.

Barrett, D. L., & Loeffler, M. (1992). The effect of depression on the manifest content of the dreams of college students. *Psychological Reports 70*, 403–406.

Beahrs, J. (1986). Multiple consciousness. In *Limits of scientific psychiatry: Role of uncertainty in mental health*, chap. 5. New York: Brunner/Mazel.

Beck, A. (1976). *Cognitive therapy and the emotional disorders*. New York: International Universities Press.

Belagrove, M. (1992). Scripts and the structural analysis of dreams. *Dreaming: The Journal of the Association for the Study of Dreams 2*, 23–38.

Berkeley, G. (1929). *Essay, principles, dialogues*. New York: Scribner.

Berkowitz, L. (1973). The case for bottling up rage. *Psychology Today 2*, 24–31.

Biddle, W. E. (1967). *Hypnosis in the psychoses*. Springfield, IL: Thomas.

Bills, I. G. (1993). The use of hypnosis in the management of dental phobia. *Australian Journal of Clinical & Experimental Hypnosis 21* (1), 13–18. Retrieved June 13, 2005, from PsycINFO (1840–Current) database.

Blanck, G., & Blanck, R. (1974). *Ego psychology: Theory and practice*. New York: Columbia University Press.

Bliss, E. L. (1986). *Multiple personality, allied disorders, and hypnosis*. New York: Oxford University Press.

Boor, M., & Coons, P. M. (1983). A comprehensive bibliography of literature pertaining to multiple personality. *Psychological Reports 53*, 295–310.

Bower, G. H. (1981). Mood and memory. *American Psychologist 36*, 129–148.

Bower, G. H., Monteiro, K. P., & Gilligan, S. G. (1978). Emotional mood as a context of learning and recall. *Journal of Verbal Learning and Verbal Behavior 17*, 573–585.

Bowers, M. K. (1961). Theoretical considerations in the use of hypnosis in the treatment of schizophrenia. *International Journal of Clinical and Experimental Hypnosis 9*, 39–46.

Brady, J., & Rosner, B. (1966). Rapid eye movements in hypnotically induced dreams. *Journal of Nervous and Mental Disease 143*, 28–35.

Braffman, W., & Kirsch, I. (1999). Imaginative suggestibility and hypnotizability: An empirical analysis. *Journal of Personality and Social Psychology 77*, 578–587.

Braun, B. G. (Ed.). (1984). *The psychiatric clinics of North America* (Vol. 7): *Symposium on multiple personality*. Philadelphia: Saunders.

Braun, B. G. (Ed.). (1986). *Treatment of multiple personality disorder*. Washington, DC: American Psychiatric Association Press.

Brenman, M., & Gill, M. M. (1947). *Hypnotherapy*. New York: International Universities Press.

Brom, D., Kleber, R. J., & Defares, P. B. (1989). Brief psychotherapy for post-traumatic stress disorders. *Journal of Consulting and Clinical Psychology 57* (5), 607–612.

Brown, D. P., Frischholtz, E., & Scheflin, A. W. (1999). Iatrogenic dissociative identity disorder—an evaluation of the scientific evidence. *The Journal of Psychiatry and Law 27*, 549–637.

Brown, ,D.P., Frischholz, E. et al. (2000). Introgenic dissociative identity disorder: An evaluation of the scientific evidence. *Journal of Psychiatry and Law 27*, 549–637.

Brown, D. P., & Fromm, Erika. (1986). *Hypnotherapy and hypnoanalysis.* Hillsdale, NJ: Lawrence Erlbaum.

Brown, D. P., & Fromm, Erika. (1987). *Hypnosis and behavioral medicine.* Hillsdale, NJ: Lawrence Erlbaum.

Brown, W. (1920). The revival of emotional memories and its therapeutic value. *British Journal of Medical Psychology 1*, 16–19.

Buber, M. (1970). *I and thou.* New York: Scribner.

Buck, J. N. (1948). The H-T-P technique: A qualitative and quantitative scoring manual. *Journal of Clinical Psychology*, Monograph Supplement No. 5.

Bugental, J. F. T. (1967). *The search for authenticity: An existential analytic approach to psychotherapy.* New York: Holt, Rinehart and Winston.

Burton, A. (1972). *Interpersonal psychotherapy.* Englewood Cliffs, NJ: Prentice Hall.

Callaway, C., Lydic, R., Baghdoyan, A., & Hobson, J. (1988). Pontogeniculoocipital waves: Spontaneous visual system activity during rapid eye movement sleep. *Cellular and Molecular Neurobiology.*

Cardeña, E. (in press). Anomalous experiences and deep hypnosis. In *Proceedings of the Conference on Developing Perspectives on Anomalous Experience.* Liverpool, U.K.

Cardeña, E., Maldonado, J., van der Hart, O., & Spiegel, D. (2000). Hypnosis. In E. B. Foa, T. M. Keane, and M. J. Friedman (Eds.), *Effective treatments for PTSD: Practice guidelines from the international society for traumatic stress studies*, pp. 247–279, 407–440. New York: Guilford Press. Retrieved June 13, 2005, from PsycINFO (1840–Current) database.

Cauttella, J. R., & Bennett, A. K. (1981). Covert conditioning. In R. J. Corsini (Ed.), *Handbook of innovative psychotherapies.* New York: Wiley.

Chambless, D., & Hollan, S. (1998). Defining empirically supported therapies. *Journal of Consulting and Clinical Psychology 66*, 7–18.

Cheek, D. B. (1962). Ideomotor questioning for investigation of subconscious "pain" and target organ vulnerability. *American Journal of Clinical Hypnosis 5*, 30–41.

Cheek, D. B., & LeCron, L. M. (1968). *Clinical hypnotherapy.* New York: Grune & Stratton.

Chu, J. A., & Dill, D. L. (1990). Dissociative symptoms in relation to childhood physical and sexual abuse. *American Journal Psychiatry 147* (7): 887–892.

Chu, J. A., Frey, L. M., et al. (1999). Memories of childhood abuse: Dissociation, amnesia, and corroboration. *American Journal of Psychiatry 156* (5): 749–755.

Christensen, C. (2005). Preferences for descriptors of hypnosis. *International Journal of Clinical and Experimental Hypnosis 53*, 3, 281–289.

Christensen, C. & Barabasz, A. (2007). Effects of a transitional object affect bridge for regression on spontaneity. Paper presented at the Annual Meeting of the Society for Clinical and Experimental Hypnosis, Anaheim, CA, October.

Comstock, C. (1986). *The therapeutic utilization of abreactive experiences in the treatment of multiple personality disorder.* Paper presented at the 3rd International Conference on Multiple Personalities and Dissociative States, Chicago: September 20.

Conn, J. (1959). Cultural and clinical aspects of suggestion. *International Journal of Clinical and Experimental Hypnosis 7*, 175–185.

Cooper, L., & London, P. (1971). The development of hypnotic susceptibility: A longitudinal (convergence) study. *Child Development 42*, 487–503.

Cooper, L., & London, P. (1973). Reactivation of memory by hypnosis and suggestion. *International Journal of Clinical and Experimental Hypnosis 21*, 312–323.

Copeland, D. R. (1986). The application of object-relations theory to the hypnotherapy of developmental arrests: The borderline patient. *International Journal of Clinical and Experimental Hypnosis 34*, 157–168.

Crawford, H. J. (1982). Hypnotizability, day dreaming styles, imagery, vividness, and absorption: A multidimensional study. *Journal of Personality & Social Psychology 42*, 915–926.

Crawford, H. J. (1991). The hypnotizable brain. Presidential address from the annual meeting of the Society for Clinical and Experimental Hypnosis, New Orleans, November.

Degun–Mather, M. (2003). Ego-state therapy in the treatment of a complex eating disorder. *Contemporary Hypnosis 20* (3), 165–173.

Dewey, J. (1916). *Democracy and education*. New York: Macmillan.

Dhanens, T., & Lundy, R. (1975). Hypnotic and waking suggestions and recall. *International Journal of Clinical and Experimental Hypnosis 23*, 68–79.

Dollinger, S. (1985). Lightning-strike disaster among children. *British Journal of Medical Psychology 58*, 4, 375–383.

Dunn, K. K., & Barrett, D. L. (1988). Characteristics of nightmares: Subjects and their nightmares. *Psychiatric Journal of the University of Ottawa 13*, 91–93.

Ellenberger, H. F. (1970). *The discovery of the unconscious*. New York: Basic Books.

Ellis, A. (1962). *Reason and emotion in psychotherapy*. New York: Lyle Stewart.

Ellis, A., & Grieger, R. (1977). *Handbook of rational-emotive therapy*. New York: Springer.

Emmerson, G. (2000a). Advanced methods in hypnotic practice. Australian Society of Clinical Hypnosis workshop conducted at Northbrook House, East Malvern, Victoria, Australia.

Emmerson, G. (2000b). The resistance bridge technique: An ego state induction that locates the origin of the problem. *Australian Journal of Clinical Hypnotherapy & Hypnosis 21* (2), 115–125. Retrieved June 13, 2005, from PsycINFO (1840–Current) database.

Emmerson, G. (2003). *Ego-state therapy*. Williston, VT: Crown.

Emmerson, G. (2006). *Advanced skills and interventions in therapeutic counseling*. Norwalk, CT: Crown House.

Emmerson, G., & Farmer, K. (1996). Ego-state therapy and menstrual migraine. *Australian Journal of Clinical Hypnotherapy and Hypnosis 17*, 17–14.

Erickson, M. (1939). An experimental investigation of the possible anti-social uses of hypnosis. *Psychiatry 2*, 391–414.

Erickson, M. (1952, 1968). Deep hypnosis and its induction. In L. M. LeCron (Ed.), *Experimental hypnosis,* pp. 70–112. New York: Macmillan.

Erickson, M. (1967). *Advanced techniques of hypnosis and therapy*. New York: Grune & Stratton.

Erickson, M. H., & Kubie, L. S. (1941). The successful treatment of a case of acute hysterical depression by return under hypnosis to a critical phase of childhood. *Psychoanalytic Quarterly 10*, 539–609.

Erikson, E. H. (1964). *Insight and responsibility*. New York: Norton.

Ewin, D. (2003). Using ideomotor signals in hypnoanalysis. Paper presented at the 54th Workshops and Scientific Program of the Society for Clinical and Experimental Hypnosis, Chicago. November 12–16.

Evans, F.J. (1979b). Hypnosis and sleep. In E. Fromm & R. Shor (Eds.) *Hypnosis: Developments in research and new perspectives*. Hawthorne, NY: Aldine Publishing.

Evans, F. J. (1979). Contextual forgetting: Posthypnotic source amnesia. *Journal of Abnormal Psychology 88*, 556–563.

Federn, P. (1952a). *Ego psychology and the psychoses*. New York: Basic Books.

Federn, P. (1952b). Narcissism in the structure of the ego. Read before the Tenth International Psychoanalytic Congress, September 1, 1927. In P. Federn & E. Weiss (Eds.), *Ego psychology and the psychoses*, pp. 38–59. New York: Basic Books.

Fenichel, O. (1941). *Problems of psychoanalytic technique*. Albany, NY: The Psychoanalytic Quarterly.

Fenichel, O. (1945). *The psychoanalytic theory of neurosis*. New York: Norton.

Fisher, C. (1974). Subliminal and supraliminal stimulation before the dream. In R. L. Woods & H. G. Greenhouse (Eds.), *The new world of dreams*, pp. 377–388. New York: Macmillan.

Fligstein, D., Barabasz, A., Barabasz, M., Trevisan, M., & Warner, D. (1998). Effects of hypnosis on recall memory: Forced and non-forced conditions. *American Journal of Clinical Hypnosis 40*, 4, 297–305.

Frankl, V. (1963). *Man's search for meaning*. New York: Simon & Schuster.

Frederick, C. (1999a). *The intelligent fellow who points: Ego-state therapy for the treatment of chronic pain*. Paper presented at the annual meeting of the American Society of Clinical Hypnosis, Philadelphia.

Frederick, C. (1999b). *Who is the dreamer? The counter-transference trance in ego-state therapy*. Paper presented at the Annual Meeting of the American Society of Clinical Hypnosis, Philadelphia.

Frederick, C. (2003a). Editorial. *American Journal of Clinical Hypnosis 46* (1), 1–2, 75–82.

Frederick, C. (2003b). *You are always in my heart: Grief as a resource*. Paper presented at the First World Congress of Ego–State Therapy, Bad Orb, Germany, March 22.

Frederick, C. (2005). Selected topics in ego-state therapy. *International Journal of Clinical and Experimental Hypnosis 53* (4) 339–429.

Frederick, C., & McNeal, S. (1999). *Inner strengths: Contemporary psychotherapy and hypnosis for ego strengthening*. Mahwah, NJ: Erlbaum.

Frederick, C., & Phillips, M. (2004). Ego-state therapy workshop. European Congress of Hypnosis. Gozo, Malta, September.

Ferenczi, S., & Rank, O. (1924). *The development of psychoanalysis*. New York: Nervous and Mental Disease Publishing.

Freeman, R., Barabasz, A., Barabasz, M., & Warner, D. (2000). Hypnosis and distraction differ in their effects on cold press or pain and EEG. *American Journal of Clinical and Experimental Hypnosis 43* (2), 137–148.

French, T. M., & Fromm, Erika. (1986). *Dream interpretation: A new approach*. New York: International Universities Press (Original work published by Basic Books, 1964).

Freud, A. (1946). *The ego and the mechanisms of defense*. New York: International Universities Press.

Freud, S. (1920). Beyond the pleasure principle. *Standard Edition* 18: 1–64.

Freud, S. (1924). Further recommendations in the technique of psycho-analysis: Observations on transference love. In *Collected papers*, Vol. 2, pp. 377–391. London: Hogarth Press and the Institute of Psycho-analysis.

Freud, S. (1933). On narcissism: An introduction. In *Collected papers,* Vol. 4, pp. 30–59. London: Hogarth Press and the Institute of Psycho-analysis.

Freud, S. (1935). A general introduction to psycho-analysis. New York: Liveright.

Freud, S. (1938). *A general introduction to psychoanalysis.* New York: Pocket.

Freud, S. (1953a). A case of paranoia (dementia paranoides). In *Collected papers,* Vol. 3, pp. 390–416. London: Hogarth Press and the Institute of Psycho–analysis.

Freud, S. (1953b). On the history of the psychoanalytic movement. In *Collected papers.* Vol. 1, pp. 287–359. London: Hogarth Press and the Institute of Psycho-analysis.

Freud, S. (1953c). The interpretation of dreams. In J. Strachey (Ed. and Trans.), *The standard edition of the complete psychological works of Sigmund Freud,* Vol. 4–5. London: Hogarth Press.

Freud, S. (1961). The dynamics of the transference. In J. Strachey (Ed. and Trans.), *The standard edition of the complete psychological works of Sigmund Freud,* Vol. 12, pp. 97–208. London: Hogarth Press (Original work published 1912).

Freud, S., & Breuer, J. (1953). On the psychical mechanism of hysterical phenomena. In S. Freud, *Collected papers* Vol. 1, pp. 24–41. London: Hogarth Press and the Institute of Psycho-analysis.

Fromm, Erich. (1951). *The forgotten language.* New York: Rinehart.

Fromm, Erich. (1973). *The anatomy of human destructiveness.* New York: Holt, Rinehart, and Winston.

Fromm, Erika. (1968). Transference and counter-transference in hypnoanalysis. *International Journal of Clinical and Experimental Hypnosis 16,* 2, 77–84.

Fromm, Erika. (1977). An ego psychological theory of altered state of consciousness. *International Journal of Clinical and Experimental Hypnosis 25,* 372–387.

Fromm, Erika. (1992). An ego-psychological theory of hypnosis. In E. Fromm & M. Nash (Eds.), *Contemporary hypnosis research,* pp. 131–148. New York: Guilford.

Fromm, Erika, & Kahn, S. (1990). *Self-hypnosis: The Chicago paradigm.* New York: Guilford.

Gabbard, G. (2000). An empirical evidence and psychotherapy: A growing scientific base. *American Journal of Psychiatry 158,* 1–3.

Gabbard, G. (2005). *Psychodynamic psychiatry in clinical practice.* Arlington, VA: American Psychiatric Publishing.

Gainer, M. (1993). Somatization of traumatic memories in a case of reflex sympathetic dystrophy. *American Journal of Clinical Hypnosis 36,* 124–131.

Gill, M. M., & Brenman, M. (1959). *Hypnosis and related states: Psychoanalytic studies in regression.* New York: International Universities Press.

Gill, M. M., & Menninger, K. (1947). Techniques of hypnoanalysis, a case report. In M. M. Gill & M. Brenman (Eds.), *Hypnotherapy: A survey of the literature,* pp. 151–174. New York: International Universities Press.

Ginandes, C. (in press). Six players on the inner stage: Using ego-state therapy with the medically ill. *International Journal of Clinical and Experimental Hypnosis.*

Glover, E. (1955). *The techniques of psychoanalysis.* New York: International Universities Press.

Gordon, M. (1973). Suggestibility of chronic schizophrenic in normal males matched for age. *International Journal of Clinical and Experimental Hypnosis 21* (4), 284–288.

Gunnison, H. (2003). *Hypnocounseling: An eclectic bridge between Milton Erickson & Carl Rodgers.* Norwalk, CT: Crown House Publishing.

Green, J., Barabasz, A., Barrett, D., & Montgomery, G. (2005). Forging ahead: The 2003 APA definition of hypnosis. *International Journal of Clinical and Experimental Hypnosis 53* (3), 259–264.

Greenberg, J. R. (1964). *I never promised you a rose garden.* New York: Signet.

Greenberg, J. R., & Mitchell, S. A. (1983). *Object relations in psychoanalytic theory.* Cambridge, MA: Harvard University Press.

Grinker, R., & Spiegel, H. (1945a). *Men under stress.* Philadelphia: Blakiston.

Grinker, R., & Spiegel, H. (1945b). *War neuroses.* Philadelphia: Blakiston.

Grof, S. (1975). *Realms of the human unconscious: Observations from LSD research.* New York: Viking Press.

Grof, S. (1980). *LSD psychotherapy.* Pomona, CA: Hunter House.

Grof, S. (1985). *Beyond the brain: Birth, death and transcendence in psychotherapy.* Albany: State University of New York Press.

Grossman, L. (2003). Can Freud get his job back? *Time,* January 20.

Gruenewald, D. (1971). Transference and counter-transference in hypnosis. *International Journal of Clinical and Experimental Hypnosis 19,* 71–82.

Gruenewald, D., Fromm, E., & Oberlander, M. (1972). Hypnosis and adaptive regression: An ego-psychological inquiry. In E. Fromm and R. Shor (Eds.), *Hypnosis: Research developments and perspectives,* pp. 495–509. Chicago: Aldine–Atherton.

Gunnison, H. (2004). *Hypnocounseling: An eclectic bridge between Milton Erickson and Carl Rogers.* Norwalk, CT: Crown House.

Guntrip, H. (1961). *Personality structure and human interaction: The developing synthesis of psychodynamic theory.* New York: International Universities Press.

Gutheil, E. A. (1970). *The handbook of dream analysis.* New York: Washington Square Press (Original work published by Liveright, 1951).

Hall, C. W. (1953). *The meaning of dreams.* New York: Harper & Bros.

Harper, R. (1959). *Psychoanalysis in psychotherapy.* Englewood Cliffs, NJ: Prentice Hall.

Hartmann, H. (1939, 1958). *Ego psychology and the problem of adaptation* (D. Rapaport, Trans.). New York: International Universities Press.

Hartmann, H. (1955). Notes on the theory of sublimation. In H. Hartmann, *Essays on ego psychology.* New York: International Universities Press.

Heaton, K., Hill, C., Petersen, D., Rochlen, A., & Zack, J. (1998). A comparison of therapist-facilitative self guided dream interpretation session. *Journal of Counseling Psychology 45,* 115–122.

Heidegger, M. (1949). *Existence and being.* Chicago: Henry Regnery.

Heisenberg, W. (1958). *Physics and philosophy.* New York: Harper.

Hilgard, E. R. (1962). Lawfulness within hypnotic phenomena. In G. H. Estabrooks (Ed.), *Hypnosis: Current problems,* pp. 1–29. New York: Harper & Row.

Hilgard, E. R. (1965). *Hypnotic susceptibility.* New York: Harcourt, Brace, and World.

Hilgard, E. R. (1977). *Divided consciousness: Multiple controls in human thought and action.* New York: John Wiley.

Hilgard, E. R. (1979). *A saga of hypnosis: Two decades of the Stanford Laboratory of Hypnosis Research 1957–1979.* Unpublished manuscript, Stanford University.

Hilgard, E. R. (1986). *Divided consciousness: Multiple controls in human thought and action* (rev. ed.). New York: Wiley.

Hilgard, E. R. (1992). Dissociation and theories of hypnosis. In E. Fromm and N. Nash (Eds.), *Contemporary hypnosis research,* pp. 69-101. New York: Guilford Press.

Hilgard, E. R., & Loftus, E. (1979). Effective interrogation of the eyewitness. *International Journal of Clinical and Experimental Hypnosis 27,* 342-357.

Hilgard, E. R., & Nowlis, D. (1972). Contents of hypnotic dreams and night dreams: An exercise in method. In E. Fromm and R. Shor (Eds.), *Hypnosis: Research, developments, and perspectives,* pp. 510-524. New York: Aldine.

Hilgard, E. R., & Tart, C. (1966). Responsiveness to suggestions following waking and imagination instructions and following induction of hypnosis. *Journal of Abnormal Psychology 71* (3), 196-208.

Hilgard, J. R. (1970). *Personality and hypnosis: A study of imaginative involvement.* Chicago: University of Chicago Press.

Hilgard, J. R. (1974). Imaginative involvement: Some characteristics of the highly hypnotizable and non-hypnotizable. *International Journal of Clinical and Experimental Hypnosis 22,* 138-156.

Hilgard, J. R. (1979). Imaginative and sensory–effective involvements in everyday life and in hypnosis. In E. Fromm & R. Shor (Eds.), *Hypnosis: Developments, research, and new perspectives,* pp. 482-517. New York: Aldine.

Hill, C., Dimer, R., Sess, S., Hillyer, A., & Seemann, R. (1993). Are the effects of dream interpretation on session quality, insight, and emotions due to the dream itself, to projection, or to the interpretation process? *Dreaming: The Journal of the Association for the Study of Dreams 3* (4).

Hill, C., Napayama, E., & Wonnell, T. (1998). Effects of description, association, or combined description/association in exploring dream images. *Dreaming: The Journal of the Association for the Study of Dreams 8,* 1-10.

Hobson, J. (1989). *Sleep.* New York: Freeman.

Hobson, J., Hoffman, S., Helfand, R., & Kostner, D. (1987). Dream design and activation–synthesis hypothesis. *Human Neurobiology 6,* 157-164.

Hobson, J., & McCarley, R. (1977). Brain as a dream state generator: An activation-synthesis hypothesis of the dream process. *American Journal of Psychology 134,* 1335-1368.

Hochberg, J. E. (1978). *Perception* (2nd ed.). Englewood Cliffs, NJ: Prentice Hall.

Horton, J. E., Crawford, H. J., Harrington, G., & Hunter-Downs, J. H. III. (2004). Increased anterior corpus callosum size associated positively with hypnotizability and the ability to control pain. *Brain 127* (8), 1741-1747.

Hume, D. (1963). *The philosophy of David Hume.* New York: Modern Library.

Hunter, M. (2004). *Understanding dissociative disorders. A guide for family physicians and health care professionals.* Williston, VT: Crown House.

Huse, B. (1930). Does the hypnotic trance favor the recall of faint memories? *Journal of Experimental Psychology 13,* 519-529.

Jacobsen, E. (1964). *The self and the object world.* New York: International Universities Press.

Janet, P. (1889). *L'automatisme psychologique.* Paris: Felix Alcan.

Janet, P. (1907). *The major symptoms of hysteria.* New York: Macmillan.

Janov, A. (1970). *The primal scream: A revolutionary cure for neurosis.* New York: Putnam.

Jourard, S. (1971). *The transparent self.* New York: Van Nostrand Reinhold.

Johnston, A. M. (1991). *Tex Johnston: Jet-age test pilot.* Washington, DC: Smithsonian Institution Press.

Jiranek, D. (1993). Hypnosis in the treatment of repressed guilt. *Australian Journal of Clinical & Experimental Hypnosis 21* (1), 61–74. Retrieved June 13, 2005, from PsycINFO (1840–Current) database.

Jung, C. G. (1916). *Psychology of the unconscious.* New York: Moffat, Yard.

Jung, C. G. (1958). *Memories, dreams, reflections.* In *Collected works, Vol. 27,* pp. 115–117. New York: Pantheon.

Jung, C. G. (1966). The eros theory. In *Two essays on analytical psychology,* chap. II. New York: Pantheon.

Jung, C. G. (1969). A review of the complex theory. In *Collected works. Vol. 8. The structure and dynamics of the psyche.* Princeton, NJ: Princeton University Press.

Kahn, D., & Hobson, J. (1993). Self-organization theory of dreaming. *Dreaming: The Journal of the Association for the Study of Dreams 3,* 3, 1993.

Kant, I. (1934). *Critique of pure reason.* New York: Dutton.

Keet, C. D. (1948). Two verbal techniques in a miniature counseling situation. *Psychological Monographs 148* (62), 294.

Kernberg, O. F. (1972). Early ego integration and object relations. *Annals of the New York Academy of Sciences 193,* 233–247.

Kernberg, O. F. (1975). *Borderline conditions and pathological narcissism.* New York: Jason Aronson.

Kernberg, O. F. (1976). *Object relations theory and clinical psychoanalysis.* New York: Jason Aronson.

Kierkegaard, S. (1954). *Fear and trembling and the sickness unto death.* Garden City, NY: Doubleday Anchor.

Kihlstrom, J. (1987). The cognitive unconscious. *Science 237,* 1445–1452.

Kihlstrom, J., & Evans, F. (1979). *Functional disorders of memory.* Hillsdale, NJ: Erlbaum.

Kihlstrom, J., & Hoyt, I. (1990). Repression, dissociation, and hypnosis. In S. Singer (Ed.), *Repression and dissociation: Implications for personality theory, psychopathology and health,* pp. 181–208. Chicago: Chicago University Press.

Kirsch, I. (1991). The social learning theory of hypnosis. In S. J. Lynn and J. W. Rhue (Eds.), *Theories of hypnosis: Current models and perspectives,* pp. 439–465. New York: Guilford Press.

Kirsch, I. (1996). Hypnotic enhancement of cognitive-behavioral weight loss treatments: Another meta–reanalysis. *Journal of Consulting and Clinical Psychology 64,* 517–519.

Kirsch, I., & Council, J. (1989). Response expectancy as a determinate of hypnotic behavior. In N. P. Spanos and J. F. Chaves (Eds.), *Hypnosis: The cognitive-behavioral perspective,* pp. 360–379. Buffalo, NY: Prometheus Books.

Kirsch, I., & Lynn, S. (1998). Dissociation theories of hypnosis. *Psychological Bulletin 123* (1): 100–115.

Kirsch, I., Montogmery, G., & Saperstein, G. (1995). Hypnosis as an adjunct to cognitive-behavioral psychotherapy: A meta–analysis. *Journal of Consulting Clinical Psychology 63* (2): 214–220.

Kleinhauz, M., Whorowitz, I., & Tobin, Y. (1977). The use of hypnosis in police investigation. *Journal of Forensic Science Society 17* (2–3), 77–80.

Kline, M. V. (1958). *Freud and hypnosis.* New York: Julian Press and the Institute for Research in Hypnosis.

Kline, M. V. (1967). Imagery, affect and perception in hypnotherapy. In M. V. Kline (Ed.), *Psychodynamics and hypnosis: New contributions to the practice and theory of hypnotherapy,* pp. 41–70. Springfield, IL: Thomas.

Kline, M. V. (1968). Sensory hypnoanalysis. *International Journal of Clinical and Experimental Hypnosis 16,* 85–100.

Kline, P. (1972). *Fact and fantasy in Freudian theory.* London: Methuen.

Kluft, R. P. (1985a). *Childhood antecedents of multiple personality.* Washington, DC: American Psychiatric Press.

Kluft, R. P. (1985b). Dissociation as a response to extreme trauma. In R. P. Kluft (Ed.), *Childhood antecedents of multiple personality,* pp. 66–97. Washington, DC: American Psychiatric Press.

Kluft, R. P. (1985c). The natural history of multiple personality disorder. In R. P. Kluft (Ed.), *Childhood antecedents of multiple personality,* pp. 197–238. Washington, DC: American Psychiatric Press.

Kluft, R. P. (1986). Clinical corner. *International Society for the Study of Multiple Personality and Dissociation Newsletter 4,* 4–5.

Kluft, R. P. (1987). On the use of hypnosis to find lost objects: A case report of a tandem hypnotic technique. *American Journal of Clinical Hypnosis 29,* 242–248.

Kluft, R. P. (1988). On treating the older patient with multiple personality disorder: "Race against time" or "Make haste slowly." *American Journal of Clinical Hypnosis 30,* 257–266.

Kluft, R. P.(1999). Current issues in dissociative identity disorder. *Journal of Practical Psychiatry and Behavioral Health 5,* 3–19.

Kluft, R. P. (1992). The use of hypnosis with dissociative disorders. *Psychiatric Medicine 10,* 4, 31–46.

Kluft, R. P. (in preparation). Dissociative identity disorder. *International Journal of Clinical and Experimental Hypnosis.*

Kluft, R. P., Frankel, F., Spiegel, D., & Orne, M. T. (1988). *Resolved: Multiple personality disorder is a true psychiatric disease entity.* (Tape cassette.) Mineola, NY: American Audio Association.

Kohut, H. (1971). *The analysis of the self.* New York: International Universities Press.

Kohut, H. (1977). *The restoration of the self.* New York: International Universities Press.

Kolb, L. C. (1988). Recovery of memory and repressed fantasy in combat-induced post–traumatic stress disorder of Vietnam veterans. In H. M. Pettinati (Ed.), *Hypnosis and memory,* pp. 265–274.

Konzag, T. A., Baandemer-Greulich, U., Bahrke, U., & Fikentscher, E. (2004). Psychotherapeutic relationship and outcome in psychotherapy of personality disorders. *Zeitzschrift fur Psychosomatische Medizin und Psychotherapies [Journal of Psychosomatic Medicine and Psychotherapy] 50* (4): 394–405.

Kroger, W. S., & Fezler, W. D. (1976). *Hypnosis and behavior modification: Imagery and conditioning.* Philadelphia: Lippincott.

Kosslyn, S., Thompson, W., Constantine-Ferrando, M., Alpert, N., & Spiegel, D. (2000). Hypnotic visual illusion alters color processing in the brain. *American Journal of Psychiatry 157,* 1279–1284.

Kramer, E. (1971). *Art therapy with children.* New York: Schocken Books.

Kris, E. (1952). *The psychology of caricature: Psychoanalytic explorations of art.* New York: International Universities Press, p. 188.

Kris, E. (1956). The recovery of childhood memories in psychoanalysis. In *The psychoanalytic study of the child*, pp. 54–88. New York: International Universities Press.

Kubovy, M., & Pomerantz, J. R. (1981). *Perceptual organization*. Hillsdale, NJ: Erlbaum.

Lang, E., & Rosen, M. (2002). Cost analysis of adjunct hypnosis with sedation during outpatient interventional radiological procedures. *Radiology 222* (2), 375–382.

Lavoie, G., & Sabourin, M. (1980). Hypnosis and schizophrenia: A review of experimental and clinical studies. In G. D. Burrows & L. Dennerstein (Eds.), *Handbook of hypnosis and psychosomatic medicine*. Amsterdam: Elsevier/North Holland Biomedical Press.

Lazar, B. S., & Dempster, C. R. (1984). Operator variables in successful hypnotherapy. *International Journal of Clinical and Experimental Hypnosis 33*, 28–40.

Lazarus, A. A. (1994). How certain boundaries and ethics diminish therapeutic effectiveness. *Ethics & Behavior 4*, 3, 255–261.

Leonard, G. (1968). *Education and ecstasy*. New York: Delta.

Levick, M. (1981). Art therapy. In R. J. Corsini (Ed.), *Handbook of innovative psychotherapies*. New York: Wiley.

Levy, J. (1974). Psychobiological implications of bilateral asymmetry. In S. J. Diamond & J. G. Beaumont (Eds.), *Hemisphere function in the human brain*. New York: Wiley.

Locke, J. (1823, 1963). *The works of John Locke*. Aalen, Germany: Scientia Verlag.

Loftus, E. F. (1979). *Eyewitness testimony*. Cambridge, MA: Harvard University Press.

Lorentzen, S. Sexton, H. C., & Hoglend, P. (2004). Therapeutic alliance, cohesion and outcome in a long-term analytic group. A preliminary study. *Nordic Journal of Psychiatry 58* (1): 33–40.

Lowen, A. (1975). *Bioenergetics*. New York: Coward.

Luborsky, L., McLelen, A., Diguer, L., Woody, G., and Seligman, M. (1997). The psychotherapist matters: Comparisons of outcomes across twenty-two therapists and seven patient samples. *Clinical Psychology: Research and Practice 4*, 53–56.

Lynn, S. J., Kirsch, I., Barabasz, A., Cardeña, E., & Patterson, D. (2000). Hypnosis as an empirically supported clinical intervention: The state of the evidence and a look to the future. *International Journal of Clinical and Experimental Hypnosis 12*, 53–66.

Machover, K. (1948). *Personality projections in the drawing of the human figure*. Springfield, IL: Thomas.

Mahler, M. S. (1972). On the first three subphases of the separation-individuation process. *International Journal of Psychoanalysis 53*, 333–338.

Mahoney, M. F. (1976). *The meaning in dreams and dreaming*. Secaucus, NJ: Citadel Press.

Malmo, C. (1990). Recovering the past: Using hypnosis to heal childhood trauma. In T. A. Laidlaw & C. Malmo (Eds.), *Healing voices: Feminist approaches to therapy with women*. The Jossey–Bass social and behavioral science series (pp. 194–220). San Francisco: Jossey–Bass.

Malmo, C. (1991). Ego-state therapy: A model for overcoming childhood trauma. *Hypnos 28*, 39–44.

Malon, D. W., & Berardi, D. (1987). Hypnosis with self-cutters. *American Journal of Psychotherapy 41* (4), 531–541.

Mamelak, A., & Hobson, J. (1989). Nightcap: A home-based sleep monitoring system. *Sleep 12*, 157–166.

Marcel, G. (1948). *The philosophy of existence*. London: Harvill.

Markowitz, J., & Street, L. (1999). NIMH propels psychotherapy research on a new court. *Psychiatric News,* October 15, 20.

Mauron, A. (2001). Is the genome the secular equivalent of the soul? *Science 291,* 831–832.

May, R. (Ed.). (1958). *Existence: A new dimension in psychiatry and psychology.* New York: Basic Books.

McKenzie, S. (1994). Hypnotherapy for vomiting phobia in a 40-year-old woman. *Contemporary Hypnosis 11* (1), 37–40.

Means, J. R., et al. (1986). Dream interpretation. *Psychotherapy 23,* 448–452.

Meares, A. (1957). *Hypnography: A study of the therapeutic use of hypnotic painting.* Springfield, IL: Thomas.

Meares, A. (1960). *Shapes of sanity.* Springfield, IL: Thomas.

Meares, A. (1976). *A system of medical hypnosis.* New York: Julian Press. (Work originally published 1961.)

Meichenbaum, D. (1977). *Cognitive behavior modification: An integrative approach.* New York: Plenum.

Meissner, W. (1991). *What is effective in psychoanalytic therapy: The move from interpretation to relation.* North Vail, NJ: Jason Aronson.

Menninger, K., & Holzman, P. S. (1973). *Theory of psychoanalytic technique* (2nd ed.). New York: Basic Books.

Messerschmidt, R. (1927–1928). A quantitative investigation of the alleged independent operation of conscious and subconscious processes. *Journal of Abnormal and Social Psychology 22,* 325–340.

Miller, M. C. (2004). Questions & answers. How important is the therapeutic alliance for the outcome of psychotherapy, and how should it affect a patient's choice of therapist? *Harvard Mental Health Letter,* September 21 (3): 7.

Miller, M. C., Barabasz, A., & Barabasz, M. (1991). Effects of active alert and relaxation hypnotic inductions on cold pressor pain. *American Psychological Association 100,* 223–226.

Milne, G. (1985). Horse sense in psychotherapy. *Australian Journal of Clinical & Experimental Hypnosis 13* (2), 132–134.

Moreno, J. L. (1946). *Psycho-drama.* New York: Random House.

Moreno, J. L., & Enneis, J. M. (1950). *Hypnodrama and psychodrama. Psychodrama Monographs, No. 27.* New York: Beacon House.

Morgan, A., & Hilgard, J. R. (1975). The Stanford Hypnotic Clinical Scale for Adults. In E. Hilgard & J. Hilgard (Eds.), *Hypnosis in the relief of pain* (pp. 134–147). Los Altos, CA: Kaufmann.

Moss, C. S. (1961). Experimental paradigms for the hypnotic investigation of dream symbolism. *International Journal of Clinical and Experimental Hypnosis, 9,* 105–117.

Moss, C. S. (1967). *The hypnotic investigation of dreams.* New York: Wiley.

Moss, C. S. (1970). *Dreams, images, and fantasy: A semantic differential casebook.* Chicago: University of Illinois Press.

Mullin, C. S. (1960). Some psychological aspects of isolated Antarctic living. *American Journal of Psychiatry 117,* 323–325.

Murray, H.A. (1943). *Thematic Apperception Test.* Cambridge: Harvard University Press.

Murray–Jobsis, J. (1984). Hypnosis with severely disturbed patients. In W. C. Wester & A. H. Smith (Eds.), *Clinical hypnosis: A multidisciplinary approach.* Philadelphia: Lippincott.

Murray-Jobsis, J. (1988). Hypnosis as a function of adaptive regression and of transference: An integrated theoretical model. *American Journal of Clinical Hypnosis 30*, 241–247.

Nash, M. (1987). What, if anything, is regressed about hypnotic age regression? A review of the empirical literature. *Psychological Bulletin 102*, 1, 42–52.

Nash, M. (2005). The importance of being earnest when crafting definitions: Science and scientism are not the same thing. *International Journal of Clinical and Experimental Hypnosis 53*, 265–280.

Nash, M., Johnson, L., & Tipton, R. (1979). Hypnotic age regression and the occurrence of transitional object relationships. *Journal of Abnormal Psychology 88*, 547–555.

Nash, M., Lynn, S., Stanley, S., Frauman, D., & Rhue, J. (1985). Hypnotic age regression and the importance of assessing interpersonally relevant affect. *International Journal of Clinical and Experimental Hypnosis 33*, 224–235.

Naumberg, M. (1947). *Studies of the free art expression of behavior problem children and adolescents as a means of diagnosis and therapy.* New York: Nervous & Mental Disease Publishing.

Naumberg, M. (1950). *Schizophrenic art: Its meaning in psychotherapy.* New York: Grune & Stratton.

Naumberg, M. (1953). *Psychoneurotic art: Its function in psychotherapy.* New York: Grune & Stratton.

Nichols, M. P., & Zax, M. (1977). *Catharsis in psychotherapy.* New York: Gardner Press.

Nunberg, H. (1932). *Allgemeine Neuronsenlehre auf psychoanalytisher Grundlage (Principles of psychoanalysis).* New York: International Universities Press.

Olsen, P. (1976). *Emotional flooding.* New York: Human Sciences Press.

Orne, M. (1951). The mechanisms of hypnotic age regression: An experimental study. *Journal of Abnormal and Social Psychology 46*, 213–225.

Orne, M. T. (1959). The nature of hypnosis: Artifact and essence. *Journal of Abnormal and Social Psychology 16*, 213–225.

Orne, M. T. (1979a). On the simulating subject as a quasi-control group in hypnosis research: What, why, and how. In E. Fromm & R. Shor (Eds.), *Hypnosis: Developments in research and new perspectives* (2nd ed., pp. 519–566). New York: Aldine.

Orne, M. T. (1979b). The use and misuse of hypnosis in court. *International Journal of Clinical and Experimental Hypnosis 27*, 311–341.

Orne, M. T., Dinges, D. F., & Orne, E. C. (1984a). On the differential diagnosis of multiple personality in the forensic context. *International Journal of Clinical and Experimental Hypnosis 32*, 118–169.

Orne, M. T., Dinges, D. F., & Orne, E. C. (1984b). *The forensic use of hypnosis.* Washington, DC: National Institute of Justice.

Orne, M. T., Whitehouse, W., Dinges, D., & Orne, E. (1988). Reconstructing memory through hypnosis: Forensic and clinical implications. In H. M. Pettinati (Ed.), *Hypnosis and memory,* pp. 21–64. New York: Guilford.

Osgood, C. & Luria, Z. (1954). A blind analysis of a case of multiple personality using the semantic differential. *Journal of Abnormal and Social Psychology 49*, 579–591.

Oster, M. I. (2003). Efficacy or effectiveness: Which comes first, the cure or the treatment? *American Journal of Clinical Hypnosis 46* (1), 10.

Palson, O. (2006). Standardized hypnosis treatment for irritable bowel syndrome: The North Carolina protocol. *International Journal of Clinical and Experimental Hypnosis 54*, 51–64.

Paulsen, S. (2007) Integrating EMDR into ego state therapy. Presented at EMDR Phase II workshop, Portland, OR.

Perls, F. S. (1969). *Gestalt therapy verbatim*. Lafayette, CA: Real People Press.

Pettinati, H. M. (1982). Measuring hypnotizability in psychotic patients. *International Journal of Clinical and Experimental Hypnosis 30*, 345–353.

Pettinati, H. M., Kogan, L., & Evans, F. (1990). Hypnotizability of psychiatric inpatients according to two different scales. *American Journal of Psychiatry 147* (1), 69–75.

Phillips, M. (1994). Developing a positive "transference" in treating posthypnotic patients. Presented at the annual meeting of the American Society of Clinical Hypnosis, Philadelphia.

Phillips, M., & Frederick, C. (1995). Healing the divided self: Clinical and Ericksonian hypnotherapy for post-traumatic and dissociative conditions. New York: Norton.

Piccone, C., Hilgard, E., & Zimbardo, P. (1989). On the degree of stability of measured hypnotizability over a 25-year period. *Journal of Personality and Social Psychology 56*, 289–206.

Pope, K. S., Sonne, J. L., & Holroyd, J. (1993). *Sexual feelings in psychotherapy: Explorations for therapists and therapists-in-training*. Washington, DC: American Psychological Association.

Prince, M. (1906). *The dissociation of a personality*. New York: Longmans–Green.

Putnam, F. W. (1989). *Diagnosis and treatment of multiple personality disorder*. New York: Guilford.

Putnam, F. (1992). Using hypnosis for therapeutic abreactions. *Psychiatric Medicine 10*, 1, 51–65.

Rado, S. (1925). The economic principle in psychoanalytic technique. *International Journal of Psychoanalysis 6*, 35–44.

Rainville, P., Duncan, G., Price, D., Carrier, B., & Bushnell, M. (1997). Pain affect encoded in human anterior cingulate but somatosensory cortex. *Science 277*, 968–971.

Rainville, P., Hofbauer, R., Paus, T., Duncan, G., Bushnell, M., & Price, D. (1999). Cerebral mechanisms of hypnotic induction and suggestion. *Journal of Cognitive Neuroscience 11*, 110–125.

Rainville, P., & Price, D. (2003). Hypnosis phenomenology and neurobiology of consciousness. *International Journal of Clinical and Experimental Hypnosis 51*, 2, 105–129.

Raginsky, B. (1961). The sensory use of plasticine in hypnoanalysis (sensory hypnoplasty). *International Journal of Clinical and Experimental Hypnosis 9*, 233–247.

Raginsky, B. (1962). Sensory hypnoplasty with case illustrations. *International Journal of Clinical and Experimental Hypnosis, 10*, 205–219.

Raginsky, B. (1963a). Hypnosis in internal medicine and general practice. In J. M. Schneck (Ed.), *Hypnosis in modern medicine*, pp. 29–99. Springfield, IL: Thomas.

Raginsky, B. (1963b). Temporary cardiac arrest under hypnosis. In M. V. Kline (Ed.), *Clinical correlations of experimental hypnosis*, pp. 434–455. Springfield, IL: Thomas.

Raginsky, B. (1967). Rapid regression to the oral and anal levels through sensory hypnoplasty. *International Journal of Clinical and Experimental Hypnosis, 15*, 19–30.

Ramonth, S. (1985a). Dissociation and self-awareness in directed day-dreaming. *Scandinavian Journal of Psychology 26*, 259–276.

Ramonth, S. (1985b). *Multilevel consciousness in meditation, hypnosis, and directed day-dreaming*. Upsalla, Sweden: University of UMEA.

Rank, O. (1932). *Art and artist, creative urge and personality development*. New York: Knopf.

Rank, O. (1952). *The trauma of birth*. New York: Brunner.

Ray, W., & De Pascalis, V. (2003). Temporal aspects of hypnotic processes. *International Journal of Clinical and Experimental Hypnosis 51* (2), 147–165.

Regardie, F. (1950). Experimentally induced dreams as psychotherapeutic aids. *American Journal of Psychotherapy 4*, 643–650.

Reich, W. (1949). *Character analysis* (3rd ed.). New York: Orgone Institute Press.

Reik, T. (1933). New ways in psychoanalytic technique. *International Journal of Psychoanalysis 14*, 321–334.

Reik, T. (1948). *Listening with the third ear*. New York: Farrar.

Reik, T. (1956). *The search within*. New York: Grove Press.

Reik, T. (1957). *Of love and lust*. New York: Farrar, Strauss & Cudahy.

Renee (Pseudonym). (1951). *Autobiography of a schizophrenic girl (with analytic interpretations by Marguerite Sechehaye)*. New York: Grune & Stratton.

Rogers, C. (1951). *Client–centered therapy*. Boston: Houghton–Mifflin.

Rogers, C. (1961). *On becoming a person: A client's view of psychotherapy*. Boston: Houghton–Mifflin.

Rolf, I. (1978). *Rolfing*. Santa Monica, CA: Dennis Landman.

Rorschach, H. (1949). *Psychodiagnostics*. New York: Grune & Stratton.

Rose, S. (1976). Intense feeling therapy. In P. Olsen (Ed.), *Emotional flooding*, pp. 80–95. New York: Human Sciences Press.

Ross, C. A. (1989). *Multiple personality disorder: Diagnosis, clinical features, and treatment*. New York: Wiley.

Rossi, E. L. (1972). *Dreams and the growth of personality*. New York: Pergammon Press.

Rossi, E. L., & Cheek, D. B. (1988). *Mind–body therapy: Methods of ideodynamic healing in hypnosis*. New York: Norton.

Rowling, J. K. (2003). *Harry Potter and the Order of the Phoenix*. Scholastic.

Rycroft, C. S. (1979). *The innocence of dreams*. New York: Pantheon.

Sacerdote, P. (1967). *Induced dreams*. New York: Vantage Press.

Sanders, S. (1986). The perceptual alteration scale: A scale measuring dissociation. *American Journal of Clinical Hypnosis 29*, 95–102.

Sanger, W. (1989). The role of acetylcholine in use-dependent plasticity of the visual cortex. In M. Steriade & D. Biesold (Eds.), *Brain cholinergic systems*. Oxford, England: Oxford University Press.

Sarbin, T. (2005). Reflections on some unresolved issues in hypnosis. *International Journal of Clinical and Experimental Hypnosis 53* (2): 119–134.

Satir, V. (1967). *Conjoint family therapy*. Palo Alto, CA: Science & Behavior Books.

Scagnelli, J. (1974). A case of hypnotherapy with an acute schizophrenic. *American Journal of Clinical Hypnosis 17*, 630–63.

Scagnelli, J. (1976). Hypnotherapy with schizophrenic and borderline patients: A summary of therapy with eight patients. *American Journal of Clinical Hypnosis 19*, 33–38.

Scagnelli, J. (1977). Hypnotic dream therapy with a borderline schizophrenic: A case study. *American Journal of Clinical Hypnosis 20*, 136–145.

Scagnelli, J. (1980). Hypnotherapy with psychotic and borderline patients: The use of trance by patient and therapist. *American Journal of Clinical Hypnosis 22*, 164–169.

Scagnelli–Jobsis, J. (1982). Hypnosis with psychotic patients: A review of the literature and presentation of a theoretical framework. *American Journal of Clinical Hypnosis 25*, 33–45.

Scagnelli–Jobsis, J. (1983). Hypnosis with psychotic patients: Response to Speigel. *American Journal of Clinical Hypnosis, 25*, 295–298.

Schafer, D. W. (1981). The recognition and hypnotherapy of patients with unrecognized altered states. *American Journal of Clinical Hypnosis 23* (3), 176–183. Retrieved June 13, 2005, from PsycINFO (1840–Current) database.

Schiff, S., Bunney, W., & Freedman, D. (1961). The study of ocular movements in hypnotically induced dreams. *Journal of Nervous and Mental Disease 133*, 59–67.

Schilder, P., & Kauders, O. (1956a). *A textbook of hypnosis.* New York: International Universities Press, p. 96.

Schilder, P., & Kauders, O. (1956b). A textbook of hypnosis. In P. Schilder (Ed.), *The nature of hypnosis.* New York: International Universities Press.

Schneck, J. M. (1965). *Principles and practice of hypnoanalysis.* Springfield, IL: Thomas.

Schneck, J. M. (1974). Observations on the hypnotic nightmare. *American Journal of Clinical Hypnosis 16*, 240–245.

Schneidman, E. S. (1947). *Make a picture story test (MAPS).* New York: Psychological Corporation.

Schreiber, F. R. (1974). *Sybil.* New York: Warner Paperback Library.

Schwing, G. (1954). *A way to the soul of the mentally ill.* New York: International Universities Press.

Sechehaye, M. (1951). *Symbolic realization.* Monograph Series on Schizophrenia, No. 2. New York: International Universities Press.

Sechehaye, M. (1956). *A new psychotherapy in schizophrenia.* New York: Grune & Stratton.

Seruda, B. (1997). *Empathic brief psychotherapy.* Northvale, NJ: Jason Aronson.

Shakow, D., & Rosenzweig, S. (1949). The use of the tautophone (verbal summator) as an auditory apperceptive test for the study of personality. *Character and Personality 8*, 216–226.

Shapiro, F. (2001). *Eye movement desensitization and reprocessing: Basic principles, protocols and procedures.* New York: Guilford.

Shaw, H. L. (1978). Hypnosis and drama: A note on a novel use of self–hypnosis. *International Journal of Clinical and Experimental Hypnosis 26*, 154–157.

Sherman, S. (1971). Very deep hypnosis: An experiential and electroencephalographic investigation. Unpublished doctoral dissertation. Stanford University.

Shevrin, H., & Luborsky, L. (1974). Subconscious stimulation before the dream. In R. L. Woods & H. B. Greenhouse (Eds.), *The new world of dreams,* pp. 371–377. New York: Macmillan.

Shor, R. (1979). A phenomenological method for the measurement of variables important to an understanding of the nature of hypnosis. In E. Fromm & R. Shor (Eds.), *Hypnosis: Developments in research and new perspectives.* New York: Aldine.

Shostrom, E. (1967). *Man the manipulator.* Nashville: Abingdon Press.

Skinner, B. F. (1939). The verbal summator and a method for the study of latent speech. *Journal of Psychology 34*, 33–38.

Smith, A. H. (1984). Sources of efficacy in the hypnotic relationship: An object relations approach. In W. C. Wester & A. H. Smith (Eds.), *Clinical hypnosis: A multidisciplinary approach,* pp. 85–114. Philadelphia: Lippincott.

Smith, J., Barabasz, A., & Barabasz, M. (1996). A comparison of hypnosis and distraction in severely ill children undergoing painful medical procedures. *Journal of Counseling Psychology 43* (2), 187–195.

Snyder, M. (1995). Self monitoring: Public appearances versus private realities. In G. Brannigan & M. Merrens (Eds.), *The social psychologist: Research adventures*, pp. 35–49. New York: McGraw-Hill.

Sonnier, I. (1982). Holistic education: Teaching in the affective domain. *Education, 103*, 11–14.

Spanos, N. P., & McPeake, J. D. (1975). Everyday imaginative activities on hypnotic susceptibility. *American Journal of Clinical Hypnosis 17*, 245–252.

Sperry, R. W. (1973). Lateral specialization of cerebral function in the surgically separated hemispheres. In F. J. McGuigan & R. A. Schoonover (Eds.), *The psychophysiology of thinking*, pp. 209–229. New York: Academic Press.

Spiegel, D. (1981). Vietnam grief work using hypnosis. *American Journal of Clinical Hypnosis 24*, 33–40.

Spiegel, D. (1983). Hypnosis with psychotic patients: Comment on Scagnelli–Jobsis. *American Journal of Clinical Hypnosis 25*, 298–294.

Spiegel, D. (1984). Multiple personality as a post-traumatic stress disorder. *Psychiatry Clinics of North America 7* (1): 101–110.

Spiegel, D. (1986a). Dissociating damage. *American Journal of Clinical Hypnosis 29* (2): 123–131.

Spiegel, D. (1986b). Dissociation, double blinds, and post–traumatic stress in multiple personality disorder. In B. Braun (Ed.), *Treatment of multiple personality disorder*, pp. 61–77. Washington, DC: American Psychiatric Press.

Spiegel, D. (1988). Dissociation and hypnosis in post–traumatic stress disorder. *Journal of Trauma Stress 1* (1): 17–33.

Spiegel, D. (1998). Hypnosis and implicit memory: Automatic processing of explicit content. *American Journal of Clinical Hypnosis 40* (3): 231–240.

Spiegel, D. (2003). Negative and positive visual hypnotic hallucinations: Attending inside and out. *International Journal of Clinical and Experimental Hypnosis 51* (2), 130–146.

Spiegel, D. (2007). Clinical hypnosis testing scales. In Barabasz, Bolland & Olness (Eds.) Proposal to the United Nations World Health Organization.

Spiegel, D., & Barabasz, A. (1988). Effects of hypnotic hallucination on P300 evoked potential amplitudes: Reconciling conflicting findings. *American Journal of Clinical Hypnosis 31*, 11–17.

Spiegel, D. & Koopman, C. (1994). Acute stress disorder and dissociation. *Australian Journal of Clinical Hypnosis 22*, (1), 11–23.

Spiegel, D., Bierre, P., & Rootenberg, J. (1989). Hypnotic alteration of somatosensory perception. *American Journal of Psychiatry 146*, 749–754.

Spiegel, D., & Cardeña, E. (1991). Disintegrated experience: The dissociative disorders revisited. *Journal of Abnormal Psychology 100* (3): 366–378.

Spiegel, D., & Classen, C. (2000). *Group therapy for cancer patients: A research-based handbook of psychosocial care.* New York: Basic Books.

Spiegel, D., Cutcomb, S., Ren, C., & Pribram, K. (1985). Hypnotic hallucinations alter evoked potentials. *Journal of Abnormal Psychology 94*, 249–255.

Spiegel, H., & Shainess, N. (1963). Operational spectrum of psychotherapeutic process. *Arch Gen Psychiatry 9*: 477–488.

Spiegel, H., Greenleaf, M. et al. Hypnosis. In B. Kaplan & V. Sadock (Eds.) *Comprehensive textbook of psychiatry*, 7th ed., Vol. 2. Philadelphia: Lippincott, Williams, & Wilkins, pp. 2128–2146.

Spiegel, H., & Spiegel, D. (2004). *Trance and treatment: Clinical uses of hypnosis* (2nd ed.). Arlington, VA: American Psychiatric Publishing.

Stampfl, T. G. (1967). Implosive therapy: The theory, the subhuman analog, the strategy, and the technique. Part I: The Theory. In S. G. Armitage (Ed.), *Behavior modification techniques in the treatment of emotional disorders*. Battle Creek, MI: V.A. Publication.

Stava, L. (1984). The use of hypnotic uncovering techniques in the treatment of pedophilia. *International Journal of Clinical & Experimental Hypnosis 32* (4), 350–355. Retrieved June 13, 2005, from PsycINFO (1840–Current) database.

Stein, C. (1970). Trance, transference and countertransferance in the resistive patient. *American Journal of Clinical Hypnosis 12*, 213–221

Soskis, D. (1986). *Teaching self-hypnosis: An introductory guide for clinicians*. NY: Norton.

Stekel, W. (1939a). *Impotence in the male* (Vol. 1–2). New York: Liveright.

Stekel, W. (1939b). *Sadism & masochism* (Vol. 1–2). New York: Liveright.

Stekel, W. (1940). *Sexual aberrations* (Vol. 1–2). New York: Liveright.

Stekel, W. (1943a). *Frigidity in women* (Vol. 1–2). New York: Liveright.

Stekel, W. (1943b). *Peculiarities of behavior* (Vol. 1–2). New York: Liveright.

Stekel, W. (1943c). *The interpretations of dreams* (Vol. 1–2). New York: Liveright.

Stekel, W. (1949). *Compulsion and doubt* (Vol. 1–2). New York: Liveright.

Stern, M. M. (1952). Art therapy. In G. Bychowski & J. L. Despert (Eds.), *Specialized techniques in psychotherapy*. New York: Grune & Stratton.

Stone, M. (1997). *Healing the mind: A history of psychology from antiquity to the present*. New York: Norton.

Strachey, J. (1934). The nature of therapeutic action of psychoanalysis. *International Journal of Psycho-analysis 15*, 127–159.

Strickgold, R., Pace-Schott, E., & Hobson, J. (1993). A new paradigm for dream research: Mentation reports following spontaneous arousal from REM and MREM sleep recorded in a home setting. *Consciousness and Cognition*, submitted.

Suedfeld, P. (1980). *Restricted environmental stimulation*. New York: Wiley.

Szechtman, H., Woody, E., Bowers, K., & Nahmias, C. (1998). Where the imaginal appears real: A positron emission tomography study of auditory hallucinations. *Proceedings of the National Academy of Sciences of the United States of America 95*, 1956–1960.

Tart, C. T. (1964). A comparison of suggested dreams occurring in hypnosis and sleep. *International Journal of Clinical and Experimental Hypnosis 12*, 263–289.

Tart, C. T. (1965). The hypnotic dream: Methodological problems and a review of the literature. *Psychological Bulletin 63*, 87–99.

Teasdale, J. D., & Fogarty, F. J. (1979). Differential effects of induced mood on retrieval of pleasant and unpleasant events from episodic memory. *Journal of Abnormal Psychology 88*, 248–257.

Tellegen, A., & Atkinson, G. (1974). Openness to absorbing and self-altering experiences ("absorption"), a trait related to hypnotic susceptibility. *Journal of Abnormal Psychology 33*, 142–148.

Thigpen, C. H., & Cleckley, H. M. (1957). *Three faces of Eve*. New York: McGraw-Hill.

Tillich, P. (1952). *The courage to be*. New Haven, CT: Yale University Press.

Tillich, P. (1960). Existentialism, psychotherapy and the nature of man. *Pastoral Psychology 11*, 10–18.

Trussell, M. A. (1939). The diagnostic value of the verbal summator. *Journal of Abnormal Social Psychology 34*, 533–538.

Tulring, E. (1983). *Elements of episodic memory.* Oxford, England: Clarendon Press.

Udolf, R. (1983). *Forensic hypnosis: Psychological and legal aspects.* Lexington, MA: D.C. Heath.

Ullman, M., & Zimmerman, N. (1979). *Working with dreams.* New York: Delacorte/ Eleanor Friede.

Vaillant, L. M. (1997). *Changing character: Short-term anxiety-regulating psychotherapy for restructuring defenses, affects, and attachment.* New York: Basic Books.

Van der Hart, O. & Brown, D. et al. (1990). Hypnotherapy for traumatic grief: Janetian and modern approaches integrated. *American Journal of Clinical Hypnosis 32*, 4, 263–271.

Wadeson, H. (1980). *Art psychotherapy.* New York: Wiley.

Wadeson, H. (1982). Art therapy. In L. E. Abt & I. R. Stuart (Eds.), *The newer therapies: A source book.* New York: Van Nostrand Reinhold.

Walker, P. C. (1984). The hypnotic dream: A reconceptualization. *American Journal of Clinical Hypnosis 16*, 246–255.

Wark, D. M. (1998). Alert hypnosis: History and applications. In W. J. Matthews & J. H. Edgette (Eds.), *Creative thinking and research in brief therapy: Solutions, strategies, narratives,* Vol. 2, pp. 287–306. Philadelphia: Brunner/Mazel.

Watkins, J. G. (1942). Offensive psychological warfare. *The Journal of Consulting Psychology 6*, 117–122.

Watkins, J. G. (1943). Further opportunities for applied psychologists in offensive warfare. *The Journal of Consulting Psychology 7*, 135–141.

Watkins, J. G. (1949). Poison-pen therapy. *American Journal of Psychotherapy 111*, 410–418.

Watkins, J. G. (1951). Hypnotherapy in the military setting. *Journal of Personality 1*, 318–325.

Watkins, H. H. (1978). Ego-state therapy. In J. G. Watkins (Ed.), *The therapeutic self.* New York: Human Sciences Press.

Watkins, H. H. (1980). The silent abreaction. *International Journal of Clinical and Experimental Hypnosis 28*, 101–113.

Watkins, H. H. (2000). Clinical trials and follow-ups using the somatic bridge. Unpublished data. Missoula, MT.

Watkins, J. G. (1949). *Hypnotherapy of war neuroses.* New York: Ronald Press.

Watkins, J. G. (1952). Projective hypnoanalysis. In L. M. LeCron (Ed.), *Experimental hypnosis,* pp. 442–462. New York: Macmillan.

Watkins, J. G. (1954). Trance and transference. *Journal of Clinical and Experimental Hypnosis 2*, 284–290.

Watkins, J. G. (1960). *General psychotherapy: An outline and study guide.* Springfield, IL: C.C. Thomas.

Watkins, J. G. (1961). El puente afectivo: Una tecincia hipnoanalitica. *Acta Hypnologica Latino Americana 2*, 323–329.

Watkins, J. G. (1963a). Transference aspects of the hypnotic relationship. In M. V. Kline (Ed.), *Clinical correlations of experimental hypnosis.* Springfield, IL: Thomas.

Watkins, J. G. (1963b). The psychodynamics of hypnotic induction and termination. In J. M. Schneck (Ed.), Hypnosis in modern medicine (3rd ed.). Springfield, IL: C.C. Thomas, pp. 363–389.

Watkins, J. G. (1967a). Hypnosis and consciousness from the viewpoint of existentialism. In M. V. Kline (Ed.), *Psychodynamics and hypnosis*, pp. 15–31. Springfield, IL: Thomas.

Watkins, J. G. (1967b). Operant approaches to existential therapy. Unpublished address presented at the International Congress for Psychosomatic Medicine and Hypnosis, Kyoto, Japan, July 12.

Watkins, J. G. (1967c). The therapeutic self. In J. Lassner, *Hypnosis and psychosomatic medicine*, Proceedings of the International Congress for Hypnosis and Psychosomatic Medicine. Berlin: Springer–Verlag, 313–320.

Watkins, J. G. (1971). The affect bridge: A hypnoanalytic technique. *International Journal of Clinical & Experimental Hypnosis 19* (1), 21–27.

Watkins, J. G. (1977). The psychodynamic manipulation of ego states in hypnotherapy. In *Therapy in psychosomatic medicine*. Vol. II, Symposia, E. Antonelli (Ed.), Rome, Italy, pp. 389–403.

Watkins, J. G. (1978). Ego states and the problem of responsibility II: The case of Patricia W. *Journal of Psychiatry and Law*, 519–535.

Watkins, J. G. (1978b). *The therapeutic self.* New York: Human Sciences Press.

Watkins, J. G. (1984). The Bianchi ("Hillside Strangler") case: Sociopath or multiple personality? *International Journal of Clinical and Experimental Hypnosis 32*, 67–111.

Watkins, J. G. (1987). *Hypnotherapeutic techniques: The practice of clinical hypnosis*, Vol. 1. New York: Irvington Publishers.

Watkins, J. G. (1989). Hypnotichypermnesia and forensic hypnosis: A cross-examination. *American Journal of Clinical Hypnosis 32*, 71–83.

Watkins, J. G. (1992a). *The practice of clinical hypnosis*. Volume II: *Hypnoanalytic techniques*. New York: Irvington.

Watkins, J. G. (1992b). Psychchoanayse hypnoanayse, Ego State Therapie: Auf dur suche nach einier effektiven therapie. *Hypnose und Kognition, 9*, 85–97.

Watkins, J. G. (1993). Dealing with the problem of "false memory" in clinic and court. *Journal of Psychiatry and Law.* 297–317.

Watkins, J. G. (1995). Hypnotic abreactions in the recovery of traumatic memories. *Newsletter of the International Society for the Study of Dissociation 13*, 1, 6.

Watkins, J. G. (2000). The psychodynamic treatment of combat neuroses with hypnosis during World War II. *International Journal of Clinical and Experimental Hypnosis 48*, 324–335. (with added commentary on J. G. Watkins' paper by W. H. Smith, 336–341).

Watkins, J. G. (2001). Commentary on "Hypnosis, the hidden observer and not so hidden informed consent" by S. J. Lynn, *American Journal of Hypnosis 43*, 293–295.

Watkins, J. G. (2001a). Ah sweet mystery: Self from the perspective of ego state therapy. In P. Howell & J. A. Hall (Eds.), *Self through art and science*. 1st Books Library, www.1stbooks.com.

Watkins, J. G. (2001b). Exploring the mysteries of self: Our conquest of the unconscious. In B. Peter, W. Bongartz, D. Revenstorf, & W. Butollo (Eds.), *Proceedings of the 15th International Congress for Hypnosis*. Munich: Oct. 4, 2000.

Watkins, J. G. (2001c). *Adventures in human understanding: Stories for exploring the self.* Wales, UK: Crown House Publishing.

Watkins, J. G. (2002). The hypnotic regression of a paranoid schizophrenic to "normalcy." *Hypnosis 29*, 6–12.

Watkins, J. G. (2003). The many faces of love: An ego state perspective. *Australian Journal of Clinical Hypnotherapy and Hypnosis*. Sept. 24, 61–66.

Watkins, J. G. (2005a). *Emotional resonance. The story of world–acclaimed psychotherapist Helen Watkins*. Boulder, CO: First Sentient Publications.

Watkins, J. G. (2005b). Editorial: Over–resonance, the emaciation and destruction of Judy's self: Modifications to ego state theory. *Journal of Trauma and Dissociation* 6, 3, pp. 1–9.

Watkins, J. G. & Johnson, R. J. (1982). *We, the divided self.* New York: Irvington.

Watkins, J. G. & Watkins, H. H. (1978). *Abreactive technique.* (Audiotape.) New York: Psychotherapy Tape Library.

Watkins, J. G. & Watkins, H. H. (1979). The theory and practice of ego–state therapy. In H. Grayson (Ed.), *Short term approaches to psychotherapy*, pp. 176–220. New York: Human Sciences Press.

Watkins, J. G. & Watkins, H. H. (1979–80). Ego states and hidden observers. *Journal of Altered States of Consciousness 5*, 3–18.

Watkins, J. G. & Watkins, H. H. (1980a). I. Ego states and hidden observers. II. Ego-state therapy: The woman in black and the lady in white. (Audio tape and transcript), NY: Jeffrey–Norton.

Watkins, J. G. & Watkins, H. H. (1980b). Teoria e pratica da terapie do estado do ego. *Revista Brasileira de Medicina*, 46–56.

Watkins, J. G. & Watkins, H. H. (1981). Ego-state therapy. In R. J. Corsini (Ed.), *Handbook of innovative psychotherapies*, pp. 252–270. New York: Wiley.

Watkins, J. G. & Watkins, H. H. (1982). Ego-state therapy. In L. E. Abt & I. R. Stuart (Eds.), *The newer therapies: A source book*, pp. 137–155. New York: Van Nostrand Reinhold.

Watkins, J. G. & Watkins, H. H. (1983). Teoria e tarapia sugli dell' io sviluppate da John e Helen Watkins. *Minerva Medica 74–N*. 2145–2146.

Watkins, J. G. & Watkins, H. H. (1984). Hazards to the therapist in treating multiple personality disorders. *Psychiatric Clinics of North America 7*, 111–119.

Watkins, J. G. & Watkins, H. H. (1986). Hypnosis, multiple personality and ego states as altered states of consciousness. In B. W. Wolman & M. Ullman (Eds.), *Handbook of states of consciousness.* New York: Van Nostrand Reinhold.

Watkins, J. G. & Watkins, H. H. (1988). The management of malevolent ego states. *Dissociation 1*, 67–72.

Watkins, J. G. & Watkins, H. H. (1990a). Ego-state transferences in the hypnoanalytic treatment of dissociative reactions. In M. L. Fass & D. Brown (Eds.), *Creative mastery in hypnosis and hypnoanalysis: A festschrift for Erika Fromm*, pp. 255–261. Hillsdale, NJ: Lawrence Erlbaum.

Watkins, J. G. & Watkins, H. H. (1990b). Dissociation and displacement: Where goes "the ouch." *American Journal of Clinical Hypnosis 33*, 1–10.

Watkins, J. G. & Watkins, H. H. (1991). Hypnosis and ego-state therapy. In P.A. Keller & S.R. Heyman (Eds.), *Innovations in clinical practice.* Sarasota, FL: Professional Resource Exchange, 23–27.

Watkins, J. G. & Watkins, H. H. (1992). A comparison of "hidden observers," ego states and multiple personalities. *Hypnos XIX*, 215–221.

Watkins, J. G. & Watkins, H. H. (1996). Over–covert dissociation and hypnotic ego-state therapy. In W.J. Ray & L. K. Michelson (Eds.), *Handbook of Dissociation*. NY: Plenum.

Watkins, J. G. & Watkins, H. H. (1997). *Ego states: Theory and therapy*. New York: Norton.

Watkins, P. C., Matthews, A., Williamson, D. A., & Fuller, R. D. (1982). Mood congruent memory in depression: Emotional priming or elaboration. *Journal of Abnormal Psychology 10*, 581–586.

Weiss, E. (1960). *The structure and dynamics of the human mind*. New York: Grune & Stratton.

Weitzenhoffer, A., & Hilgard, E. (1959). *Stanford Hypnotic Susceptibility Scale Forms A & B*. Palo Alto, CA: Consulting Psychologists Press.

Weitzenhoffer, A., & Hilgard, E. (1962). *Stanford Hypnotic Susceptibility Scale: Form C*. Palo Alto, CA: Consulting Psychologists Press.

Whalen, J. E., & Nash, M. (1996). Hypnosis and dissociation: Theoretical, empirical, and clinical perspectives. In L. K. Michelson & W. J. Ray (Eds.), *Handbook of dissociation: Theoretical, empirical, and clinical perspectives*, pp. 191–206. New York: Plenum.

Wilbur, C. B. (1988). Multiple personality disorder and transference. *Dissociation 1*, 73–76.

Wilson, T. (1986). Effect of holistic and non-holistic teaching strategies on cerebral hemispheric laterality. Unpublished dissertation, Washington State University.

Winnicott, D. (1965). *The maturational processes and the facilitation environment*. New York: International Universities Press.

Wolberg, L. R. (1945). *Hypnoanalysis*. New York: Grune & Stratton.

Wolberg, L. R. (1948). *Medical hypnosis: Vol. I. Principles of hypnotherapy*. Vol. II: *Practice of hypnotherapy*. New York: Grune & Stratton.

Wolman, M. M. (Ed.). (1979). *Handbook of dreams: Research, theories and applications*. New York: Van Nostrand Reinhold.

Wolpe, J., & Lazarus, A. (1966). *Techniques of behavior therapy*. Oxford, England: Pergamon Press.

Woods, R. L., & Greenhouse, H. B. (1974). *The new world of dreams*. New York: Macmillan.

Woody, R. (1973). Clinical suggestion and systematic desensitization. *American Journal of Clinical Hypnosis 15*, 250–257.

Wright, M. E. (with B. A. Wright). (1987). *Clinical practice of hypnotherapy*. New York: Guilford Press.

Yalom, I. D. (1980). *Existential psychotherapy*. New York: Basic Books.

Zamore, N., & Barrett, D. L. (1989). Hypnotic susceptibility and dream characteristics. *Psychiatric Journal of the University of Ottawa*. November 14 (4): 572–4.

Zeig, J. (1974). Hypnotherapy techniques with psychotic in–patients. *American Journal of Clinical Hypnosis 17*, 56–59.

Index

A

Abandonment, 228
Abreactive techniques, 3, 15, 57
    abreactive inductions and, 66–69, 228
    affect bridge and, 72–78
    corrective emotional experience and,
      82–86
    criticisms of, 86–90
    indicators for, 65–66
    Kluft's Fractionated Abreaction, 91–92
    poison pen therapy and, 86
    release abreactions in, 63
    silent abreaction and, 69–72
    slow-release–slow-burn procedure,
      90–91
    somatic bridge and, 78
    split-screen technique, 92–93
    summary of, 93–94
Active imagination, 145, 147, 153
Adaptive regression, 3, 278
Adler, Alfred, 133
The Affect Bridge, 73
Affective resonance, 309
Age regression, 47, 51, 149, 152
Alert hypnosis induction, 109
American Psychiatric Association, 221
Amnesia, 141, 202–215
Antarctic isolation, 127
Anxiety, 196
Archaic involvement, 278
Archetypes, 111, 236
Atavistic regression, 278
Autohypnosis, 298
Automatic messages, 201
Automatic writing, 200
Awareness, total alert, 8, 10

B

Barabasz, M., 98
Barabasz technique, 109
Barrett, Deirdre, 129
Beck, Aaron, 84
Behavioral contracts, 222
Bipolar disorder, 221, 230

Birth abreactions, 93
Borderline personality disorder, 242, 252
Bound effects, release of, 15
Brown, Daniel, 63
Brown, William, 59

C

Castration anxiety, 189
Cathartic therapy, 64
Cathexes (energies), 20
Cholinergic pontogeniculoocipital (PGO)
    system, 130
Clay model, 106
Cognitive behavioral hypnotherapy, 5
Cognitive behavioral insight, 5
Cognitive behavior modification, 126
Cognitive insight, 5
Cognitive resonance, 309
Cognitive therapy, 84
Colored clays (plasticine), 113
Combat fatigue, 59
Condensation, process of, 132
Conflict, areas of, 113, 132
Conscious expression, 132
Consciousness, level of, 132
Coping mechanisms, 236
Counter transference, 2, 14, 18

D

Death, fears of, 24–25
Defense mechanisms, 10, 48
Defensive processes, 292
Dehypnotizing suggestions, 32
Depersonalized, 296
Depression, treatment of, 84
Diagnostic evaluation, 231
*Diagnostic Statistical Manual of Mental
    Disorders* (DSM-IVTR), 35, 62
DID treatment strategies, implementing,
    226–230
Differentiation, 249, 251–253
Digital photographic hypnography, 112
Displacement, process of, 132